NEW HORIZONS: EXPANDED EDITION

ON PLUTO

Inside the Mind of Alzheimer's

GREG O'BRIEN

Foreword by Lisa Genova
Epilogue by David Shenk

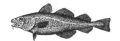

Codfish Press
Brewster, MA

© 2018 Greg O'Brien, Codfish Press, Brewster, MA

ISBN 978-0-9913401-8-7 paperback, expanded edition
2018, Revised/expanded edition
Initial book design/page layout, Joe Gallante,
Coysbrook Studio, Harwich, MA
Initial cover design, Brandy Polay
On Pluto revised/expanded edition interior design,
Paraclete Multimedia, Orleans, MA

Cover design, Brad Harris
Research assistance, Conor O'Brien
Creative direction, Brendan O'Brien
Printed by Paraclete Press, Brewster, MA
Distributed by Penguin Random House Publisher Services

In Praise of *On Pluto:*
Inside the Mind of Alzheimer's

"Told with extraordinary vulnerability, grace, humor, and profound insight, *On Pluto* is an intimate look inside the mind of Greg O'Brien, a journalist diagnosed with early-onset Alzheimer's. But the real gem of *On Pluto* lies in its unflinching look inside Greg's heart. If you're trying to understand what it feels like to live with Alzheimer's, and you are because you're reading these words, then you need to read this book."

—LISA GENOVA, *New York Times* bestselling author of *Still Alice, Left Neglected, Love Anthony,* and *Inside the O'Briens*

"With a wicked sense of humor and a journalist's curiosity, Greg O'Brien reports from the front lines of his own battlefield. Much like Glen Campbell whose artistry shined in the face of his disease, Greg is in full control of his craft. In spite of being in the grip of Alzheimer's disease, Greg's storytelling is beautifully crafted, insightful, and at times transcendent."

—TREVOR ALBERT, producer, *Glen Campbell: I'll Be Me, Groundhog Day,* and *Multiplicity*

"A more eloquent, witty, and honest spokesperson, this horrible disease will never see. Greg O'Brien is my hero, and will soon be yours after reading his groundbreaking book!"

—DR. RUDY TANZI, vice-chair of Neurology and director of the Genetics and Aging Research Unit at Massachusetts General Hospital, the Joseph P. and Rose F. Kennedy Professor of Neurology at Harvard Medical School, and chair of the Cure Alzheimer's Fund Research Consortium

"A brilliant journalist, Greg O'Brien has bravely chosen to live his life out of the shadows and in the spotlight. To say Greg is a writer is like saying Fred Astaire did a two-step or that Thomas Edison was a tinkerer. Greg is eloquent, insightful, spiritual, humorous, and visionary. He is the Poet Laureate of Alzheimer's. There are few pluses to Alzheimer's, but getting to know and work with Greg is at the top of that list."

—GEORGE & TRISH VRADENBURG,
co-founders, UsAgainstAlzheimer's

"Greg O'Brien's *On Pluto: Inside the Mind of Alzheimer's* is the most compelling, honest, and complete 360-degree narrative out there on how Alzheimer's disease impacts a family. This expanded edition updates us on Greg's personal AD journey and includes chapters written by his wife and children with great honesty and humor. As Greg says the Irish way, 'Never get mad. Get even!' Greg compels us to fight Alzheimer's not for ourselves, but for our children and grandchildren, and generations to come."

—MERYL COMER, advocate and author, *Slow Dancing with a Stranger*

"In *On Pluto*, Greg O'Brien has given us a priceless gift: an honest, funny, heartbreaking, and powerfully poignant look into the world of an Alzheimer's sufferer by a man who lives with it. Greg O'Brien is a brilliant observer and superb writer, and he is at the top of his game in this book. It's as if he has willingly dropped himself into a kind of mental tornado, so that he can tell us what he sees from inside. You have never read a book quite like it, and probably never will again."

—WILLIAM MARTIN, *New York Times* bestselling author of *Cape Cod,
Back Bay*, and *The Lincoln Letter*

"Greg O'Brien writes with the consummate knowledge of a guide and the courage of a pioneer. In this important and transcendent book, he serves both roles as he folds back the veils of fear and traverses the treacherous territory of early-onset Alzheimer's. *On Pluto: Inside the Mind of Alzheimer's* glows with honesty, intelligence, and compassion, and, given the subject, is a surprisingly spirit-renewing book."

—ANNE D. LECLAIRE, author of bestselling *Listening Below the Noise,
Leaving Eden*, and *The Lavender Hour*

"Most sufferers of early-onset Alzheimer's do their very best to hide it from everyone, sometimes even themselves. Greg O'Brien has chosen to look the beast in the eyes, and give us a candid, unflinching portrait of his family's tragic history of the disease, as well as his own determination to not go down without a fight."

—S T E V E J A M E S, producer of the short film *A Place Called Pluto* and considered among the most acclaimed documentary producers with noted works: *Hoop Dreams, Life Itself, Stevie, The New Americans, The War Tapes, At the Death House Door,* and *The Interpreters*

"Alzheimer's messed with the wrong man. If there's anyone who can stand up to this awful disease with the right blend of eloquence, anger, and honesty, it is the defiant and profound Greg O'Brien. This book is a beacon of hope for anyone who can read or listen."

—D A V I D S H E N K, author of *The Forgetting*, a *New York Times* bestseller, and creator of *Living with Alzheimer's* film project

"Greg O'Brien's daily movements now include, he tells us, periodic trips to Pluto, a dark and distant planet off the grid of enduring memory. But Greg's story of his life has mapped for us an inner space that is as light and present as Pluto is bleak and lonely. The courage of this book lies in the way that Greg speaks his peace into the dark. The hope of this book lies in the way that the dark, in the least expected of moments, seems to be listening to Greg, in inextinguishable love."

—M I C H A E L V E R D E, founder, Memory Bridge, the Foundation for Alzheimer's and Cultural Memory

"Greg O'Brien takes us on a personal journey into Alzheimer's disease and marks the trail for others traveling this treacherous path. At once fighting and accepting his fate, he eloquently describes the delicate balance between living and dying with this mind-robbing disease. As his mind fails and his wisdom grows, he is teaching us to defy the popular notion that memory is everything."

— D A N I E L K U H N, MSW, author of *Alzheimer's Early Stages: First Steps for Family, Friends, and Caregivers*

"Never before have we been offered such a clear understanding of how Alzheimer's disease affects day-to-day perceptions. Greg O'Brien's first-hand account of his own disease process will force us all to rethink the way we deliver care, and is a must addition to the libraries of all professional and family caregivers."

—S U Z A N N E F A I T H, RN psych, clinical director,
Hope Dementia & Alzheimer's Services

"As a clinician working daily with families and individuals dealing with Alzheimer's and dementia, the question we most often grapple with is how does one live well with the disease? Greg O'Brien's book, *On Pluto: Inside the Mind of Alzheimer's,* offers an answer, rich in wit, courage, and a precision of detail that makes the book not only informative, but an extremely satisfying read. For the 5.5 million American families currently dealing with dementia, and for those of us who serve them, *On Pluto* is a critical and groundbreaking book. We are fortunate to have Greg's voice and spirit among us; he is a true American hero."

—D R. M O L L Y P E R D U E, PhD, director of
Family Services, Hope Health of Cape Cod

"Greg O'Brien's personal battle against Alzheimer's is an everyman's fight; he is the quintessence of the lead character in the epic Alzheimer's novel, *Still Alice.* O'Brien, through faith, humor, and journalistic grit, is able, like a master artist, to paint a gripping, naked word picture of this progressive, chronic disease for which there is no cure—a sickness that will swamp a generation. O'Brien bluntly offers Baby Boomers and generations to come a riveting guide of how to live with Alzheimer's, rather than dying with it."

—A L I S A M. G A L A Z Z I, co-founder of Dementia Care Academy,
former executive director, Alzheimer's Services of Cape Cod and the Islands

About *On Pluto:*
Inside the Mind of Alzheimer's

On Pluto: Inside the Mind of Alzheimer's has won the 2015 Beverly Hills International Book Award for Medicine, the 2015 International Book Award for Health, and was an Eric Hoffer International Book Award finalist, as well as a finalist for USA Best Book Awards.

Author and longtime journalist Greg O'Brien also is the subject of the short film *A Place Called Pluto*, directed by award-winning filmmaker Steve James, available online at livingwithalz.org. NPR's *All Things Considered* has run a series about O'Brien's journey, and PBS/NOVA followed the *Pluto* journey in its groundbreaking Alzheimer's documentary, *Can Alzheimer's Be Stopped?* O'Brien has been part of many regional and national interviews.

O'Brien has served on the national Alzheimer's Association Early Stage Advisory Group; is an advisor to the Cure Alzheimer's Fund of Boston; and is a board member of the Washington, D.C.-based advocacy organization UsAgainstAlzheimer's.

CONTENTS

PART ONE:

On Pluto: Inside the Mind of Alzheimer's

DEDICATION

To my mother, Virginia Brown O'Brien, whose
courageous battle with Alzheimer's taught me how to stand
firm in faith against a demon of a disease.

Romans 5:3-5—"We exalt in our tribulations, knowing
that tribulation brings about perseverance; and
perseverance, proven character; and proven character,
hope; and hope does not disappoint."

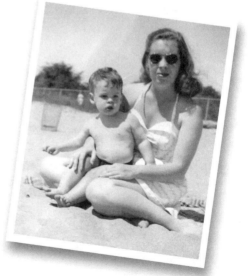

Age of innocence, 1953:
Virginia Loretta Brown O'Brien,
Rye Beach, Westchester County, NY, with son, Greg.

FOREWORD
ORIGINAL EDITION

Lisa Genova

Every story has a beginning, middle, and end. I met Greg O'Brien somewhere in the middle. I received an email from him at the end of March 2011. He introduced himself as a journalist, a fellow Cape Codder, and a fan of *Still Alice*.

It was an email aimed to woo and impress me, and just as I was thinking this, I read:

"Don't be overly impressed by the articulation of this email. It took about two hours to write. Years ago, I would have written this in five minutes or less. But it was worth the time."

Like his mother and maternal grandfather before him, Greg had been diagnosed with early-onset Alzheimer's. He wanted to know if we could meet and talk. I get this kind of email a lot and do my best to offer an ear, encouragement, advice, and connections for further support. It's typically a sincere but brief relationship, most often limited to a few email exchanges. I had no idea when I agreed to meet Greg that he'd be on my mind pretty much every day since then, that he'd become a close friend and personal hero.

Since I've known Greg, he's been fighting through the drifting fogs of dementia, determined to press on, drawing on everything he is—brilliant journalist, adoring and faithful family man, generous and lovable Irishman with a great sense of humor, masterful storyteller—to write *On Pluto*. Greg is the author of four Cape Cod–related books, and has won many prestigious awards for journalism over a thirty-year career, but I believe this book is Greg's greatest achievement and contribution, not to the cure for Alzheimer's (at least not directly), but to our understanding of how to live and love in the presence of Alzheimer's.

In his own words, "While I have the facility to do so, I want to communicate to others, to those who will face this demon some day and those who love them, that with the proper medical direction, life strategies, faith, and humor one can prevail in the moment and lead a productive life for as long as possible."

Understanding the scientific pathology of Alzheimer's is critically important for improving diagnostic imaging, developing more effective treatments, and someday, discovering a cure. Understanding the science—the accumulation of amyloid and tau, identifying genetic risk factors, elucidating NMDA receptor regulation—is necessary and will take time and money. But equally important to furthering research for a future cure is an understanding of the human experience of Alzheimer's now. What does it feel like to live with Alzheimer's? This kind of knowledge is also necessary, but it requires a different kind of investment. It takes courage and empathy.

We're all terrified of Alzheimer's. The fortress of fear, shame, stigma, alienation, and isolation that surrounds Alzheimer's today is not unlike what we saw with cancer forty to fifty years ago. We didn't even say the word "cancer." Instead we called it "the big C" in hushed voices. But something changed. We began talking openly about cancer. We began wearing looped ribbons and walking to raise awareness and money, and as communities, we began rallying around our neighbors with cancer, offering dinners and carpools and support.

We acknowledged the human experience of living with cancer. And now we have treatments for cancer. We have cancer survivors.

Right now, we have no Alzheimer's survivors. We need to find the courage to talk about Alzheimer's, to acknowledge not just the end of this disease, but also the beginning and the middle. We need to change the image of this disease, which tends to depict only an elderly person in end stage, "an empty shell," someone dying from Alzheimer's. Someone who is, perhaps, easier to ignore. This image excludes the millions of people LIVING with Alzheimer's, people newly diagnosed in their forties, fifties, sixties, and seventies; people living somewhere in the beginning and the middle. People like Greg O'Brien.

What does it feel like to live with Alzheimer's? What does that image look like?

This is what Greg O'Brien so bravely, intimately, and beautifully shares with us. Recounting memories of his mother and grandfather, the day of his own diagnosis, symptoms of disorientation, stories of forgetting names and faces—even his wife—told with unflinching truth, grace, and humor, Greg shares with us what it feels like to live with Alzheimer's in the hope that we will better understand it. Understanding is the path to empathy. Empathy is the key to human connection.

Greg and I met a few years ago to talk about Alzheimer's. I expected to listen to this stranger, tell him what I knew, and help him out if I could. Then he'd be on his way, and I'd go back to my life without Greg O'Brien. Instead, I sat with a man so open and real, a man fighting to be present and live every single day to the fullest, with everything he's still got, a man who could find humor in the ugliest and scariest of moments. I was captivated, enamored, inspired. Surprised.

Since that day, Greg's Alzheimer's continues to advance, but the man I met more than three years ago is still here. He's tenacious, funny as hell, generous, incredibly smart, and brave. He's still open and real. He loves his family, his friends, and Cape Cod with a huge heart. He's a man I'm proud to call my friend.

Greg has told me many times that he believes his purpose is to share this story, that it might reach and improve the lives of millions of people traveling a similar journey.

I believe it will, Greg.

Lisa Genova is the *New York Times* bestselling author of *Still Alice, Love Anthony, Left Neglected, Inside the O'Briens,* and a fifth book to be released soon about ALS (amyotrophic lateral sclerosis).

FOREWORD
NEW HORIZONS

Lisa Genova

For over thirty-five years, Greg has been a writer for various local and national newspapers and magazines. He's been an editor, an investigative reporter, and a publisher. You can hear him regularly on NPR and see him on TV shows like *Chronicle* and *NOVA*. He's even a bit of a movie star, featured in the documentary film *A Place Called Pluto*, directed by Steve James. He's also one of the best friends I'll know in this lifetime.

Greg's first email to me was in March of 2011. He introduced himself, told me that his mother had died of Alzheimer's three years ago and that he was her caregiver. And now he'd been diagnosed with early-onset Alzheimer's. Greg told me that he knew about me because his neurologist from Tufts suggested that he read *Still Alice*. God bless that neurologist. He told me he was experiencing symptoms of memory loss, loss of place, loss of balance, hallucinations, depression, rage, loss of self.

As the part of his brain responsible for his memory was shutting down, he said he was determined to carry on, to protect and use the part of his brain responsible for his creativity, his writing, his "sweet spot," with every instinct left for as long as he could.

He told me that he wanted to take all that he is—all his experience as a writer, as a caregiver to his mom, as an investigative reporter—and write a book, a first-person account about what it's like to live with Alzheimer's from the inside out. He said he wanted to use the time he had left and his cognitive reserve to speak out about this disease, to change the public perception. Basically, he wanted to share the scariest, most vulnerable, personal experience of his life with the world. He always downplays how heroic this is.

I encouraged him, but not knowing him well yet, I didn't have a whole lot of confidence that he could finish such a book. I meet so many people who say they want to write a book, and they never do. They have all kinds of excuses—excuses far less daunting than Alzheimer's.

It didn't take long in knowing Greg for me to realize that not only would he finish this book—but that it would be brilliant, important, and deeply meaningful to people all over the world.

He and I spend a lot of time traveling the world separately but with the same mission—speaking about Alzheimer's, trying to educate, raise money for care and research, break down the fear and the stigma and the shame, show people that this is not simply a disease of the dying elderly, that millions of people are LIVING with Alzheimer's, people who look like Julianne Moore and Greg O'Brien.

I love when I go to give a talk somewhere and I learn from the audience that Greg has been there before me. They rave about his talk, about how funny and smart and generous he is. They tell me how much his talk has helped them. They tell me they LOVE him. I always smile, so proud, and say, "I love him, too."

People all over this world love you, Greg, because you let us in, you let us see you without barriers or pretense, you let us know the real you. And the real you is a beautiful, stubborn, amazing badass.

Lisa Genova is the *New York Times* bestselling author of *Still Alice*, *Love Anthony*, *Left Neglected*, *Inside the O'Briens*, and a fifth book to be released soon about ALS (amyotrophic lateral sclerosis).

The Nun Study

Molly Perdue

Family is an extended circle, and I'm a part of Greg's extended family on Cape Cod. What I respect most about him is his open, accepting love and his God-given faith to reach beyond boundaries. We share Alzheimer's as a common thread.

Years ago, it didn't matter how many times I patiently walked the Provincetown flats at the Cape's tip to prove to my mother that what she was seeing were not drowning nuns, as she was convinced in her Alzheimer's, but black buoys bouncing in the bay.

My partner, Melanie Braverman, and I had moved my mother, Virginia, to Cape Cod from Central Florida just before Mother's Day in 2002, after it had become clear that she needed our help. A Navy WAVE in World War II, then a homemaker and realtor, my mother always had a stubborn streak. With the progression of her Alzheimer's symptoms, that streak took on a life of its own.

"The nuns are drowning!" she would shout. "Drowning! We have to call the police!" To calm her, I would pretend to phone the Provincetown police chief, alerting him to the drama unfolding in the harbor as my mother listened.

"They're coming," I told her. "The police are coming. Help is on the way!"

More often than not, this reassured her enough to turn her attention back to Oprah, until the tide went out and the "nun buoys" were revealed once more.

In the summer of 2009 on a misty afternoon, shortly before my mother's death, the phone rang from beneath a stack of papers. I shuffled through the pile to retrieve it. I was in the midst of completing my doctorate from Northeastern University, as my inexhaustible 5-year-old Sam raced from one room to the next, while our 4-year-old, Jonah, played tug of war with his grandmother. Giggling filled the living room until a switch flipped inside my mom's head, causing her to believe the toy belonged to her, not Jonah. I could hear Jonah scolding her:

"That's my ducky, Gaga, give it back!" Both of their vice grips tightened on the toy duck's slight neck before I interceded.

Exasperated, I groped for my ringing phone, as my mother glared at me.

"HELLO!" I nearly shouted into the phone.

It was Greg O'Brien. He had read a recent Alzheimer's article I had written for the *Cape Cod Times*, and wanted to talk to me about the disease: my mom, his mom, and caregiving. Greg had recently been diagnosed with early-onset Alzheimer's, following in the footsteps of several family members. It was the first time we had ever spoken, and I was struck by how forthright he was about a disease process that usually begins in denial. As a long-time journalist, he was contemplating writing a book about living with Alzheimer's. He saw himself, given his family history and his training as a veteran reporter, as a window into the disease, fully aware that Alzheimer's strikes women, blacks, and Hispanics in higher numbers than white males. Alzheimer's, he said, respects no demographics, no gender, color, preference, religion, or political party. The disease is as "bipartisan" as it gets, Greg said.

"*Start it now,*" I told him. And so we set up a meeting.

Today, close to eight years later, Greg continues to be irreverent in the face of his Alzheimer's in this revised, expanded edition of *On Pluto: Inside the Mind of Alzheimer's*. Through the many national radio shows and public appearances we've done together, I have watched Greg adapt his considerable strategies to keep working, speaking, and writing despite his intense short-term memory loss, his growing intolerance of large crowds, his inability to manage airports or recognize familiar faces, and the terrifying hallucinations and rage. Greg is forging his life into the future with the fire and force of a blacksmith, affronted by the very notion that he might have to give more of himself to a disease that has already taken so much.

Why should he? Why should anyone? Alzheimer's is a disease of the mind and the body, not of the soul. In spite of my mother's Alzheimer's, she taught me how to soothe our colicky first child; it was her arms into which he took his first steps. Over the years, our family, with my mother in tow, took road trips that would have made less hearty individuals' heads spin, pulling our clown car minivan up in front of random hotels and spilling our multigenerational chaos onto the curb: strollers, portable commodes, and my mother in her wheelchair buried beneath babies and piles of coats.

Although my mother is gone now, it's through my friendship with Greg, and his ability to show us the world through his lens, that helps me understand the complexity of living with Alzheimer's. Life doesn't end after diagnosis; it just gets more complicated, as Greg details in this edition.

What makes Alzheimer's disease different than other illnesses are the significant behavioral and psychiatric changes that accompany the loss of memory. Will a cure for Alzheimer's ever be found? If Greg has anything to say about it, yes. In spite of all we've learned, Alzheimer's remains a mystery. Why do some, like Greg, seem to progress more slowly than others? The answer may lay deep in the brain itself. The notion of "idea density" in writing and language could be a predictor of Alzheimer's and the capacity to fight the disease after onset. The belief comes out of seminal research referred to as "The Nun Study," an ongoing longitudinal study, begun in 1986, to examine Alzheimer's disease. In brief, the more ideas one can express in as few words as possible, the higher one's "idea density" and projected intellect—thus greater ability to battle diseases of the mind. The Nun Study, driven by the work of founding investigator David Snowden that began at the University of Minnesota, measured the density of ideas and "linguistic density" in writing samples from Catholic Sisters of Notre Dame as they entered the convent in their late teens, and continued such examination of cognitive abilities until their deaths. Most of the nuns had agreed to bestow their brains for further scientific research.

According to results, study experts have linked positive emotions to a longer life, mirroring corresponding studies and illustrating that depression increases risk of cardiovascular and cognitive disease. Individuals rated as optimists on personality tests were more likely than doomsayers to live longer lives. Greg clearly straddles the dividing line on this. In typical ethnic humor, Greg told me recently that a first-generation Italian friend of his passed along that his immigrant father had instructed him as a young boy: "Don't mess with the Irish. They don't know how to fucking die!"

Perhaps early on, the grammar school letters the nuns had assigned Greg to write to the Blessed Virgin on May Day, a day in the Catholic liturgical calendar of devotion to the mother of Jesus, not only increased his idea density and writing skills, but provided, as well, some fortification for the future from Alzheimer's. I can only imagine what was in those notes. We'll never know. They were set ablaze soon after they were written, along with the scribblings of other students, in a ceremonial fire with smoke drifting to heaven. The only place they might remain is in Greg's memory, which is slowly but surely fading. This is the tricky part of the disease. As the clock ticks, life is filled with uncertainty, and imbued with unpredictable, incremental loss. We search in this disease for the gift of time. For me, it was potluck dinners with mom and neighbors, her dancing at a friend's wedding, and summer deck parties. Even at sundown when my mother's confusion peaked, or later when she was wheelchair-bound, Gaga retained her ability to have fun, and so did we, even as those moments in living with this disease grew further and further apart.

The day after the 2016 presidential election, a high anxiety moment for all, Greg, his son Conor (his day-to-day family caregiver), and I were driving back to the Cape from a speaking engagement in Bangor, Maine. Conor was stretched out in the back, and Greg was sitting in the passenger seat as I drove. Greg's gaze trained resolutely forward. He was on Pluto. In seconds, an enormous billow of gasoline smoke wafted from the side of the road. About a mile or so later, Greg intoned, "Wow, must be a car on fire?" rubbing his eyes. I smiled reassuringly at him, aware of how long it had taken him to smell the smoke, to absorb the accident. His sense of smell, along with taste, is fading in this disease.

"Yes, it's on fire all right," I said, having sped past the wreck a while back, knowing that if we hesitated we'd get stopped in a long line of traffic, waiting for someone to put out the fire.

Despite the roadside drama, the feeling of our trip that day was nothing short of exuberant. The adoration Conor has for his dad was palpable, even dozing off in the back seat, periodically reviving to check his phone for messages from his mother, Mary Catherine, his sister, Colleen, and his brother, Brendan. The O'Briens are proof that Alzheimer's is a disease not of an individual, but of a family. There's a clip from an incredible on-line film about the O'Brien family journey called *A Place Called Pluto*, produced by award-winning filmmaker Steve James, a snapshot of the family's ongoing struggle to understand what Alzheimer's means in their lives. During my remarks that morning I talked about the clip in which the entire O'Brien clan discusses with disarming honesty their worries about what might lie ahead: Greg's cessation of work, bankruptcy, loneliness, loss of self, all of it laid out on the table in front of them. Unlike other progressive, terminal diseases, Alzheimer's confronts us in our most intimate places, in bedrooms and bathrooms, in church, or in line at the bank, or the grocery store. What seems like the most ordinary part of the film to me is the most revolutionary: a family sitting down at a kitchen table to talk.

When I explain to audiences what can be accomplished in the truly daunting face of this disease, I talk about the reason my partner and I created the nonprofit Alzheimer's Family Support Center of Cape Cod. The premise of the center is simple: we help families like the O'Briens, caregivers, and individuals with the disease, to begin a conversation, bringing Alzheimer's out of the darkness. Our goal is to help families navigate the complexities and challenges they face across the span of the disease by providing free of charge a research-based family and community-centered social model.

Alzheimer's is an enormous, uncontrollable, expensive disease with the power to overwhelm an individual or family with the stereotype that nothing can be done to make it easier, but we know that this is not true. We know that the earlier families connect, the better off they will fare. We know that most family caregivers are untrained in how to help a loved one navigate hallucinations or deal with abrupt mood changes, or how to respond to someone who has lost their sense of place and time. So we teach them. We commit to providing support over what can be a long haul, and we help families make the long haul worth living. Greg O'Brien is proof that we don't have to live in the shadows of our fears. He and his family are at the forefront of bringing the phenomena of Alzheimer's into the light.

That morning in Maine, in his usual disarming manner, Greg spoke candidly of his journey. A woman with Alzheimer's sitting in the front row began to weep as he spoke. Watching her husband comfort her, I felt the familiar wash of hope and sadness as I stood next to Greg. Thanks to his unwavering perseverance and leadership, more and more people with Alzheimer's are seeing their disease as something to live with, rather than to die from. The dying part, Greg says, comes later.

Greg has told me many times that he now has to rely more on his heart than his brain. In every sentence of *On Pluto* he exposes his heart to us, challenging us as he lives his life with meaning and purpose despite his Alzheimer's, not by denying it, but by meeting it head-on. Surely this is a message that resonates in *all* of us, whether we are battling Alzheimer's or not.

Dr. Molly Perdue, MA, MS, PhD, author of *Exploring the Experiences of Family Caregivers: Cape Cod's Invisible Workforce, Upholding the Promise of Olmstead for People with Alzheimer's and Dementia-related Disease* (Northeastern University, 2012), has worked with thousands of families and individuals dealing with dementia. As co-founder and executive director of the Alzheimer's Family Support Center, Perdue continues her work as an educator, clinician, researcher, and advocate for families and individuals living with Alzheimer's and dementia-related diseases.

ACKNOWLEDGMENTS

O n *Pluto: Inside the Mind of Alzheimer's* has required more than six years of reporting, three years of writing, editing, and revisions, and more than two score of advisors, colleagues, family, and friends. This book would only be a concept without them. First of all, I would like to thank my wife of thirty-eight years, Mary Catherine, and my children: Brendan, Colleen, and Conor, who sustain me and encouraged me to complete this work. Mary Catherine has been my mooring on this project; Brendan my mentor; Colleen my soul, who has opened many doors nationwide in the Alzheimer's community through her selfless volunteering; Conor my rudder, keeping me grounded with his Celtic humor; and granddaughter Adeline my ballast. Secondly, I would like to thank close friend and celebrated author Lisa Genova, whose inspiration, encouragement, and guidance kept me on track, steadied me along the way, and pushed me when I needed to be pushed. Thank you! Her epic novel, *Still Alice*, has given voice and clarity beyond measure to those with Alzheimer's. She is a hero to the cause.

I am also grateful for a gifted team of advisors, writers, and editors who steered me along this twisting path: Alzheimer's expert Dr. Rudy Tanzi of Massachusetts General Hospital, Harvard, and the Cure Alzheimer's Fund of Boston; George Vradenburg and his late wife, Trish, co-founders of the Washington, D.C.-based UsAgainstAlzheimer's; Alzheimer's Association president and CEO

Harry Johns and associates Monica Moreno and Emily Shubeck; Elizabeth Gelfand Sterns, chair of the Alzheimer's Association Judy Fund, producer of the Academy Award-winning movie *Still Alice*, and a former senior vice president at Universal Studios; Maria Shriver for her persevering and powerful advocacy in fighting Alzheimer's; Cure Alzheimer's Fund executive director Tim Armour; U.S. Senator Ed Markey, champion for the cause of Alzheimer's on Capitol Hill; Congressman Bill Keating; National Public Radio (NPR) reporter and producer Rebecca Hersher; Pluto project directors and close friends Ken Sommers, chief operating officer of PayPal for Europe, Middle East and Africa; Paul Tingley of Paraclete Press; editorial advisor Alisa Galazzi; author and mentor Skip Rosen; *New York Times* bestselling authors Meryl Comer, Anne LeClaire, and William Martin; editors Jon Sweeney and Victoria Anderson; writer/editor Gerald Cousens; my personal physician Dr. Barry Conant, an inspiration to me; retired *Providence Journal* editorial page editor Robert Whitcomb, a former editor at *The Wall Street Journal* and *International Herald Tribune*; documentary producer George Pakenham, *Idle Threat*; author Ira Wood, founder of Leapfrog Press; Charlie Henderson; Terry and Jan Hoeschler and family; Mike Saint and Steve Shepherd; and the support of Sam Lorusso and Dave and Laura Peterson; Robert McGeorge; Ron Rudnick; Jim Botsford; Bill, Jonathan, and Betina Todd; Eric and Terri Guichet; Howard Hayes; Rick and Ella Leavitt; editorial advisors George Pakenham; as well as close friends Kristi Tyldesley, Paul and Leslie Durgin, Lindsay, Harry, and Coley Durgin, Braedy Taugher, Nancy O'Malley, Martha Hunter Henderson, Pam Hait, Mark Forest, Traci Longa; Scott Farmelant; and my nephew Kenny McGeorge for his soulful, never-say-die inspiration in his daily battle against advanced autism, a life lesson for me. Kenny keeps me fighting.

My sincere thanks also to close friends Patti Branca, Mary Valentine, Ann Branca, and the late Ralph Branca; Dan and Kathleen Murphy; former *Cape Cod Today* publisher Walter Brooks; attorneys John Twohig, Susan Nicastro, Jack Eiferman, and Teresa Foley of Goulston & Storrs of Boston, and Duane Landreth, Chris Ward, and Melanie O'Keefe of La Tanzi, Spaulding & Landreth on Cape Cod;

Meryl Moss and Carole Claps of Meryl Moss Media of Westport, CT; Bill Gladstone and Kimberly Brabec of Waterstone Productions of Cardiff, CA; author and CNBC television commentator Tom Casey; Ray Artigue, president of the Artigue Agency in Phoenix; Ed Lambert, WXTK-FM; Kevin O'Reilly, president of Creative Strategies & Communications; former *Arizona Republic* editorial writer Joel Nilsson and investigative reporter Chuck Kelly; writer John Lipman; *Cape Cod Times* publisher Peter Meyer and editorial page editor William Mills, and Carol Dumas, former editor of *The Cape Codder* for pressing me to persevere; and Vicky Bijur and Deborah Schneider.

Also, deep appreciation to Robert Kraft and Jonathan Kraft who taught me, through example, to find a way to win.

Much credit goes to legendary documentary director and producer Steve James *(Hoop Dreams, Stevie, Interrupters,* and *Life Itself)*; *New York Times* bestselling author David Shenk *(The Forgetting, Alzheimer's: Portrait of an Epidemic, The Genius in All of Us,* and *Data Smog)*, a former advisor to the President's Council on Bioethics and a senior advisor to the Cure Alzheimer's Fund in Boston; and to Julia Pacetti of JMP Verdant Communications in Brooklyn. The Cure Alzheimer's Fund, in association with the MetLife Foundation, sponsored the production, with Shenk as executive producer of four short films on the stages of Alzheimer's (livingwithalz.org), produced by world-class documentary producers. *A Place Called Pluto,* one of the films documenting my own family's journey in this disease, was produced by James. The films can be accessed on livingwithalz.org.

In addition, I would like to thank Kim Campbell, wife of legendary singer Glen Campbell; Sean Corcoran, senior managing editor at WGBH News, Boston's PBS station; Arun Rath at WGBH; WCAI radio producer Mindy Todd; Sam Broun of WCAI; UsAgainstAlzhiemer's board members, staff and supporters Sally Sachar, Ginny Biggar, John Dwyer, Karen Segal, Drew Holzapfel, Brooks Kenny, Jill Lesser, Elizabeth Plant, and Jason Resendez; and Adam Gamble, publisher of On Cape Publications, for his steady direction; his skilled associate and author Mark Jasper; Mark Suchomel and Jeff Tegge of Legato Publishers Group; Joe Gallante of Coy's Brook Studio for his impressive initial layout and design; Paraclete Multimedia for interior design of revised/expanded edition; and artist/graphic designer Brandy Polay for her stunning original cover design and Brad Harris for his incisive cover design of the expanded *On Pluto* edition.

The Alzheimer's community on Cape Cod and the Islands was instrumental in guiding me and inspiring me along the process; among them: Dr. Molly Purdue and Melanie Braverman of Alzheimer's Family Support Center of Cape Cod; Suzanne Faith, RN psych, clinical director, Hope Dementia & Alzheimer's Services; and Pat Collins, a key Hope Dementia & Alzheimer's Services associate. Hope Dementia & Alzheimer's Services of Cape Cod and the Islands (hopedementia.org) has been a lifeline in providing services to me and my family.

Speaking of family, in addition to my mother, I thank my father, Francis Xavier O'Brien, for pushing me, through his own example, to pursue a career in journalism. I thank my brothers and sisters: Maureen, Lauren, Justine, Paul, Bernadette, Tim, Andy, and deceased brothers Gerard and Martin for their love and hope at all celestial levels. I also thank the late Carl Maresca, Suzanne O'Brien, Peter O'Brien, Scott O'Brien, "Uncle" Mark O'Brien, Stephen and Melina Maresca, Lou McGeorge, Tommy and Barb McGeorge, Jerry Reardon and family, Larry O'Malley, Barbara Anne Newbury, Jeanne O'Brien, Sally O'Brien and family, David Thompson, Matt Everett, author John Everett, and Laken Ferreira. Also, I thank my forty-four nieces and nephews; it might sound like a Gaelic cult, but family is the core of existence. Also, special thanks to Ray Hunter; Tom and Kathleen Henze and family; Bob and Gretchen Kelly and family; Buzz Keefe; Greg Keefe; Brendan Bruder; special friend Marcia Calasio; Lisa Cooper; Terry Stewart; Dave Baby; Marty Hinds; Dave Ernest; Harry and Gena Bonsall; Adria Renke; Scott Burns; Jim Burns; and Tom and Debbie Woods.

Special recognition also to close friend and college buddy Pat Calihan, who died recently of dementia; to his devoted wife, Becky, and all of Pat's family. Pat, we will never forget you. Promise!

Finally, I thank friends and colleagues for their love and support, in no particular order: Peter, Aaron, and Matt Polhemus, and Francie

Joseph; Jess Ritchie; Augusta Hixon; Bobby and Susan Norton; Tom and Peg Ryan; John and Katie Piekarski; Matt Everett; Tim and Maggie Everett; Mark St. John; Billy and Nancy St. John; Tony and Karen Keating; Jimmy and Debbie Dianni; Vinny and Kim Dempsey; Dickie O'Connell; Joe and Cathy Lewis of Joe's Beach Road Bar & Grille in East Orleans for their ongoing support; John Murphy and his family of the Land Ho! in Orleans; the gang at Mahoney's; close friends and supporters Dick and Nancy Koch; Charlie and Cindy Sumner; Dana and Gayle Conduit; Steve Shepherd; Mark and Anne Ohrenberger; Uncle Cody Morrow, Tim Whelan, and John Terrio; Cape Cod Museum of Natural History executive director Bob Dwyer; Anne Saint; Frank Andrews; Pat Fox; Ricky Weeks; Frank and Carolyn Dranginis; Mike Gradone; Mark Mathison; Brian Kavanaugh; Geoff and Rebecca Smith; Vern and Missy Smith; Barry, Nancy, and Kristin Souder; Barbara and Matt Losordo; Pastor Doug Scalise; former *Martha's Vineyard Times* editor Doug Cabral; Eileen and Jeff Smith; Paul and Mitzi Daley; Donald and Jack Shea; Bill O'Brien; Joe Penney; Sarah Alger; Wally Steinkrauss; Deb Farr; Tim Mahoney; Guy Stutz; Linda Figueiredo; Dave Taglianetti; Randy Hart; Mike Ford; Jeff Ford; Rob Chamberlain; Tammy Glivinski; Steve Boyson; Lynda Walsh; Debbie Stewart; Joanne and Len Hensas; Melissa and Nathaniel Philbrick; Linda Edson; Libby Gibson, Andrew Vorce, Leslie Snell, Linda Williams; Nat Lowell; Rick Turer; Barry and Joanne Powers; Sean Summers, Linda Apsey; producer Trevor Albert, and director/producer James Keach.

On Pluto would not be possible without the love and support of close friends and newspaper colleagues Bill Elfers, Chuck Goodrich, and their families. In ways they may never have realized in the moment, they encouraged me to reach for the best in this journey. Thank you.

In addition, I would also like to thank my close Fairfield University alumnus friends and other college buddies who contributed to an *On Pluto* GoFundMe page (www.gofundme.com/rallyforGOB); among us, we have more secrets about each other than the origins of the universe: Bob Kelly, Buzz Keenen, Bill Rogers, Ted Martens, Bill

Martin, Mike Kitson, Joe Berardino, Joe Moore, Greg McGrath, Dr. Terry Sacchi, George Groom, Matt Grasberger, Gary Bowen, David Baby, Paul Hoffman, Jack Keough, John Ryan, Dennis Gallagher, Skip Pakenham, George Romeo, Bill Kruse, Beth Kruse, Jim Clarke, Bob Pellegrino, Don Salomone, Kurt Raschi, Tom Kerwin, Scotty Burns, Tom Woods, Jim Burns, Peter Callagy, Ellen Kruse, and Ed Sapeta.

Thanks, also in my long-term memory to: Gail Lenihan Perry, Kerry Mahoney-Brown, Barbara Roe-Jamison, Linda Stamford-Changarelli, Judy Warren-Aufuso, Mary Obeck, Virginia Armando, Mary Devanney, and Donna DiCarlo.

Finally, I want to thank close friend and surrogate brother Bob Newman, general manager of magnificent Ocean Edge Resort in Brewster for allowing me to write a good part of this expanded *On Pluto* edition from the beautiful terrace at Ocean Edge overlooking Cape Cod Bay, an inspiration that carried me in the process.

In reading this litany initially, my brother-in-law Carl joked, "*Really!* You could have included the Red Chinese and the Bolsheviks."

Well, it takes a village with Alzheimer's.

In closing, I thank retired U.S. Supreme Court Justice Sandra Day O'Connor, whose husband, John, died of Alzheimer's. Justice O'Connor instructed me many years ago in the art of court reporting when I was a cub reporter at *The Arizona Republic* and she was a Maricopa County Superior Court judge. Justice O'Connor has been an enduring inspiration for families battling Alzheimer's.

ON PLUTO

Inside the Mind of Alzheimer's

INTRODUCTION

Living with Alzheimer's

Greg O'Brien

"As I look back over a misspent youth, I find myself more and more convinced that I had more fun doing news reporting than any other enterprise. It really is the life of kings."

—H.L. MENCKEN

A scribe is nothing without good notes. For years I've taken detailed notes as an embedded reporter inside the mind of Alzheimer's, chronicling the progression of this monster disease. Ever since I knew that something was terribly wrong after serious head injuries had "unmasked" a disease in the making, my reporting instincts, working off what doctors call a cognitive reserve, compelled me to document.

Like the word guessing game charades, I often use Google when I can't find the right words. "Sounds like," I type, describing the elusive word or action in the broadest of terms, then through a prolonged process of elimination, on a good day I find the word I was searching for, an agonizing process that drains. On bad days, I punt. For this expanded edition, I drafted daily over time thousands of pages of additional notes and journals as symptoms progress, to compile a blueprint of strategies, faith, and humor, a day-to-day focus on living with Alzheimer's, not dying with it—a hope that all is not lost when it appears to be.

1

The dictionary defines hope as confidence in the future; the Bible calls it faith. Collectively, we will need every ounce of hope in fighting Alzheimer's, a disease that stole my maternal grandfather, my mother, and my paternal uncle. Shortly before my father died of complications from circulation disorders, he, too, was diagnosed with dementia. Now Alzheimer's has come for me. In so many ways, those with Alzheimer's are like a dandelion—born as a flower, becoming a weed, then dying from the head down.

The numbers across the nation and the world are numbing. According to the Alzheimer's Association International, every three seconds someone in the world develops dementia. The Centers for Disease Control and Prevention has reported that the death rate from Alzheimer's in the United States rose an average 55 percent from 1999 to 2014, and is expected to increase precipitously in years to come. There are now 5.5 million Americans diagnosed with the disease, a number that does not take into consideration those who haven't sought a diagnosis or diagnoses that have not been properly reported. Worldwide, close to 30 million people have been diagnosed with Alzheimer's. By the year 2050, the number of Alzheimer's diagnoses in the U.S. is expected to more than double to 13.8 million people, and worldwide more than 135 million are projected to have some form of dementia.

The disease, statistics confirm, affects woman, Hispanics, African Americans, and Asians in greater numbers than white males. From 1999 to 2014, the death rate in the U.S. from Alzheimer's rose more than 43 percent for white males, 62 percent for women, 99 percent for African Americans, 107 percent for Hispanics, and 151 percent for Asians.

Alzheimer's, which slowly robs one of self and destroys mental and physical capacity, is the sixth-leading cause of death in U.S., and the only leading killer for which there is no cure or no means of slowing the progression. In England and Wales, Alzheimer's and other dementias have now challenged heart disease as the leading cause of death, and other countries are reporting similar rises.

The scourge of the Baby Boom generation in the U.S. and those 65 or older worldwide is cresting. The epidemic is no longer a threat; it is in play. In the next 15 years, Alzheimer's and other forms of dementia are expected to exceed cancer and heart disease sevenfold, and without a cure, it will bankrupt Medicare.

"There's the cruel fact that as we become more sophisticated in our ability to operate and medicate away physical issues associated with aging—such as heart disease and stroke—there is more time for something to go awry in our minds," the *Washington Post* observed recently.

And then there's the lurching cost. Soaring health costs for long-term care and hospice for those with Alzheimer's and other dementias are projected to increase from $259 billion in 2017 to $1.1 trillion in 2050. The impact on caregivers is equally staggering. When one in the family has Alzheimer's, the entire family suffers from it. The Centers for Disease Control and Prevention reports that caregivers of persons with dementia, including Alzheimer's, provide billions of hours annually of unpaid assistance. The effort creates ineffable financial and medical strain among selfless caregivers, who are more prone to deep depression and a breakdown of their immune systems.

"These findings raise needed public awareness of how fast this disease is growing and destroying families, and how we must stand firm against any action that reduces the nation's ability to innovate and speed cures," says George Vradenburg, co-founder with his late wife, Trish, of the distinguished Washington, D.C.-based advocacy group UsAgainstAlzheimer's.

To raise such awareness, new horizons are needed to probe the depths of the unimaginable, as NASA's intrepid spacecraft New Horizons explored beyond imaginable reach with a historic flyby in July 2015 of the dwarf planet Pluto, coming within 7,700 miles of the icy sphere after traveling 4.6 billion miles, and now heading deeper into the Kuiper Belt, then out into interstellar space, drifting in an endless sea of the cosmos in the hopes, perhaps, of landing in the palm of God's hands. There are remarkable parallels between Alzheimer's and Pluto: dense isolation, penetrating silence, a harsh environment, and a world of unthinkable contrasts.

On Pluto: Inside the Mind of Alzheimer's is the first book written by an investigative reporter embedded inside the mind of Alzheimer's chronicling the progression of his own disease. This expanded edition explores a sequence of progressions, the narratives of others in this disease, and first-person reflections from family and caregivers about the hope of living with Alzheimer's. The dying part comes later. The first section of *On Pluto*, the initial edition, probes the diagnosis of Alzheimer's and its stinging aftermath; the second section, part of the new expanded edition, delves into strategies for living with the disease and chronicles the narratives of others; the third section offers first-person family reflections on caregiving, the struggles of the journey, and the peace of unconditional love.

As the great Bugs Bunny once opined, "Don't take life too seriously, 'cause no one gets out alive." As a weathered reporter, I see myself in this journey as a narrator for the Baby Boom generation struggling with Alzheimer's. My story is their story; their story in my story. There is an old axiom in the newspaper business: if you don't tell your own story, someone else tells it for you. For many years, doctors, scholars, and medical experts, God bless them, have been telling the story of Alzheimer's. Now it's time for those in the cusp of this disease to speak out. *On Pluto* seeks to hold a mirror to a generation in crisis, akin perhaps, in historical terms, to holding a lantern in Revolutionary times at the top of the old North Church steeple in Boston's North End, "One if by land, and two if by sea." Today worldwide, those in the disease, their families, and their caregivers are holding two lanterns in this midnight ride. As Henry Wadsworth Longfellow so beautifully wrote:

"A voice in the darkness, a knock at the door,
And a word that shall echo for evermore!"

Death comes to all. While we have little influence over time and place, we can choose our attitudes as we head through the tunnel to a brighter light. As Leonardo da Vinci observed in the fifteenth century: "While I thought that I was learning how to live, I have been learning how to die." Aren't we all, if we lift the thin veil of denial?

So, we press on in the shadows of role models. One of the most inspiring to me is a man called "Sweetness." He taught us legions on the gridiron about perseverance. The late Hall of Fame Chicago Bears legend, Walter Payton, nine times an All Pro, was one of the most prolific running backs in NFL history; he died too young at age forty-five of cancer. Toward the end of his extraordinary career, a sports commentator declared on air in full reverence: "Walter Payton has run for more than nine miles!" To which his co-anchor replied intuitively, "Yes, and Payton did that getting knocked down every 4.6 yards, and getting back up again!"

If anyone had true grit in the fight against Alzheimer's, it was Glen Campbell. Diagnosed with the disease in 2011, he refused to retreat, courageously relying on his muscle memory as one of the nation's greatest songwriters and country pop singers, teaching the rest of us along the way how to shine when the stage lights go dim.

While the lights now have gone dark for Campbell, his spirit and the faith of the man endures—a beacon for the world.

In Campbell's fight against this demon, he was not "shackled by forgotten words and bonds." While the words early on eluded him at times, the bonds were never-ending with his faithful family, friends, and anyone who cared to embrace the vision of a man comfortable enough in his own skin years ago to have taken an immeasurable risk on a national stage as a daring role model living with Alzheimer's, until the end.

Upon announcing his diagnosis, akin to a death sentence, Campbell, along with his courageous wife, Kim, and three of his gifted children, daughter Ashley and sons Cal and Shannon, launched an intrepid "Goodbye Tour"—151 inspiring concerts throughout the nation. The Goodbye Tour, subject of an inspiring film by award-winning filmmakers James Keach and Trevor Albert, was a labor of love for Campbell, a labor that would have tested a man half his age, unfettered by disease.

Director Keach called Campbell "a Rocky with a guitar."

I've been blessed to know Kim Campbell, along with filmmakers Keach and Albert. They are soldiers on the front lines in this lonely fight, and have inspired me in my own journey with Alzheimer's. As Campbell took to his heart with music, he motivated me to continue writing for as long as it is possible.

Campbell was a lamppost earlier in my life. I was drawn to his music as a young man on cross-country trips from Westchester County in New York, to the University of Arizona in Tucson, where I studied journalism. Campbell's sweet, often raw and throaty voice, resonating from a vintage eight-track tape cartridge, offered the verve to keep me focused while driving my yellow Opel Kadett. The two of us were worlds apart, yet unknowingly headed on a collision course with Alzheimer's.

On the road, I memorized just about every lyric of his *Greatest Hits* album, produced in 1971, never forgetting to hit the replay: "Wichita Lineman" as I crossed Kansas; "By the Time I Get to Phoenix," as I drove through the Petrified Forest in remote northeastern Arizona, often at 2 a.m. with moonlight glistening off the semi-desert shrub steppes and colorful badlands; and "Gentle on My Mind" as I passed the graceful Santa Catalina Mountains, rising from the valley on the outskirts of Tucson. I can still hear Campbell's voice.

And then there's Pat Summitt, the legendary retired coach of the Tennessee women's basketball team, who told the *Knoxville News Sentinel*, after announcing her diagnosis of early-onset Alzheimer's and finishing out the 2011–12 season: "There's not going to be any pity party, and I'll make sure of that . . . Obviously, I realize I may have some limitations with this condition since there will be some good days and some bad days."

And so it is with chronic illness, good days and bad days. You get knocked down, you get back up. Again and again. You find a way to win—as New England Patriots coach Bill Belichick would insist— on the playing field, on the job, in the home, or in a fight against cancer, heart disease, AIDS, Parkinson's, autism, depression, diabetes, dementia, or any number of vile illnesses. Lying down in football, as it is in wrestling, is a position of defeat. That's not a good place for any of us. As a famed billboard on Boston's Southeast Expressway proclaimed in the early '70s about Boston Bruin premier center Phil Esposito: "Jesus Saves. But Esposito scores on the rebound!"

My place today is with early-onset Alzheimer's; it's a death in slow motion. A freeze frame at times.

Doctors tell me I'm working off a "cognitive reserve," a backup tank of inherited intellect that will carry me in cycles for years to come. They tell me to slow down, conserve the tank. It's lights out, they warn, when the tank goes dry, just as it was for my mother. In laymen's terms, the right side of my brain—the creative, sweet spot— is intact, for the most part, although the writing and communication process now takes exponentially longer. The left side, the area of the brain reserved for executive functions, judgment, balance, continence, short-term memory, financial analysis, and recognition of friends and colleagues is, at times, in a free fall. Doctors advise that I will likely write and communicate with declining articulation, until the lights dim, but other functions will continue to ebb. Daily exercise and writing are my succor, helping me reboot and reduce confusion. I try to stay locked in, as a missile is on target, but "locked in" likewise is a medical disorder in which an individual who cannot speak because of paralysis communicates through a blink of an eye. Some days, I find myself between definitions—using every available memory device and strategy, cerebral and handheld, to communicate.

More recently, I've experienced blackouts and the right side of my body collapsing without notice, as brain signals fail to connect. I've now lost my right to drive, and I've lost senses of taste and smelling, along with a greater loss of balance and continence.

All the darkness in the world, my mother taught me, cannot snuff out a single candle. I know that darkness. It's a place I call "Pluto," in allegorical terms, a reference from my early days as an investigative reporter when I went deep "off-the-record" with sources. "We're heading out to Pluto," I would say, "where no one can see you or can hear what is said."

The Pluto metaphor still works for me, more than ever, as I seek the peace of isolation and pursue the urge to drift out as Alzheimer's overcomes at intervals. Pluto is the perfect place to get lost. Formerly the ninth planet, it is now relegated to "dwarf planet" status. Pluto's orbit, like Alzheimer's, is chaotic; its tiny size makes it sensitive to immeasurably small particles of the solar system, hard-to-predict factors that will gradually disrupt an orbit. Over the years, I've taken close family, colleagues, and clients "out to Pluto" to discuss off-record unmentionables of life in a place without oxygen. There will come a day when, like my grandfather and my mother before me, I won't return from this dark, icy place; and when that happens, I want family and friends to know where I am. The Irish like to say, "Never get mad, get even." And so, I'm getting even with Alzheimer's—not for me, but for my children, for you and your children, and for a generation of Baby Boomers, their families and loved ones, who face this demon prowling like Abaddon.

On Pluto: Inside the Mind of Alzheimer's is not a pity party or a misery memoir. It is an insider's guide, a generational road map of how to battle this cunning killer for as long as possible. To fight an enemy, one must study the enemy, and have working strategies in place. As the great ancient Chinese general Sun Tzu, assumed author of *The Art of War*, once counseled, "Tactics without strategy is the noise before defeat."

There is plenty of noise on the Alzheimer's front today, much defeat, and hardly enough funding for a cure. Not even close.

Alzheimer's, named for Dr. Aloysius "Alois" Alzheimer, who in 1906 first identified amyloid plaques and neurofibrillary tangles that rob the brain of identity, is the most common form of dementia— an umbrella term for irreversible cognitive collapse. Alzheimer's progresses slowly in stages, slaying neurons in the brain. The early stage is marked with increasing impairment of learning and short-term memory with some language challenges. The moderate stage is a progressive deterioration that leads to incapacity to perform certain common daily functions: short-term memory worsens, filter is lost, rage is intense, inability at times to recognize familiar places and people; some urinary and bowel incontinence; and at times, "illusionary misidentifications," which the layman, less politely, would term hallucinations.

I'm slowly moving toward the moderate stage, doctors say. The advanced stage—the stereotypical perception of Alzheimer's—is characterized by wandering and a complete shutdown of cognitive and body functions. Collectively, this slow demise can take up to two decades or more once it's been diagnosed, and can begin in pathology fifteen years before diagnosis. With some, the progression, for reasons unknown, is far quicker.

This is not your grandfather's disease; it is fast becoming a disease of the young or young at heart. It's been said that Alzheimer's is like having a thin sliver of your brain shaved off every day.

Stephen King couldn't have devised a better plot.

Should you be frightened if you frequently forget where you put your keys? Maybe it's nothing, perhaps a "senior moment," or maybe it is the start of something. There is a clear distinction between forgetting where you parked your car and forgetting what your car looks like; forgetting where you put your glasses, and forgetting that you have glasses; getting lost on familiar roads because you've been daydreaming, and getting lost because your brain's capacity to store information is greatly diminished.

On Pluto: Inside the Mind of Alzheimer's is a story that might be yours one day, or the story of a close friend or loved one; please don't assume it won't. Some of the language within is raw, full of rage, but real in its pain and fear. In full candor, we can all assist future generations in the hand-off of a cure for Alzheimer's and other dementias, with a greater collective understanding of the disease, more resources, and a worldwide commitment to find a cure. My hope is that we all listen more. A pebble tossed into a placid pond ripples far more than in roiling waters. In the pages to follow, I offer a front-row seat into the mysteries of this disease, an out-of-body experience on a trajectory to Pluto.

To understand this disease, one must step outside to see inside.

Ernest Hemingway once wrote, "The world breaks everyone, and afterward, some are strong in the broken places."

Be strong in the broken places . . .

PART ONE

ON PLUTO
Inside the Mind of Alzheimer's

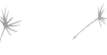

1

A Place of Recall

The wind has shifted on Cape Cod. A rusted iron cod on the weathervane at the gable end of the barn is pointing southwest, a warning of foul weather fast approaching from the nor'east. The weathered New England cedar shingles at a precise nine-inch pitch are wet with a fine mist. Near a side door, framed by lobster buoys washed up on the shoreline, a simple white dory window box is filled with colorful perennials. The barn has the feel of a dune shack, a writer's retreat at the end of a barrier beach—all of it natural, a reflection of the man and his memories snug within.

The door is open, revealing a time capsule of newspaper and magazine clippings, shelves of books, photos of the renowned, the infamous, and other memorabilia. I am innately connected to this man within and to his memories. In his sixties, he is well-kept, the product of running four miles a day; his horn-rimmed glasses and long tufts of graying hair evoke the look of a college professor. He strikes me as a bit of a prick, yet engaging. I know him, yet I can't relate in the moment. He's not the person I remember.

"Memory is deceptive, colored by today's events," Albert Einstein once observed.

Today's events are a flash, fully an out-of-body encounter, a flood of disconnected synapses, as I discern a flickering picture as if

13

maneuvering rabbit ears on a vintage black-and-white TV, trying to get the focus just right. The human brain, a fragile organ that inaugurates connectivity the first week *in utero*, contains 100 billion neurons—16 billion times the number of people on Earth—with each neuron igniting more than 10,000 synaptic connections to other neurons, totaling more than a trillion connections that store memories. If your brain functioned like a digital video recorder, it could hold more than three million hours of TV shows, enough video storage for 300 years. Not bad for a mass the size of an average head of cabbage, with the encoding, storage, and retrieval capacity to determine, on a good day, how many angels can dance on the head of a pin. So, why can't I get a clear picture today? The image is out of focus. When I look through this prism of an altered state, the picture is muddled. I press on for affirmation.

The man is the essence of a Baby Boomer—an over-achiever, an individual of purpose, gregarious, the oldest boy in an Irish Catholic family of ten, a father of three, husband of a virtuous wife for forty years, the patriarchal uncle to forty-four nieces and nephews, and a man who always thought, until now, that better days lay ahead. That's the way it is with Boomers, the invincible generation—sons and daughters of the Greatest Generation whose grandparents endured World War I, and whose parents then survived the Great Depression and World War II, perhaps the last world conflagration until Armageddon. These Boomers, a record 75 million of them born between 1946 and 1964, first played by the rules, then broke the rules, then made new rules. Boomers grew up in a time when we thought shit didn't happen.

I look to the walls around my office in order to connect the dots. The writer within grew up in the 1950s, formative years when Einstein was still thinking, Hemingway was still writing, and Sinatra was still crooning. Like all Boomers of the day, the man's early life reflects history: the long, fading shadow of Franklin Delano Roosevelt; the dropping of hellish atomic bombs on Hiroshima and Nagasaki; the Korean War; the election of presidents Dwight Eisenhower, John F. Kennedy, Lyndon B. Johnson, Richard Nixon, and all the baggage; the apocalyptic Cuban Missile Crisis; the Vietnam War; Woodstock; the birth of free love; and the death of innocence. It was a revolutionary time that spanned perhaps more cultural shifts than any other generation with writers, artists, and musicians who still define this country's political, secular, and artistic persona.

Like the Beatles' *Nowhere Man*, "Isn't he a bit like you and me." Looking around a room, one can learn legions from what's displayed on the walls. They paint "word pictures." Everywhere, there are historical, framed front-page stories and magazine covers from *The New York Times*, *The New Yorker*, *Washington Post*, the *Daily News*, the *Los Angeles Times*, the old *Boston Herald Traveler*, *Boston Record*, and one from the *Yarmouth Register*, dated July 12, 1861, reporting Abraham Lincoln's declaration to Congress of the Civil War. The office is a news museum of sorts, with news clippings of the firing on Fort Sumter, JFK's assassination, Nixon's resignation, Anwar Sadat's murder, the shooting of Pope John Paul II, the Shuttle explosion, the 9/11 attacks on the World Trade Center and Pentagon, and much more. In a corner is a frayed copy of the July 21, 1969 *Burlington Free Press* announcing that man has walked on the moon. Below the fold, toward the bottom of the page, is a photo of a 1968 Oldsmobile Delmont 88 that took a horrible turn for the worse into history off a narrow dike bridge on Martha's Vineyard. The caption directs readers to an inside story, the luck of the tragic Irish: Ted Kennedy's "Chappaquiddick incident," the death of Mary Jo Kopechne, buried on page six.

On the walls are news reports and magazine stories the man wrote years ago for publications—stories on Tip O'Neill, Jimmy Carter, the Kennedy family, Bill Clinton, the federal court system, political corruption, and investigative stories on the mafia. On a wicker chair nearby is a profile of a former Phoenix Superior Court judge, who in the late '70s mentored him at *The Arizona Republic* in the art of court reporting—Sandra Day O'Connor. Years later, President Ronald Reagan appointed the Stanford Law School graduate who grew up on an Arizona cattle ranch as the nation's first woman Supreme Court Justice. Judge O'Connor had urged her student repeatedly before leaving for Washington to keep asking questions.

"Keep at it until you get the answers!" she counseled. And he does today.

Everything in this room tells a story, purposefully arranged in almost chronological order, as if to remind, almost reassure, its occupant of a timeline, a collective long-term memory, the hard drive of one's life, the answers—from historic events, to family photos, to memorabilia. In a curious contradiction, there's a hint of eclectic New York and Boston family roots, which clash over sports: framed headlines of the New England Patriots, Red Sox, Boston Celtics, and Boston Bruins, alongside classic black-and-white photos of a young Mickey Mantle, Yogi Berra, Joe DiMaggio, and Lou Gehrig. On a shelf below, a 1917 photograph of a sullen Babe Ruth in a Boston Red Sox uniform stares out blankly. There is a quote of Ruth's below it: "Never let the fear of striking out get in your way."

Curiously enough, tacked to an adjacent wall is a tale, author unknown, of an Irishman's dying wish with two strikes against him.

His Irish friends relate:

An elderly gentleman lay dying in bed. While suffering the agonies of a pending death, he suddenly smelled the aroma of his favorite chocolate chip cookies, wafting up the stairs. He gathered his remaining strength and lifted himself in the bed. Leaning against the wall, he slowly made his way out of the bedroom and with even greater effort, gripping the railing with both hands, he crawled downstairs. With labored breath, he leaned against the door-frame and gazed into the kitchen. Were it not for death's agony, he would have thought himself already in Heaven for there spread out on wax paper on the kitchen table were literally hundreds of his favorite chocolate chip cookies.

Was the elderly Irishman in Heaven or was it one final act of heroic love from his Irish wife of sixty years, seeing to it that he left this world a happy man?

Mustering one great final effort, he threw himself towards the table, landing on his knees in a rumpled posture. His parched lips parted; the wondrous taste of the cookie was already in his mouth, seemingly bringing him back to life.

The aging and withered hand trembled on its way to a cookie on the edge of the table when he was suddenly smacked with a spatula by his wife ...

Fuck off, they're for the funeral!

There will be no funeral today, only an epiphany of what's to come, and with the luck of the Irish, maybe a few steaming hot chocolate chip cookies, as denial gradually gives way, over time, to reality. Stephen Stills had it right: "Love the one you're with."

I do.

For I must.

For this man is me.

2

Mr. Potato Head

A sea of spring dandelions outside the barn is leaning toward the bay in a stiff wind, a wave of yellow. They capture my attention. I am drawn to the cluster. The dandelion—a French derivative for "*dent de lion*," the tooth of a lion, with its sharp yellow leaves and believed to date back 30 million years—is born as a flower, becomes a weed, dies slowly from the head down; then its white, fluffy seeds, gentle blowballs, genetically identical to the parent plant, blow away to pollinate the world.

And so it is with Alzheimer's.

Ralph Waldo Emerson wrote in his essay *Fortune of the Republic*, "What is a weed? A plant whose virtues have not yet been discovered." Perhaps Emerson, who succumbed to Alzheimer's-like symptoms, was contemplating the dandelion—a free-spirit of a plant, a symbol of courage and hope, with relevance in medicine, legend, and in Christianity. In medieval times, the dandelion, a bitter herb, was a symbol for the crucifixion of Christ.

The virtue of Alzheimer's is a hope for redemption—not here for now, but beyond.

Sitting alone in my office, deep in thought, looking out over an acre of overgrown lawn, sprinkled with dandelions, and surrounded inside by the hard copy of long-term memory, a place where confusion gives way to clarity and humor resurrects, I remember the yarn of the septuagenarian who reluctantly arranged a medical exam after years of denial:

"I have some bad news for you," the doctor says after a battery of tests. "You have cancer!"

"That's dreadful," the man replies.

"It gets worse," the doctor notes.

"You have Alzheimer's!"

The man pauses to collect his thoughts, then says with full confidence, "Thank God, I don't have cancer!"

I laugh, but it's more an enigma than a joke.

Some inherit stock portfolios and buckets of cash. Others, hand-me-downs. I've inherited my folks' medical records: my late father, Francis Xavier O'Brien, a mulish second-generation Irish American and a Bronx boy, had prostate cancer, complicated by critical circulation disease and an onslaught in his final days of dementia; my mother, Virginia Brown O'Brien, with second-generation Irish roots as well, the hero of my life, died of Alzheimer's in a bruising, knockdown prizefight of a battle, as her father had decades earlier.

I have been diagnosed with both—cancer and Alzheimer's.

I've declined cancer treatment for now, on grounds that no one by choice wants to go to a nursing home. I saw what Alzheimer's robbed from my grandfather and my mother, and learned earlier in life about "exit strategies" from seasoned venture capitalists in New York and Boston. Alzheimer's, to me, is far more distressing than my cancer. I'm looking now for an exit strategy.

You can't remove a brain.

Daily, I return to my office on the Cape in search of a past that has more relevance to me than the present or a future. There is great peace here among the elements of history, humor, and faith—cornerstones in my life. I look for strength from mentors, past and present, referenced in those clips and photos on the walls: celebrated country editors like the late Malcolm Hobbs of *The Cape Codder*, a surrogate father figure, the distinguished Henry Beetle Hough of the *Martha's Vineyard Gazette*, and my late neighbor John Hay, considered among the nation's finest nature writers, on par with Henry David Thoreau. Hay was a man who could paint brilliant word pictures with the stroke of a typewriter key as a master does with a brush. I was blessed in spending time with them, absorbing like a sea sponge as they taught me to write. They all have become an enduring part of what I believe a good writer, a persevering individual, ought to be. Perseverance separates the artist from the dabbler, editor Hobbs once told me. So it is with life; you press on.

Near my writing desk is a copy of the bestseller *The Perfect Storm*, known in these parts as the Halloween Nor'easter of 1991. I first met author Sebastian Junger as a young man when he was a budding scribbler, soon to be star, and I was an editor at *The Cape Codder*, instructing the freelancer in the art of reporting, letting a good story tell itself. Junger, an excellent student with extraordinary drive, excelled beyond all expectation. I find myself today in the midst of my own perfect storm—a rogue wave of fear, perhaps a life unfulfilled.

On a bookcase in the corner are photographs of my children— Brendan, Colleen, and Conor, and my wife Mary Catherine—all reminders of a past and a fleeting present. There is a recent precious photograph taken by Colleen at an Alzheimer's fundraising marathon that she ran in Boston. The photo is of a pure white running cap alongside two purple wrist bands, the symbolic color of the battle against Alzheimer's, all arranged on a stark linen table cloth. She wore them in the race.

The cap is inscribed, "Dad, this is for you."

Dementia runs in my family, practically gallops on some branches of the family tree. My maternal grandfather, George Brown, died decades ago of "hardening of the arteries," a precursor for Alzheimer's, now considered a code word for Alzheimer's or vascular dementia. I had a chilling front-row seat as a child, and later, head-on with my mother's slow progression of a death in slow motion. My dad, in the waning months of a complicated medical history, was also diagnosed with dementia, and his only brother, my uncle, now suffers from a variant of Alzheimer's. The images are piercing.

It was in 2009 when I was diagnosed with early-onset Alzheimer's, several years after first experiencing early symptoms and after a horrific head injury sustained years earlier in a bicycle accident that doctors say "unmasked" a disease in the making. Head injuries, experts say, can precipitate Alzheimer's and other dementias when one is predisposed to the disease. Years later, I sustained a second tramautic head injury in a car crash, in addition to all the concussions sustained playing baseball and football in high school and college.

According to the Mayo Clinic, one is at greatest risk of developing dementia, Alzheimer's, or CTE (chronic traumatic encephalopathy) after head injuries, particularly if one has other risk factors, like a family history, carrying the Alzheimer's marker gene, or sport injuries. A recent study, for example, published in *JAMA* (*Journal of the American Medical Association*) found that 99 percent of deceased National Football Association players who had donated their brains to scientific research were found to have CTE, a neurodegenerative brain disease found in individuals with repeated head injuries. "The disease," CNN reports, "is pathologically marked by a buildup of abnormal tau protein in the brain that can disable neuropathways and lead to a variety of clinical symptoms. These include memory loss, confusion, impaired judgment, aggression, depression, anxiety, impulse control issues and sometimes suicidal behavior."

Dumbass that I was with the bike accident, I wasn't wearing a helmet at the time. Repeated clinical tests, an MRI, and a brain scan confirmed the diagnosis. The brain (SPECT) scan revealed "a large deficit involving the temporal parietal and also occipital lobes bilaterally," as noted in the blunt eighty pages of my medical records. That's code for pack your bags, buddy. Another test revealed that I carry a gene called ApoE4. Present in about fourteen percent of the population and implicated in Alzheimer's, ApoE4 is a known genetic risk for the disease. Inheritance indeed is a mixed bag. Doctors tell me that I'm working off a "cognitive reserve," a reservoir of inherited intellect that will carry me in cycles for years to come. They tell me to slow down, conserve the tank. I'm not sure how much reserve remains; I guess I'll find out how smart my mother was. I'm hoping she was a genius. The brain I inherited is like an old Porsche engine. It has to crank at high speeds, or it sputters. When I run out of gas someday, I hope I pull off the road to a place with a water view. For now, I keep driving, foot to the floor.

I strive to keep the focus today on *living* with Alzheimer's, not dying with it.

But the view within is out of sync many days. The "right side" of my brain—the creative sweet spot—is mostly intact, although the writing and communication process now takes much longer. The left side, reserved for judgment, executive functions, and financial analysis, is in a free fall on bad days. Doctors advise that I will likely write and communicate, with diminishing articulation, until the lights go out, as other functions continue to wane, an idiot-savant syndrome, I suppose.

"Plan for it," they have advised me.

But as the Great Bambino once said, "You can't beat the person who won't give up."

These demons, I keep telling myself, *don't know who they're fucking with!*

Years ago, I thought I was Clark Kent, but today I feel more like a baffled Jimmy Olsen. And on days of muddle, more like Mr. Magoo, the wispy cartoon character, created in 1949, who couldn't see straight, exacerbated by his stubbornness to acknowledge a problem, or like Mr. Potato Head, with the wacky pushpins and all. The genius of Brooklyn-born investor George Lerner in the early '50s, the original Mr. Potato Head sold for ninety-eight cents, was the first toy ever advertised on television, and came with pushpin plastic hands, feet, ears, two mouths, two pairs of eyes, four noses, three hats, eyeglasses, a pipe, and eight felt pieces resembling facial hair. Fifty years ago, Hasbro provided a plastic potato body, given complaints of rotting vegetables. I think of myself now as Mr. Potato Head with a rotting head and stick-on body parts, depending on my mood and the brain's diminishing ability to function.

Before the onset of Alzheimer's, I thought of my brain as a large depository, a dumping ground of sorts, a large storage bin for stashing a cornucopia of politics, current events, sports, trivia, and points of view that nobody really cares about but me. In Alzheimer's, the brain atrophies; it shrinks radically, a shrinkage of brain tissue. And I always thought shrinkage was what happened to guys after a dip in a cold ocean.

"Getting old ain't for sissies," Bette Davis once opined. She was spot on. We all need to put on our big boy and big girl pants.

Daily medications serve to keep my engine in tune and slow a progression of the disease: twenty-three milligrams daily of Aricept, the commonly prescribed Alzheimer's medication, the legal limit; twenty milligrams of Namenda in a combined therapy that serves to reboot the brain; fifty milligrams of Trazodone to help me sleep; and twenty milligrams of Celexa (Citalopram) to help control the rage on days when I hurl the phone across the room, a perfect strike to the sink, because in the moment I can't remember how to dial, or when I smash the lawn sprinkler against an oak tree in the backyard because I can't recall how it works, or when I push open the flaming hot glass door to the family room wood stove barehanded to stoke the fire just because I thought it was a good idea until the skin melts in a third-degree burn, or simply when I cry privately, the tears of a little boy, because I fear that I'm alone, nobody cares, and the innings are starting to fade. Hey, I'm not stupid, nor are the millions of others with Alzheimer's; we just have a disease.

But on particularly down days, in between moments of focus, I feel a bit like a svelte stand-in for Curly Howard of *The Three Stooges*, lots of running in circles—"nyuk-nyuk-nyuk ... woob-woob-woob!" Alzheimer's is a sickness that runs in circles or meanders for an eventual kill. It's analogous to the prototypical arcade game Pac-Man in which a pie-faced yellow icon navigates a maze of challenges, eating Pac-dots to get to the next level. While the iconic video game was designed to have no ending, there are no "power pellets" in Alzheimer's to consume the enemies of ghosts, goblins, and monsters, as this Pac-Man in slow motion consumes brain cells, one by one.

Game over! At some point you run out of quarters.

"You're a pioneer," a counselor once urged me in a men's early-onset Alzheimer's support group, speaking before a gathering of lawyers, engineers, architects, and a minister—all diagnosed with the disease, and individuals as accomplished as one would find anywhere. "Take good notes," he urged us.

I have.

Having witnessed the demise of family members, seen the anguish firsthand inside nursing homes, felt the disconnect of dementia in intimate terms, I've overcome a reticence to speak out. There was a time when I worried about what family, friends, colleagues, and clients would think or say. No longer. I suppose one could say that I'm outing myself now. Gore Vidal once observed, "Style is knowing who you are, what you want to say, and not giving a damn."

I don't give a damn, if that's what it takes to get the word out.

As any writer knows, solid reporting follows a stock of knowledge. So, I've studied the brain to the extent that I can and have learned, over time, that it is the most energy-consuming part of the body; it represents about two percent of the body's weight, but has the raw computer power of more than 16 billion times the number of people on Earth. Without sufficient brain power, some suggest, we're like astronauts on a space walk whose lifeline has just been cut. We drift to the ends of the universe. Out beyond, to Pluto.

Boomers will drift, facing an unimaginable epidemic of Alzheimer's and related dementias, in projected numbers seven times greater than cancer or heart disease, whose critical research and funding starkly outpaces Alzheimer's tenfold. There are an estimated 35 million people worldwide today diagnosed with Alzheimer's or a related dementia, an estimated five million in the U.S. afflicted with Alzheimer's, and predictions of up to 13.8 million Americans diagnosed with the disease by 2050 (www.alz.org).

Yes, I realize that that's the second time I've quoted those statistics to you, dear reader, but they bear repeating.

Researchers suggest new ways of combating the disease. Alzheimer's in the making must be stopped long before it damages the brain, doctors say. Research shows that once an individual begins to lose synapse (the brain structure allowing a neuron, a nerve cell, to pass an electrical or chemical signal to another cell), and once neurons are lost, the brain cannot recover. Alzheimer's starts long before symptoms are apparent to others, perhaps ten or more years earlier, and if diagnosed early and treated with medications before loss of synapse, the progression may be slowed, although it cannot be stopped, as doctors are learning.

Part of living with Alzheimer's and slowing the progression is in the daily training regimen to accelerate synapse. Consider the jaggy dendrite we learned about in high school biology—a spine or tree-like projection of a neuron that passes signals to other brain cells. Exercising the brain, experts say, builds new dendrites, pathways that create alternate routes for synapse that can help one function with Alzheimer's for longer periods, while other neurons are dying off. In short, I believe, one can re-circuit the brain to receive and transmit information, staving off, for a time, some of the more horrific symptoms of this disease. But in the end, the neurons go dead.

This is the place I find myself today, pushing back daily against a loss of synapse that is progressing, as neurons go dead. The challenge with public perception of Alzheimer's is that few want to embrace the disease, take it seriously, at least not until a family member or close friend is found in a nursing home sleeping in urine and talking to the walls. Public awareness of this disease, a balance between science, medicine, and faith, needs to change dramatically in anticipation of an Alzheimer's epidemic for Baby Boomers and others to come. In a snapshot, Alzheimer's is not the stereotypical end stage; it is the journey from the diagnosis to the grave.

There is an upside: you can get out of jury duty in a New York minute!

Does loss of brain function render loss of self; can we thrive in spiritual terms when the mind begins to fail? While the brain can be dissected, the soul is far more elusive, a place where sparks can miraculously shine through dysfunction. The balance between science and religion constitutes the essence of life, as we all struggle with this. "Death is not extinguishing the light. It is putting out the lamp before the dawn has come," wrote Rabindranath Tagore, the noted early twentieth century Bengali poet, philosopher, and thinker, the first non-European to win the Nobel Prize in Literature. Tagore and Einstein, among the brightest minds of the last millennium, both wrestled with concepts of the mind, life, death, and beyond: can the essence of a person survive without full function of the brain? It is a question probed daily by experts in the field of Alzheimer's, other forms of dementia, autism, and a range of brain disorders. It is a question for which those with Alzheimer's seek an answer. Tagore suggested the answer is "no" when the two met on July 14, 1930 at Einstein's home on the outskirts of Berlin, thought to be one of the most stimulating, intellectually riveting conversations in history, exploring the gap between the mind and the soul. The encounter was recorded.

"If there be some truth which has no sensuous or rational relation to the human mind, it will ever remain as nothing so long as we remain as human beings," Tagore told Einstein.

Replied Einstein bluntly, "Then I am more religious than you are!"

Out of the mouth of babes, six years later, a Manhattan sixth grader named Phyllis pursued the answer further after a question was posed in her Sunday School class on the truth between science and belief in God—the dividing line between the brain and the soul.

Moved by the query, Phyllis wrote Einstein, and he replied candidly: "Everyone who is seriously involved in the pursuit of science becomes convinced that some spirit is manifest in the laws of the universe, one that is vastly superior to that of man."

Einstein later said, "Before God we are all equally wise—and equally foolish."

3

Hell No!

The journey through Alzheimer's is a marathon, if one chooses to run it. It is exhausting, fully fatiguing, just staying in the moment and fighting to remember like an elephant, the largest land animal on Earth.

Elephants are my favorite. They have documented long-term memory, coveted today by Boomers. On a shelf in my office is a small ceramic elephant holding a fishing pole. I purchased it years ago from a gallery in Santa Fe, a cerebral place of awe-inspiring natural light. The ceramic serves to remind me daily of the need for retention and focus. The artwork has a place of prominence: It is the elephant in the room.

The word "dementia" is onomatopoeia for many, a word that conjures up a sound—in this case, a howl in the night or biblical imageries of a demonic maniac, a portrait no one wants to own.

Dementia is derived from the Latin root word for madness, "out of one's mind," an irreversible cognitive dysfunction, a walking nightmare in which you can't escape the bogeyman no matter how fast you run. Alzheimer's is a marathon against time, and so I keep running to outpace this disease that ultimately will overtake me.

Symbolic of the race, I run three to four miles a day, some of them at a pace of five- to six-minute miles on a treadmill, not bad for a man in his seventh decade. The rage within drives me to outrun the disease, but the sprinting will not halt the advance of ongoing memory loss, poor judgment, loss of self and problem solving, confusion with time, place, and words, withdrawal, abrupt changes in mood, and yes, the flat-out, earsplitting rage.

Words are the core of my life, and they are now lost on me at times. I often transpose words in what some medical professionals call an "attentional dyslexia." Public restrooms can be a problem. I look for the word "men," but at times, delete other letters around it, entering on occasion the "wo-men's" room, like a deer caught in headlights. The astonished look upon my face belies the innocence of my brain.

I think of my brain today, once a prized possession, as an iPhone: still a sophisticated device, but one that freezes up, shuts down without notice, drops calls, pocket dials with random or inappropriate conversation, and has a small battery that takes forever to charge. The inner anger is intense and manifests with Tourette's-like expletives and curses, involuntarily at times and in primordial fury over what is happening to me. I try to hide it from family and friends; often I can't. I've spoken to priests and ministers about the guilt of taking the Lord's name in vain; they tell me that God is resilient, everlastingly forgiving; that the Lord has wide shoulders. While we have free will, in God, there are no secrets.

Always persevere, the late legendary Brooklyn Dodgers pitcher Ralph Branca, a mentor and father figure, instructed me as a youth. Branca, who tossed the fabled home run pitch to New York Giant Bobby Thomson at the Polo Grounds on October 3, 1951, once told me, "God doesn't give you more than you can handle."

I never forgot that. Yet in a moment of doubt, I wonder. The fight against this disease consumes me, as with others, seven days a week, twenty-four hours a day mostly, often intentionally outside the wheelhouse of observers, but more and more in an embarrassment of lapses when one side of the brain, the frontal lobe that directs executive functions, continually wants to shut down, while the occipital lobe, the rear-most portion of the brain that controls creative intellect, declares: *Hell no!* The battle is numbing, like witnessing a head-on crash in slow motion when one can't remember how to find the brakes.

Today, I have little short-term memory, a progression of blanks; close to sixty percent of what I take in now is gone in seconds. It is dispiriting to lose a thought in a second, 72,000 seconds a day in a twenty-hour period of consciousness; to stand exposed, and yet stand one's ground, to begin to grasp in fundamental, naked terms, who one really is—the good, the bad, and the ugly. The ugly is haunting to me; the many things one would like to take back over the years, but cannot—feelings of failure and transgression.

I rely on copious notes and my iPhone with endless email reminders. I am startled when my inbox tells me I have forty new emails, then I realize that thirty-five of them are from me. The reminders help, though often I have no sense of time or place, and there are moments when I don't recognize people I've known most of my life—close friends, business acquaintances, and even my wife on two occasions. Sometimes, my mind plays games and paints other faces on people. Rather than panic, I just keep asking questions until I get some answers, or at least avoid yet another awkward episode. I work hard at deflecting the loss of judgment and filter. I find myself becoming more childlike, curiously enjoying the moments of innocence and potty talk. It's a reversal of fortune. In college, I was a history major, an honor student, good at rote memory. *Fuggedaboutit* now, Mr. Potato Head!

The most disturbing symptoms in my private darkness are the visual misperceptions, the playful but sometimes disturbing hallucinations—seeing, hearing, smelling, tasting, and feeling things that aren't there, as my mother once did. There was a time in Boston, for example, after a late business meeting when I retrieved my car on the third floor of a parking garage near Boston City Hall, only to find that a thick, grated metal wall had been pulled down to block my path. I feared I was locked in for the night. Walking toward the obstruction, the wall suddenly disappeared. It wasn't real.

Then there are those crawling, spider, and insect-like creatures that crawl regularly, some in sprays of blood, along the ceiling at different times of the day, sometimes in a platoon, that turn at ninety-degree angles, then inch a third of the way down the wall before floating toward me. I brush them away, almost in amusement, knowing now that they are not real, yet fearful of the cognitive decline. On a recent morning, I saw a bird in my bedroom circling above me in ever tighter orbits, then precipitously, the bird dove to my chest in a suicide mission. I screamed in horror. But there was no bird, no suicide mission, only my hallucination. And I was thankful for that.

To add to this mix, in what may be a brush with vascular dementia, I haven't had feeling in parts of my feet, hands, and lower-arm extremities for almost three years. Doctors are running tests. At least in the summer, out on my boat on Pleasant Bay, I don't feel the bites of greenheads—those nasty, stinging saltmarsh flies that draw blood.

Most diseases attack the body, but Alzheimer's attacks the mind, then the body. At sixty-five, I am reasonably trim with a reflection of muscle memory, but doctors have told me that beneath the surface, I might have the body of an eighty-year-old—a view confirmed in a recent New England Baptist Hospital diagnosis of acute spinal stenosis, scoliosis, and a further degeneration of the spine. Expect more breakdowns, they say. Bring on those greenheads!

Every night now, I sleep in my clothes; it feels more secure that way, often in sneakers tied tightly at my ankles so I can feel pressure below. Feet, don't fail me now. As the brain shrinks, it instinctively makes decisions, experts say, on what functions to power and what functions to power down to preserve fuel—much like the diabolical HAL 9000, the heuristically programmed computer on the spaceship *Discovery One* bound for Jupiter in Stanley Kubrick's *2001 Space Odyssey*.

"I'm sorry, Greg, I'm afraid I can't do that," my HAL-like brain seems to be saying. Pardon the paraphrase, Hal, but in your own words: *"I'm afraid. I'm afraid... the mind is going. I can feel it. I can feel it. My mind is going. There is no question about it. I can feel it. I can feel it... My instructor... taught me to sing a song. If you'd like to hear it I can sing it for you."*

There is no singing today, no artificial intelligence; I'm preserving fuel in my brain and limb-to-limb. I still have feeling on the bottoms of my feet for walking and running, yet no feeling on the tops of my feet. I still have feeling on the bottoms of my fingers for keyboarding, but little or no feeling on the tops of my hands, often at times up to my elbows. The tops of my feet and hands are dispensable, I suppose. My brain, a.k.a. HAL, may be conserving power, I've been advised—a sort of a cerebral brownout, akin to a calculated reduction in big city voltage to prevent electrical blackout in a deep sea of confusion.

A fish rots from the head down.

My brain was once a file cabinet, carefully arranged in categories, but at night as I sleep, it's as if someone has ransacked the files, dumping everything onto a cluttered floor. Before I get out of bed each morning, I have to pick up the "files" and arrange them in the correct order—envelopes of awareness, reality, family, work, and other elements in my life. Then it's off for coffee.

Ah, my caffeine friend. I love coffee, practically inhale it—a habit from my old days in the *Boston Herald American* newsroom when I would grab cups of coffee, hot and fresh, and walk from the newsroom down to the press room and back to work out the organization of a story. In my office, there is a retro vintage red tin sign that reads: *"Coffee! You can sleep when you're dead!"* But there are moments when I get confused about coffee, too, particularly on certain days walking from my office to the house with my laptop and empty coffee cup in hand. I know I'm supposed to do something with both. My brain sometimes tells me to put the laptop in the microwave and connect the cup to the printer. My spirit says otherwise: *Bad dog!*

I've been a bad dog lately. The disconnects continue exponentially, and they are alarming. Alone in my office a year ago when my brain froze up, I began screaming at God.

"You don't give a shit about me," I yelled. "Where the hell are you? I thought you're supposed to be here for me! I'm trying to do the best I can!"

Moments later, realizing I had to meet with someone, I rushed out to the car, only to find the back left tire as flat as a spatula.

Great, just fucking great, I yelled in rage. *God damn it, you just don't give a shit about me, Lord!*

I limped in the car about three miles down winding country roads to Brewster Mobil, in a Tourette's of swears the entire way.

"Got a problem," I told the attendant abruptly. "Fix it."

The sympathetic attendant, a kid who had graduated from high school years ago with one of my sons, said dutifully that he'd patch the tire right away—working his pliers to pull out the obstruction that had sent me into chaos. He returned in short order.

"You might want to look at this," he told me.

I stared intently at the culprit with astonishment. I couldn't believe what I saw. "Believe it," he said.

The culprit was a small, narrow piece of scrap metal, bent into a cross.

A perfect cross.

4

Heading Out to Pluto

My private darkness is, as I've explained, like an allegorical Pluto, a reference from my early days as an investigative reporter when I went deep "off-the-record" with sources. "We're heading out to Pluto," I would say, "where no one can hear what is said."

Now relegated to "dwarf planet" status, a sixth the mass of the moon and a third its volume, a "plutoid," given it is one of the bodies within the Kuiper Belt, a dense cluster of rock and ice. Pluto is a fine place to get lost metaphorically. Pluto's orbit, like mine at times, is chaotic; its tiny size makes it sensitive to immeasurably small particles of the solar system, hard-to-predict factors that will gradually disrupt an orbit—the perfect place to have a conversation that "never existed" or a conversation one can't recall. Over the years, I have often taken close family, colleagues, and clients "out to Pluto" to discuss unmentionables of life, revelations, and comments that need to stay in a place without oxygen. Many have been there and back with me, allegorically. I want them to be familiar with the planet. One day, like my mom, I won't return from this dark, icy place, and I want my family and friends to know where I am.

Then, as I've learned from observing my grandfather and mother, it's off even further beyond Pluto to Sedna for the final journey, the end staging of Alzheimer's. Sedna, a far more desolate place, the so-called dwarf tenth planet orbiting the sun beyond Pluto, was discovered in 2003. It is the coldest, darkest, most distant known body in our solar system—84 billion miles from the light of the sun, with an exceptionally long and elongated orbit, taking approximately 11,400 years to complete. It's a place where the temperature never rises above minus 240 degrees Celsius, minus 464 Fahrenheit.

That's consummate isolation; the word picture helps me relate. Distant heavenly bodies are far less intimidating to me than the realities of the end stage of Alzheimer's. Completion of the journey brings one to a far better, more peaceful place—Heaven, or however you want to define it. Family is waiting for me there, and there are days I can't wait to join them.

In the meantime, I see a lot of smart doctors and counselors with a range of connections to top Boston area hospitals and an assortment of coping mechanisms. But I crave the simple touch—an earnest smile, a hug, a touch of the hand—far more than a medical prescription or a clinical trial. A simple touch increases body awareness and alertness for those with Alzheimer's, and reduces feelings of confusion and anxiety. My general practitioner, Dr. Barry Conant, a close friend, an extraordinary man, and a better golfer than I, has offered the best advice to date. He has urged me, on numerous occasions, to stop assaulting Alzheimer's head-on.

"You can't win in a head butt," he has said with great insight. "That doesn't work."

"You just have to learn to dance with it!"

Perhaps Robert Frost said it best: "In three words, I can sum up everything I've learned about life: *It goes on.*"

Life goes on. Even on Pluto. The unnerving reality of Alzheimer's—the "he is me" part—resonates every day in fear, hope, humor, fundamental anger, challenge, and faith. No one wants to talk about Alzheimer's, but Alzheimer's doesn't play favorites. Just ask the families of individuals like Ronald Reagan, Norman Rockwell, E. B. White, former British prime ministers Harold Wilson and Margaret Thatcher, Barry Goldwater, Charlton Heston, Rita Hayworth, Otto Preminger, Aaron Copland, Sugar Ray Robinson, Burgess Meredith, civil rights defender Rosa Parks, Glen Campbell, Peter Falk, Pat Summit, Barbara Smith (B. Smith)—restaurateur, author, model, and television host, and the millions more afflicted with the disease or about to grapple with it—a spouse, family member, or close friend. A grim prognosis.

But laughter can be a powerful antidote to dementia—the pain, conflict, and stress of it. A good laugh, doctors say, reduces tension and can leave muscles relaxed for up to forty-five minutes. Laughter boosts the immune system, decreases stress hormones, and triggers the release of endorphins—the natural drug of choice.

Siri, my droll personal assistant and the knowledge navigator for my indispensable iPhone 5, is getting into the act.

Ask Siri, "Tell me a joke about Alzheimer's?"

"I can't," she often responds. "I forget the punch line."

Peter Falk never forgot a punch line. As a young investigative reporter for *The Arizona Republic* in the late 1970s, I modeled myself after the enigmatic Columbo—disheveled, wry, iconic, and exceeding expectations that had been intentionally lowered, yet always a city block ahead of others in his thinking.

"Aahhhh, there's just one more thing ... There's something that bothers me."

Early on in my marriage, I told my wife, Mary Catherine McGeorge (MC, as she is called today, given that the name is a mouthful or sounds like I married a nun), that all I had hoped to amount to in life was embodied, not in the riches of a lawyer, banker, or stock broker, but in the genius of Columbo—his meandering way of getting to the point, catching the detached off guard, breaking the story. Most women would have run for the hills, but MC bought into it—trench coat, spilled coffee, and ultimately, index finger to the frontal lobe.

Be careful what you wish for. I've become Columbo—the wily investigator, the cross-examiner par excellence, the reporter in wrinkled khakis, the guy who retells his stories, the man with Alzheimer's. Congratulations! What is Mary Catherine thinking now? God bless you, Peter Falk.

When MC and I first met at the University of Arizona in Tucson in 1971, she was thinking she wanted little to do with me. No surprise there. I was a court-jester type and accustomed to such rebuffs; never took them personally, actually fed off them. A carpetbagger from the East, I was best friends and roommates with her brothers, Tommy and Louie, and I was always good for laughs, not bad in sports, got good grades, and generally easy on the eyes in a crowded, smoky college bar, but no matinee idol. MC, in contrast, was stunningly beautiful in a natural way—Jennifer Aniston-like. Still is.

When she arrived in Tucson from California, guys lined up to date her, as if the Ark of the Covenant had been unearthed. Looking back, the queues were reminiscent of the conga line of headlights at the conclusion of the movie *Field of Dreams*. Tommy and Louie, on military orders from their father, Ken, who was the spitting image of John Wayne, were sentries at the guard, protecting their little sister at all costs. I respected and admired Ken, yet mostly feared him terribly; he was a tall, broad, sturdy rancher, a member then of the Arizona sheriff's posse, and a retired lieutenant colonel under General George Patton. Nobody messed with this guy. Nobody. While the bad dog in me wanted to date MC, the smart guy in me knew I didn't have a chance. I'm a smart guy for the most part. Or used to be.

So we became friends. Good friends in time. After graduation, when I was a cub reporter at *The Cape Codder* newspaper in Orleans, Massachusetts, I spent some holidays with the McGeorges—all nine of them—in Bakersfield, California. MC and I had a common thread in journalism, her college major. She had the distinction of writing for the *Tombstone Epitaph*, which in 1882 chronicled Deputy U.S. Marshal Wyatt Earp's shootout at the O.K. Corral in the "town too tough to die."

In June 1975, brother Louie came to the Cape for a visit. Little sister Mary Catherine tagged along. I showed them the country newsroom where I worked, the wide beaches of the Outer Cape with shifting sand dunes that rise to the skies, fresh, clear kettle pond remnants from the last great ice age, the great marshes of Wellfleet, the moors of Truro, and the eclectic vibe of Provincetown. Louie, one of my best friends, but a lightweight of a guy, was easily drained; his sister was full of verve. One night after a dinner of fresh cod landed on the Chatham docks, we were chatting it up late beside a fireplace, stoked with fresh-cut oak, in the living room of my parents' Eastham summer home where I lived alone. Louie dozed off early in typical fashion, then went to bed. MC and I continued to talk. At about 3:45 a.m. there wasn't much else to say, so intuitively, I reached over in the moment and kissed her. An innocent kiss, stretched as long as I thought proper. We laughed. I felt as though I had just kissed my kid sister. Bad dog!

But I got over it, and asked her if she wanted to watch the sun rise over Nauset Beach in Orleans. We headed, hand-in-hand, out to my beat-up Triumph TR6 parked in the driveway—top down, doors ajar, a rusted muffler, and drove to the beach. The night was ablaze in light, as if the Lord had flecked the heavens with a paintbrush of bright white. The rolling cadence of a gentle surf was soothing, and barefoot, you could almost count the grains of sand beneath us. On cue, at 4:52 a.m., rays of sunlight sprung from a horizon of deep, opaque blue and began to bleach the lower sky. As the sun slowly emerged from its slumber, we turned and kissed again. It was innocent, but it was love. You never forget real love.

As we slowly walked back to the car, I was fully captivated by the moment, then whammo! It hit me. I began to think of Louie.

Holy shit, I thought. *How do I explain this?*

I had broken the code.

Semper fi with the brothers and Ken no more. A court martial, death before a firing squad, a public hanging at the O.K. Corral, perhaps all of the above, awaited me.

I didn't want to show fear with Mary Catherine, so I kept the conversation to lighter issues and drove home in denial. As I was about to turn the corner down my dead-end street on Cestaro Way in Eastham, I could hear my muffler roaring. I gunned the engine like a NASCAR champion, popped the gear into neutral, then slowly and silently coasted to the driveway. Run silent, run deep.

"Louie can't know about this, not yet," I finally told MC, as we kissed again.

She agreed. *Semper Fi.*

But I was in a panic about what John Wayne might think. Those daunting words from the classic movie *Sands of Iwo Jima* raced through my head, "Tomorrow we're gonna take Iwo Jima, and some of you guys might not be coming back." Frankly, I thought some friendly fire was in line from the brothers.

MC and I promptly walked to our respective bedrooms, and within a half hour, Louie, an early rising farm boy, came to my door and promptly threw a pillow at my head.

"Time to get up, asshole," he said.

"Ohhhhh, is it morning yet?" I replied after ten minutes of sleep.

Hours later, Louie began to put the pieces together after MC and I fell asleep at the beach at 11 a.m.

I made it back safely from Iwo Jima, and two years later, we were married in Bakersfield where MC's folks lived then. Louie and Tommy were in the wedding party. And I was on decent terms with John Wayne, but in time, I was to have a geography lesson that I will never forget.

Following the love of my life, I relocated from Cape Cod to Phoenix, to an investigative reporting job at *The Arizona Republic*, but my heart was for newspapering in the East. We returned three years later after I was hired as a political reporter at the *Boston Herald American*, turning down an opportunity for a reporting job with the *LA Times* in its newly created San Diego bureau, but after all, East is East and West is West. I'm a homeboy.

MC was ambivalent about the relocation; while the romance to date was enticing, the thought of leaving close family was not. For most of our marriage, we have agreed on just about everything, from raising the kids to closely held beliefs, but on geography, we are planets apart. You say "aunt," I say "ont." In retrospect, neither of us is right; in fact, my wife now says "ont," but you couldn't fool her dad with a copy of Rand McNally.

We spent our first Christmas after marriage with MC's family in the majestic snow-country Pinetop mountains of northern Arizona. At a well-appointed, long, and narrow dinner table at a mountaintop lodge where whispers could be overheard, Louie and Tommy, after a few beers, played me like a harp with the old man.

"So, Greg, when are you and MC moving back East?" they asked on cue.

My father-in-law dropped his fork and stared at me, as if I had just burned down a convent full of nuns.

"So, what's *this* all about?" he inquired.

When you're halfway across the river, you have two choices: retreat or forge forward. I chose to drown.

"Well, Ken," I said. "Many years ago, you took your bride Mary Ellen from Kansas City all the way to Arizona."

Without breaking a stride, he bellowed, *"Yeah, but at least I kept her on this side of the Mississippi!"*

Silence. Deafening silence. No one dared speak to the Wizard of Oz; *just follow the yellow brick road*, I kept telling myself. I should have listened to Voltaire, who observed in the 1600s, "Behind every successful man stands … a surprised mother-in-law."

Over time, life for MC and me was blissful in the East for the most part, but life can change. Thirty-eight years of marriage, three children, careers, the ups and downs, and life-altering moments are change agents.

So is health.

As you cross the Sagamore Bridge over the Cape Cod Canal, heading to the mainland, far from the Mississippi, the view to the starboard is startling in its natural beauty, its expanse of sapphire shoreline, and soul-searching mood for deep reflection. On an incoming ocean tide, the roiling waters of the canal spill out into Cape Cod Bay with the force of a rip, rushing to a horizon where water flushes up against the sky. At the crest of the bridge, with 135 feet of ship's clearance below, you can see a swath of blue for miles, as it meanders up the coast toward Plymouth, "America's Hometown."

The 17.4 mile canal—a part of the Atlantic Intracoastal Waterway, a freighter bypass that connects Cape Cod Bay to the north with Buzzard's Bay to the south—was the revelation of Pilgrim Miles Standish, who in 1623, explored this low-lying stretch of land between the Manomet and Scusset rivers in search of a trading route that would forever isolate the Cape from the rest of Massachusetts, in both geography and in spirit. Negotiating the Sagamore Bridge and its sibling, the Bourne Bridge, is symbolic to the locals: a route on-Cape and off-Cape, a passageway to different states of mind. Coming or going, the bridge is always pause for reflection about what draws one so closely to this fragile spit of sand, a possession that began in me as a young boy in the early '50s and has gripped me since.

Heading off-Cape on Thursday, July 2, 2009 in my sunbleached, yellow Jeep with Mary Catherine in the passenger seat was a particularly potent time of a weighing up of life—a moment, I considered, of fleeting independence as we made our way toward Plymouth to a life-altering appointment with a neurologist on referral, a specialist in the care of Alzheimer's disease. I looked to the starboard from the peak of the bridge, as I usually do, but staring this time through the empty expression of my wife. Her focus, like a faithful mariner, was due north, just getting there. The morning was brilliant, on the lip of the ceremonial July 4th weekend, the ritual start of the Cape and Islands "season." In less than twenty-four hours, miles of campers, SUVs, and Beamers would be queued up in traffic for a summer fix, but on this otherwise bracing day, all the buzz of the solstice was lost on me. Fixed in thought, a carousel of images of innocent days on pastoral Coast Guard Beach and Nauset Light Beach flashed through my head—images of raising our three children in a place far more a privilege than just a street address. I've always believed that on Cape Cod, Nantucket, and Martha's Vineyard, we are privileged just to live here, but not privileged for being here. The place is far larger, more inspiring in the natural, than we. I thought, driving in my Jeep, about the promise of the past, the potential that I had once felt, and the resolve to persevere on a still dazzling, yet dead-end peninsula with one way on and one way off. My life at this point seemed to mirror this.

As we negotiated the Sagamore to the realities of the mainland, I thought of recent roadblocks in my life, the unexpected detours on the day calendar. In so many ways, I had taken a privileged past, a presumptive future, and God-given talents all for granted. Like an enduring lobsterman in the fertile currents of Pleasant Bay, I had been pulling full pots all my life, loaded with an abundance of blessings, and now the pots were coming up empty. Over time, I had lost my bearing—adrift in unchartered waters in a place where I could once spot channel buoys by instinct. The realization was as chilling to me as the ocean current off Chatham in February. I had tried in the recent past to conceal the cold truth from others, to work the spin of distraction—the so-called Wizard of Oz strategy, *Pay no attention to the man behind the screen!* I was always good at deflecting. But no longer; not with family, close friends, and some colleagues who have known me for years, and now had begun to realize that something might be terribly wrong. The curtain was drawn in Oz. There was no wizard.

I began to think about the unsettling memory loss over the last few years: the loss of self and place; the piss-poor judgment; a wholesale loss of filter; the visual impairments; the incontinence, often after performing like a puppet before clients; the mental numbness; a complete loss of self-esteem; and the agitation of clinical depression that began as a boy. I thought about that horrifying dislocation months ago while Christmas shopping with my son Conor in a Providence mall, not knowing for a half hour where I was or who I was. I thought about that serious head injury years ago that doctors say likely accelerated the dementia symptoms, and about my recent diagnosis of prostate cancer—another medical hand-me-down most likely from my parents. I thought about the rage I felt within.

"So, what's next?" my wife asked, as if I knew.

I kept staring. We all deal differently with challenging times; not sure there is a correct way. Some exhale, some inhale, some just deflect and probe in more pragmatic ways. My wife is a goalie with her emotions. She can deflect, at least externally, the best slap shot drilled at her. It's a survival mechanism that she has passed down to some of our children. But all those emotional pucks, all that vulcanized rubber of denial, mount up and never decay. They just sit there, consuming space.

Mary Catherine was in the nets again this day.

In the back seat, there were some answers, but not the kind built on hope.

"Thanks for your kind referral of Mr. O'Brien," clinical neuropsychologist Gerald Elovitz of the Memory Center wrote just days earlier to my personal physician, Dr. Conant. "I know from him that you spent much time discussing his cognitive changes, and the test results here show that they are real."

Elovitz, who years earlier had diagnosed my late mother with Alzheimer's disease, went on to note, with reference to awaited test results of a brain SPECT scan, "I suspect an emerging frontotemporal dementia becoming more significant over the past eighteen months and likely to progress … If there is no frontotemporal dementia, I would then suspect an early-onset Alzheimer's-type dementia."

In a seven-page medical report, with terrifying cognitive test performance graphs, Elovitz described a person I would have never recognized, but yet had become—all results in analysis in the probable dementia range:

"Mr. O'Brien is younger than ninety-eight percent of the mean norm group age [for dementia], so his below average performance is very problematic … [His] results fell within the range of cognitive impairment … His seriously impaired score indicates a significant cognitive deficit in learning capacity for new information, and he needed cues on more than half of the test items to obtain the score. General function levels fell in the very poor general function consistent with dementia. Mr. O'Brien's very high agitation level merits concern. The findings here reveal short-term memory function within the first-stage dementia range."

Some denouement, I thought. What a freakin' loser I am! I had always been an A-brain guy, a good provider, a decent husband, a caring father, and beyond that, a high-functioning, creative mind. For me, it was never about the money; it was all about succeeding in life—paying the bills, taking care of family, and the process of intense thought, problem solving, and inspiration. The Jesuit logic, as my father used to say. Doctors, in follow-up medical reports, noted a "superior intelligence," a nice shout out, I suppose, but perhaps I could have done more with it. Shame on me for that, all the more, shame now that the dots were not connecting, a disconnect at intervals of alarming proportion. My prized possession was heading to a state of atrophy.

Shit, this sucks!

The pretext was over; strategies and disguises for overcompensating in recent years exposed. But I was aversely at peace with it. Someone was finally listening. Maybe I wasn't alone, home alone. Mary Catherine, meanwhile, wobbly on her emotional skates, stood as firm as she could in the crease of the net, awaiting the next shot. Her head was in the game; protective mask down and no time for small talk.

Elovitz had observed in his report, "I went over these [dementia] possibilities with both the patient and his wife, and he told me frankly, 'I am not surprised,' and seems relieved that we at least are addressing them head-on."

Head-on is the only way I've known since I slid down the birth canal. The prone position. The oldest boy in a family of ten, I learned early on, for example, that if you don't grab for food, face-first, head-on at the dinner table, there will be nothing left. No one is going to feed you.

My mother was never a great cook. A second-generation Irish American with close ties to County Wexford, she boiled everything gray. We used salt, pounds of it, as seasoning, and ketchup, poured liberally for supplemental flavoring, just to kill the taste. In the cluttered kitchen of our family home at 25 Brookdale Place in Rye, New York—not far from the Upper East Side of Manhattan where my mother grew up—the pot roast simmered on Sundays from morning Mass until early evening. The hoary smell that wafted through the three-story stucco home still makes me nauseous today; I'm sure the scent still emanates from the walls. You had to cut the pot roast with a chainsaw.

Mom used to call me a "lazy chewer," but the meat was rawhide-tough laced with fat. With all those mouths to feed, she knew how to stretch a dollar like it was Gumby.

As a teenager, I noticed her often standing at the kitchen window overlooking a corn patch with Rye Brook in the distance, meandering out to Long Island Sound. She was talking to herself, fully engaged in conversation. I wasn't sure with whom. At first, I thought it was a way of deflecting the stress of raising a brood of kids with a collective attention span of a young yellow lab. The disengaging increased: misplacing objects, loss of memory, poor judgment, and yes, the rage—warning signs years later that I began noticing in myself.

After my father, a small man with the heady name of Francis Xavier O'Brien, had retired as director of pensions for Pan Am, and my mom left her teaching job, my parents sold the house in Rye in the early 1990s and moved to the Cape. They settled into our Eastham summer home, not far from Coast Guard Beach on the Cape Cod National Seashore, where daring lifesavers once plied the stormy surf to rescue shipwrecked sailors. The lure of the sea was intoxicating to my father. He had always sought retirement to Cape Cod and my mom, the dutiful wife, came along for the ride, ultimately a body and mind thrashing against the surf. Those early retirement years on the Cape were blissful—an opportunity for me, living just two towns away in Brewster, to spend time with my folks. I felt privileged that I was the only sibling on the Cape, but with favor comes responsibility. My dad, in time, had severe circulation disorders requiring several life-threatening operations, rendering him to a wheelchair. My mother progressively continued her cognitive decline, but fought off the symptoms like a champion to care for my father.

"I can't get sick," she kept saying when all the siblings urged her to see a doctor. "I can't get sick," as if saying the words made her whole.

Yet, she was sick, and she knew it.

The forewarning signs were textbook, but we were all in denial, as is often the case with dementia, for both the patient as well as the extended family. No one wanted to go there, particularly my dad, who feared a trip to the nursing home, a lights-out nightmare for him and my mom.

Over time, Mom began sticking knives into sockets, misplacing money, brushing her teeth with liquid soap, refusing to shower, not recognizing people she knew, hallucinating, and raging at others, often directly at me.

Unremittingly, she cared for my dad, always refusing to succumb to disability. She encouraged me in my own progression; she taught me how to fight, how to live with Alzheimer's, how never to give into it. At times, we even took our Aricept together. I worked diligently at rebonding with my mother, restoring a relationship that had gone sour earlier, perhaps because she saw too much of my father in me. She knew and I knew, but we didn't talk about it much. I was a father's son in every way; he was my idol. Yet, my mother became my role model in the resolute life she lived. St. Francis of Assisi once said, "Preach the Gospel at all times, and when necessary, use words." My mother preached with her courage.

Out of a gut necessity and an innate love for one another, my parents ultimately morphed into one. Mom became my father's legs, fetching for him what he needed while in his wheelchair; Dad became her intellect, her *raison d'être*. It was a *Love Story* of Erich

Segal proportions. My siblings and I watched this slow-motion train wreck with bewilderment and with awe.

Then, one late Sunday afternoon in 2006 on a visit with my parents, I finally got it. Hit me like a dummy in a crash test. I brought my mother a photo of all her children from a recent family reception, and she couldn't name one of them, including me. She had no clue, and was still driving at the time. As I left my parents' home that night, I could only think of the jarring interjection in the movie *Jaws* when Chief Brody first encountered the mammoth shark: *"We're gonna need a bigger boat!"*

We had a leaking dinghy at the time. Two weeks later, ironically Independence Day, 4th of July weekend—with my dad continuing to suffer from acute circulation disorders and internal bleeding after numerous fire drill ambulance runs to the hospital with Mom in tow—my mother took me aside and said she was about done.

"I don't know how much longer I can do this," she told me. "I'm not sure how long I can hold on."

Instinctively, I reassured her that the family had her back, all of us, but I felt this penetrating sinking feeling that we were at the precipice of a steep cliff and ground was giving way. Hours later, I got an emergency call that Dad once again had been rushed to Cape Cod Hospital in Hyannis. Mom was with him, yet another fire drill. The nurse told me to hurry.

I met my parents in the emergency room, filled to the brim with the walking wounded of summer. It took thirty-six hours to get my father into a hospital room. About twenty-eight hours into the ordeal, I noticed that my father, sitting in his wheelchair in an emergency room cubicle, was bleeding onto the floor. In a panic, I tried to divert my mom's attention from the pool of blood. It was too late. She was horrified. I could see it in her face; she was done.

"I'll get the doctor, Mom, don't worry," I said as I raced for the door.

She grabbed my right elbow from behind.

"Greg, would you take over," she asked quietly and in unusual peace.

"Yeah, Mom, I'm getting the doctor now," I said. "I'm getting the doctor."

"*No,*" she replied as I continued for the door. "*Would you PLEASE take over?*"

I stopped in my tracks.

Something inside me said that she was saying goodbye. I turned and looked into her eyes. It was as if someone had pulled down a curtain. As I watched her, I had the feeling of seeing a person, who had been holding on to a dock on an outgoing tide, let go.

I saw her drift. Within ten minutes, she curled up like a kitten in my dad's hospital bed, while he sat unconscious, bleeding in his chair.

Who are the parents now, I thought?

My wife finally broke the silence.

"Do you know where you are going?" she asked.

I wasn't sure on a number of fronts. So, I just kept driving.

The exit for Plymouth came up quickly, an anesthetizing ride north on Route 3 past miles of scrub oaks and pines. I had to call several times to the office of neurologist Dr. Donald Marks to get the directions straight. I was a bit on edge, awaiting results of a SPECT scan brain image test.

On the third floor of a boxy red brick building, Dr. Marks's office had all the ambiance and accoutrements of a hospital waiting room. Opening the door, I felt as though I were slipping into Lewis Carroll's *Alice in Wonderland* where "nothing would be what it is, because everything would be what it isn't."

I was dizzy with delusions of what could lie ahead. The office was filled with decent individuals, mostly in their eighties, all with cognitive impairments picking their way through the perplexities of age and a maze of cruel games the mind can play. At fifty-nine, I was the only "young" man in the room (yikes!), and saw myself outside the box of dementia, yet felt trapped within it. I glanced at my wife.

Like most couples, we've had our ups and down in marriage, more ups, hopefully, than downs. I felt badly for her. Today was a trip down.

I was told earlier that Dr. Marks, an expert in the study of the mind, gets right to the point. "He's precisely what you need; a skilled neurologist who will speak directly, no bullshit," Dr. Conant had advised me earlier, sounding a bit like my dad, who delighted in telling others that he customarily had to drill a piece of granite between my ears just to get my attention.

Dr. Marks lived up to the billing. Knowledgeable, cerebral, and caring in a clinical way, he put me through the paces of more clinical tests: word recall, various supplementary checks on short-term and long-term memory, category naming, visuospatial skills, and other evaluations. I flunked them all. Bottom line: the clinical tests reinforced Elovitz's forthright assessments, and the SPECT scan identified a brain in progressive decline. His formal diagnosis: "EOAD," as he wrote in his report. I glanced at it quickly, inverting the first letter, dealing with some related dyslexia, and thought for a moment that he had written, "TOAD."

"No," he said, "Early-onset Alzheimer's disease." The words cut into me like a drill press.

"I can deal with this," I said defensively. "This is not a surprise. I can fight it."

My reporter instincts kicked in. I showed little emotion, just digested the diagnosis on a self-imposed deadline. Facts, get the facts straight. I first thought about my mom, about my grandfather; I knew the deal. I wanted more facts. This was no time for emotion. The vital questions of who, what, when, where, why, and how flashed through my head, which felt little sensation at the moment. I was afraid now to look at my wife, so I stared at Dr. Marks, trying to remain in a state of control that I had just realized was beyond me. After all, I'm a Baby Boomer and we're all in control. At least, we suppose.

Finally, I gave into the emotion.

I felt Mary Catherine staring at me. I think she must have known all along.

"What do we tell the kids?" I asked her. My voice splintered. When you're married to someone for close to four decades—when you've been through all the "for better and for worse" throes of marriage, when you have a partner who knows you almost as well as you know yourself, when you've been in love, fallen out of love, fallen back into love, and drifted, then at a time like this, little needs to be said. We both knew what the future held. No one had to sky write. We were all about the kids.

Mary Catherine grabbed my hand, we nodded, and then listened to the doctor. The moment is embedded in my mind in a freeze frame.

Dr. Marks, a man of great compassion and incredible intellect, offered support, but got right to the point.

"You need to take the diagnosis seriously," he counseled me in front of my wife, having been prepped in advance on my aversion to reality. "You have a battle ahead of you. I'm speaking to you as if you were terminal. Are you getting this?"

I was. There was hardly a tone of political correctness in his voice; I needed the reality check. You must know your enemy—study with military precision—to fight your enemy.

Alzheimer's is a death sentence. The words resonated throughout my mind. I stared at Dr. Marks with the same vacant expression of looking out from the Sagamore. I felt the tears running down the sides of my face. My eyes didn't blink.

"A most unusual situation of a bright man who had the opportunity to witness dementia in a parent ... with self-awareness of early symptoms within himself," Marks wrote in his initial report, dictated on voice recognition software as if the report were being written in slow motion before me. Marks also observed that a previous brain MRI revealed some "frontal Flair/T2 changes, consistent with a previous head injury."

"This may have 'unmasked' Alzheimer's pathology," he added, "but his genetic loading is striking ... The brain SPECT scan is most compelling in clinical context for Alzheimer's."

Marks encouraged me to remain as physically fit as possible "as he is to keep his cerebral blood flow out. I suspect he is exhibiting the phenomenon of 'cognitive reserve' in which case he may tolerate on a functional basis impairments further into the baseline underlying pathophysiology of the disease longer than one who does not have the same cognitive reserve."

"The diagnosis has been made, in my opinion," he concluded in his report. "I am not sure how much longer he has in terms of being able to reliably and meaningfully provide the quality of work he has put out in the past. The general point is there needs to be balance between a healthy desire to overcome obstacles and yet acknowledge fundamental reality."

A final word of advice, Marks urged me to meet as quickly as possible with an estate attorney to protect family assets, given the statutory five-year "look back" during which a nursing home can attach personal properties and bank accounts. He also recommended that I designate a healthcare proxy, future caregivers, and assign power of attorney.

In the space of a bleak afternoon, my identity in the real world— my mind, along with the cherished red cedar shingle home that I had built for the family about thirty years ago, the one with the high-pitched, red cedar wood roof on about two acres of farmland off a winding country road that was now a part of a National Register of Historic Places—was on hold.

There wasn't much more to hear or to say. We left the office, and drove home in silence most of the way. The stillness spoke legions. I couldn't wait to get back over the bridge, my Linus security blanket. Lots to digest quietly in a forty-five-minute ride home. The assimilation of urgency was choking—bucket lists of cleaning up relationships, end-time planning that we all like to put off, and the strategies of surviving financially, physically, and emotionally. Many before me and many today, I thought, have been captive in such a contorting state of affairs with a range of disabilities, health issues, and timelines. I wasn't alone. Yet, I felt so isolated.

I felt sad for my Mary Catherine. This wasn't fair to her. And I couldn't fix it.

Dammit, I couldn't fix it!

The tool box was empty. I couldn't repair my brain. Ever. Not even with duct tape. All my adult life, I had relied on duct tape to fix leaks from the upstairs bathroom in the kitchen ceiling, "repair" broken appliances, hang posters, fix a tail light, repair a garden hose, act as a big Band-Aid, steady a cabinet door, fix a hole in the wall, hold a car door shut or a car window in place, fix a toilet seat cover, hold a choke in place on an outboard engine for the boat, as a Wiffle ball, a tool belt, and once, as a last resort, as an ace bandage for a pulled groin to get through the 5K Brew Run one hot August day in Brewster.

"How are you doing?" I finally asked, as if from Mars.

My wife, as author John Gray might put it, is from Venus. I love Mary Catherine, but often she doesn't want to be confused with the facts; she seeks a safe harbor, as any good sailor does. I fly by the seat of my pants. I find reality far below the surface, bottom fishing for answers. My wife, to the contrary, is more comfortable at sea level. You say "tomato," I say "to-mado." A fixture in our marriage, but we ain't calling the whole thing off! "Well, we have a lot to consider," she said; an understatement that could fill the Grand Canyon.

I knew. Like me, she felt alone.

Then we came upon the Sagamore Bridge. That's when the faith kicked in—a bridge to a new reality, a new hope for me. I was going home, sanguine about the fact that I had some answers in hand. But for MC, it was new isolation this side of the Mississippi. Maybe her father was right. As we coasted to the crest of the Sagamore, "the seventh bridge of Dublin," as it's called Éire, given the number of emerald transplants on the Cape, I thought of John Belushi in the classic movie *Animal House*.

"What? Over? Did you say 'over'?" the unrelenting Bluto Blukarsky declared at the Delta House, urging his brothers to fight on. "Nothing is over until we decide it is! Was it over when the Germans bombed Pearl Harbor? Hell no!"

Germans?

Hey, I was on a roll. So I charged over the Sagamore Bridge with a satchel of denial.

Life goes on, doesn't it?

5

"Denial Ain't a River in Egypt"

Sigmund Freud had much to say about denial. Among the most influential and controversial thinkers of the twentieth century, his work and theories helped shape our views of childhood, personality, memory, sexuality, and therapy. Denial (Freud called it abnegation) is a defense mechanism for one faced with a fact too uncomfortable or overwhelming, which one rejects—insisting reality is not true, in spite of crushing evidence. There are three fundamental types of denial, Freud suggests: simple denial, denying the reality of an unpleasant fact or situation; minimization, admitting a fact, but denying its seriousness; and projection, admission of both a fact and its seriousness, but denial of any responsibility in it.

Denial is a Rosetta Stone of modern life. When in doubt: deny, deny, deny. We see it in politics, in business, at home, and then in the confessional. To précis Mark Twain in a Bronx tongue: *Da Nile ain't just a river in Egypt.*

After my diagnosis, I was in full-throttle denial, responding to a five-alarm call to arms: protect my wife, my children, myself, my business, and my friends. I had learned at the knee of my father, a master of denial, the Zen of creative drift. My dad brought denial to an art form with my mother in her Alzheimer's; it was a De Niro-like performance, struggling himself with circulation disorders, cancer, and early symptoms of dementia. In his eighties, he was driven by the fear that if my mother died—*Black Hawk Down*—no one would care for him, and that he'd be carted off to a nursing home, a dread dating back to the loss of his parents as a boy. And so he contrived a patchwork quilt of my mom—sort of a Stepford wife, the perfect caregiver. As the 1975 classic movie based on Ira Levin's novel, *The Stepford Wives,* declared in promos: *"Something strange is happening in the Town of Stepford ... where a young woman watches the dream become a nightmare ... and realizes that at any moment, any second— her turn is coming."*

So was mine.

I hate suits. They make me uncomfortable, the corporate image, as well as the clothing. Particularly on a stuffy summer morning in June 2010 at the law firm of La Tanzi, Spaulding & Landreth in Orleans on the Cape. The building was filled with suits, a striking contrast just up the street from postcard perfect Rock Harbor in Orleans where charter fishing boats spill out into Cape Cod Bay to ply the rich fishing grounds of Eastham, Wellfleet, and Provincetown. As the lawyers plied their trade in designer attire, fishing boat captains minutes away, clad in bulky sweatshirts and faded jeans stained with fish guts and seagull poop, picked their way out of a narrow channel at dead low tide, searching for stripers and schools of blues on the horizon. The contrast in cultures of the Outer Cape, one that gives definition to eclectic, was not lost on me. Nor was the moment.

In a small, lawyerly-appointed conference room on the west side of the building, the kind of gathering space that makes one imagine they are queued up for a fiscal colostomy, I sat next to my wife with a pile of legal documents awaiting my signature. I was here to sign my life away, a hand-off of assets—everything I owned, everything in the secular world that makes a male whole. In short, my identity—my material umbilical cord, as short as it is.

I felt like telling the suits in a quiet rage: *I can now say with great confidence on any given subject that I will forget more than you'll ever know!*

For close to a year, I had been dragging my sorry ass on this hand-off, deflecting the well-intentioned counsel of financial, legal, and medical advisors. Legally, I had to consider the five-year "look back" policy on admission to a nursing home. In summary, if a person doesn't own assets for at least five years, a nursing home, by law, must enroll the individual as he or she is—in my case, as a destitute dumbass, just a step above a ward of the state. For such people, there is no encumbering the assets of other family members, even a wife. Point made, point accepted, life today sucks.

It wasn't as though I was flush with cash: a nice Cape home; a $1.2 million term life insurance policy (some "retirement plan"); a decent salary for someone independently employed on a short medical tether; and big long-term debt, enough to choke a Clydesdale. Not the kind of particulars for an obsequious profile on the business pages of the *Boston Globe*. When one gets to a certain stage in life, individuals often contemplate the contents of an obituary more than a résumé. An obit is more enduring. My obit bucket list is formal appointment to the Brewster's Alewife Committee—the old salts of the town that annually prepare the town's ancient herring run for the arrival in early spring of thousands of herring (called alewives), navigating the churning waters of Cape Cod Bay to swim upstream and spawn in inland mill ponds. Legend has it that the name "ale-wife" comes from comparison generations ago with a corpulent female tavern keeper in Nova Scotia. Just sayin'.

"But don't be a dumbass," good, loving friends had counseled me. "Swallow your damn Mick pride and just sign the documents. Hand your wife the keys, the kitchen sink, and everything else. You owe that to your family."

I fully understood that, but knowledge often collides with emotion, and on this afternoon, I was adrift in doubt. The lawyers were resolute that all provisions must be properly in place, initialed, and signed correctly, so I could have the proper legal protections in place.

I was ready, somewhat kicking and screaming, having just read *Still Alice* on advice of my doctor, who called the Lisa Genova best-selling novel "remarkable" in its insight, yet chilling in its supposition. I had put off the reading for almost a year, fearing the story of fictional Alice Howland, happily married with three grown children and a second home on the Cape, a distinguished Harvard professor who noticed that the forgetfulness creeping into her life had given way to wholesale confusion, then the devastating diagnosis: early-onset Alzheimer's disease. I couldn't put the book down—inspiring, edifying, and a forbidding reality check, all at once. I was looking into a mirror. I was Alice, *sans* the dress. I keep the book on my desk for reinforcement. I was now ready to let go of the minutia of life. At least trying.

My attorneys were pleased all this was finally in place, but I was having a problem with the upside of it. In my gut, I knew it was the right thing to do; shoulda done it a year ago. Just swallow the pride, sign the damn documents: the Last Will and Testament, the Durable Power of Attorney, the Healthcare Proxy, and the DNR, "Do Not Resuscitate." I kidded with my wife beforehand that I should be signing a DNS, "Do Not Salvage"—a Black Irish reference about taking my boat out into the Atlantic one day when the brain cells drain, and rolling off the bow.

I hit for the cycle this day, as they say in baseball, then sat disorientated at a mahogany conference table that I'd already stained with hot coffee leaking from my Styrofoam cup. I felt naked, fully exposed.

"I know this is difficult," attorney Chris Ward told me. Four years earlier, I had engaged Ward in a Cape Cod Hospital room in Hyannis in the same legal procedure for my parents. What comes around goes around, I thought, reflecting back on my appointment as their power of attorney and healthcare proxy. Now my wife was next in succession. It was a humbling experience.

Page by page, I initialed all the particulars of documents that rendered me—the so-called bread-winning family patriarch—to the status, I felt, of Clarabell the Clown. Honk the horn for Howdy

Doody! I tried desperately to deflect the inner humility. I felt my self-worth ebbing like the tide. The Brewster house, my alter ego, a place where perhaps Henry David Thoreau might have felt at home, was transferred with the swing of a pen to my wife. Don't mean to be melodramatic, but it wasn't about the assets; it was about my profound connection to a place sacred to me—a home, not a house, where we all became a family. Now, I felt like a renter.

So much for any control in life, as we are all conditioned to covet. It had never been about a hand-off to my wife and kids, wholly and happy to do so, but one of losing a sense of self. I felt vacant. No one in the room, including my wife, my best friend, could understand this. I was alone, searching for the humor in it, vowing to find it.

"Yes, Chris," I replied, in understatement. "This is difficult."

After the swell of documents had been signed, Mary Catherine and I walked quietly to the parking lot and left in separate cars.

She went home to the house. Her house. I went to Willy's Gym, the usual, to run off five miles of mental numbness. Now we had to tell the kids. I had put that off, as well.

Months earlier, I first raised the issue with my oldest boy, Brendan, on a drive to the western part of the state. Brendan—now a writer/producer in the Boston area—was working with me at the time as a political/communications strategy consultant. On a three-hour drive to meet with a client, Brendan at the wheel, we talked about the Patriots, Celtics, Red Sox, Bruins, all the small talk I could conjure, then got to the point. I had been probing for just the right words, but was coming up empty. How do you tell the first among equals in the family, *primus inter pares*, that he has to row a little harder? I kept thinking back to the day he was born twenty-nine years earlier at Boston's Brigham and Women's Hospital after Mary Catherine's agonizing twenty-three-hour labor. She's right about the pain of delivery; men have no freakin' clue. So typical of the gender, I tried to comfort her, telling her how to breathe, as if you needed to go to Harvard to figure that out. When Brendan finally emerged, I counted fingers, toes, and then saw a tiny wiener. I sobbed like a baby, held my newborn son, comforted my wife, and then like a proud father, darted off to Fenway Park, to the official souvenir shop on Lansdowne Street, to buy up every infant Red Sox apparel I could find.

"I need to talk to you about something," I told Brendan, as we passed the exit for Lakeville on Route 495, heading for the Mass Pike. "It's about my health. I've been meaning to talk to you for a while."

"Sure," he said in an uneasy tone that reminded me of his mood when I told him many years ago there was no Santa Claus. "I'm fumbling for the right words here, but … ahh, I've been having serious memory problems for some time," I said.

"What's up, Dad?" he asked candidly, focused on the road and what may lay ahead.

"Well, I've been getting lost often, confused about the time and place, my judgment has been lacking at times, I'm having difficulties problem solving, and experiencing much rage. Kinda like Gam, you know."

"What do the doctors say?" he asked. "No bullshit, Dad. What's up?"

"It's not the final act I was expecting at this stage in life," I said. "I thought I'd bow out more gracefully. But recently, I've had a batch of clinical tests and a brain scan."

"So what's up, Dad?" he asked again, more to the point.

"I've just been diagnosed with early-onset Alzheimer's."

Brendan kept driving, his eyes fixed on the road. He was absorbing, then finally said, "That explains a lot."

He, like others, had noticed the early symptoms, but passed it off as my eccentricities—creativity—over time. We talked about it for several miles; he asked questions about the diagnosis, what it meant, and about the future for both me and the family. Brendan had more questions; I was getting uneasy with the conversation, thinking about the classic Jon Lovitz line in the movie *City Slickers*, "Too much information!" I shut down. So we drove on, talking about other things, the usual father/son stuff—work, sports, and politics of the day. Brendan reinforced his love and full support, but was predictably guarded in emotion as he digested the conversation—a shield he would drop soon.

I was looking forward weeks later to a July 4th-weekend trip to bucolic Coronado Island off San Diego, trying not to focus on seminal moments in my life that all seemed to be happening near Independence Day. Coronado, five miles off the port of San Diego, is a paradise of a place—an out-of-body, other-world experience, a place where one can forget.

But first there was unfinished business. I had to speak with the other kids. I learned early on in journalism that if you don't tell your story, someone else will tell it for you. That wouldn't have been right here.

My daughter, Colleen, was on the Cape on a short break from her duties in Washington, D.C. as a communications analyst on contract with Homeland Security. She now teaches underprivileged kids in a Baltimore elementary school. Conor, a junior at the time, studying sports management at Johnson & Wales University in Providence, was hanging at the house. So, we asked Brendan to come down from Boston for a family conference, under the guise that we'd all go to dinner, which eventually we did—a great meal at Joe's Tavern in East Orleans, a local family hangout on the way to Nauset Beach.

I've always been late, and this time was no exception, as the kids waited with inevitable annoyance for me in the living room, as I contemplated in earshot in my bathroom what I was about to tell them. My ears were burning. I was looking for the right words.

"So, anyone want a drink?" I asked, as I finally emerged. "Daaaaad, let's get going," Colleen said, with nodding assurance from Brendan and Conor. "It's getting late."

"I'm having a glass of red wine. Who wants one?" I said in yet another attempt at delay.

The kids, eyes rolling, obliged. My wife, knowing the script, already had hers in hand. Maybe a double or a triple.

"Your father has something to tell you," she prompted me.

All eyes were in my direction. Stage fright has never been an issue for me, but the words were not flowing, as I was accustomed in life. *Get to the freakin' point*, I thought, assuming that Brendan might already have passed some of our conversation along to his siblings.

It was an awkward talk, one couched with language that explained the diagnosis, the need for the family to buckle up, but left hope in the room. There were questions, tears, and hugs. I think, at some level, they all knew. No one really wanted to talk about it. Finally, Conor broke the ice, as the youngest of the family can often do.

"So, Dad, you're losing your mind!" he said. "You might say so," I replied.

We all laughed; there was no comeback. We all seemed to understand. Now, on to dinner and talk of the Patriots, Red Sox, Celtics, Bruins, Pluto, and the Milky Way. Life goes on, as Robert Frost said, particularly if we seek to move forward; times to share, bills to pay. Woody Allen in a wry exchange in the movie *Annie Hall* put an exclamation point on survival instincts in an anecdote about a guy who goes to a psychiatrist, complaining about his brother who thinks he's a chicken. When the doctor suggests he turn his brother in, the man replies, "I would, but I need the eggs!"

My family needs the eggs.

The flight to San Diego was peaceful; departing Boston and flying high above the jagged harbor islands, I tried to leave my baggage behind. I've always been captivated, flying coast to coast, watching this magnificent country unfold beneath me. Good thinking weather. Hours later, as the plane banked a right over the Pacific Ocean to line up with a runway, I felt cleansed. But as the great Roman Empire scribe Publius Flavius Vegetius Renatus cautioned centuries ago, "In time of peace, prepare for war!"

Coronado, connected to San Diego by a ten-mile isthmus called the Silver Strand, offers some of the nation's finest beaches and enough natural beauty and gawking potential to satisfy the most judicious traveler. Spanish for "the crowned one," Coronado is a jewel of an isle. I couldn't wait.

The first night, Brendan, my brother-in-law, Louie, and I stayed at the Coronado Island Marriott Resort, overlooking the pristine San Diego Bay and the downtown. My wife, who had arrived earlier, spent the evening at the Hotel del Coronado with her sister, Nancy, who had been named in my will as special family medical consultant; I knew Nancy would always have my best interest at heart, and wouldn't dispatch me prematurely to a nursing home.

After a late afternoon swim, a fresh fish dinner, and a walk along the boardwalk, Brendan, Lou, and I went back to the hotel. Lou, a great guy, but a lard ass of a night owl, wanted to go to bed again, so Brendan and I walked to a bar for a beer. There was still some unfinished business between us. He had no clue. Timing can be terrible, particularly on a flee from reality; it often has no respect for timelines.

I had brought with me all the signed legal documents naming Brendan as my power of attorney and my legal guardian, should something ever happen to Mary Catherine. All assets, if anything left, would pass to him to be distributed to the kids. I was to have nothing, just as the lawyers wanted. Brendan needed to know this. Now was the time. Timing often sucks, even on placid Coronado.

Once again, I couldn't find the right words over a Blue Moon, even with a slice of orange on the lip of a chilled glass. So, we walked back to the hotel and I engaged him in conversation on the second-floor balcony outside our room, above what seemed to be a plantation of palms and tropical flowers, sifting in the sultry Coronado ocean breeze.

I showed him the documents. He wanted nothing to do with it. Nothing.

"I don't want to talk about it!" he shouted. *"I don't want to fucking talk about it!"*

"But you gotta," I said. "You have to know, Brendan. We have to talk. You're the oldest boy and you have to start acting like it. I need you! Get it!"

It was the most powerful confrontation I've ever had with any of my children, one I hope never to repeat.

I showed him the documents again. He pushed them away.

"This is bullshit! It's fucking bullshit!" he screamed.

"Fine, then you need to see something else," I replied, opening the door to the hotel room to bring out another pile of papers. They were my medical records, a word picture of a swan dive off a cliff.

"Read 'em," I said, waving the papers in front of his face. "Look at them. They're right here!"

We were both in rage. My brother-in-law woke up, poked his head out to the balcony, and asked if everything was alright. "It's fine, Lou," I said, motioning him quickly back into the room.

Brendan grabbed the papers, about thirty pages in all, and began to read.

He stopped at a page that summarized the neurologist's finding.

"The diagnosis has been made in my opinion," the doctor's report said. "I am not sure how much longer he has in terms of being able to reliably and meaningfully provide the quality of work he has put out in the past. It may also be helpful if his counselor would help in negotiating more open discussion of his growing limitations with other family members so he suffers less isolation."

Brendan was stunned.

"This is bullshit! This is bullshit!" he yelled in a voice that pierced within.

In primal anger, he ripped the documents into pieces, then tossed them off the balcony. The chunks of paper—my personal, naked, and wrenching medical reports—fell among the palms like a blanket of snow.

"This is bullshit! That's what I think. It's bullshit!" he yelled even louder, his eyes now tearing up.

He paused for a second to catch his breath. "It's bullshit, Dad. It's just fucking BULLSHIT!" He stopped again, sobbed, and then said in a lowered voice, "It's bullshit because I know it's true!"

He then fell into my arms and cried like a baby. We hugged, talked some more, and then went to bed.

I didn't sleep well that night. I awoke at first light to the realization, the horror, that my medical records—documentation that I was losing my mind, as Conor had pointed out days earlier—were strewn among paradise, all throughout the tropical plants, near the pool.

I grabbed a plastic trash bag, and picked up as many pieces of the clinical reports, test results, and medical comments as I could. My past and my future were now in the trash.

6

The Wayback Machine

Mister Peabody was the smartest beagle ever to walk the Earth. Everyone over fifty-five knows this. In cartoon terms, he was an inventor, entrepreneur, scientist, Nobel Laureate, and a two-time Olympic medalist. Impressive for a member of the humble hound group.

Appearing in the late 1950s and early '60s as the erudite canine of *Rocky and His Friends* and *The Bullwinkle Show*, Mister Peabody, in benevolence, adopted a dorky, orange-haired orphan named Sherman. In a moment of dog genius, Mr. Peabody invented the "WABAC" Machine as a birthday gift for his surrogate "son," a rejiggered "should-have-been-machine," in modern culture often referred to as the Wayback Machine, a convenient way to reintroduce issues or events of the past, as we would like to view them.

I suspect Mister Peabody in his self-referential humor might have had early-onset Alzheimer's; yet, he was a virtuoso in his day. I find that Mr. Peabody's WABAC Machine, a time tunnel, has greater relevance in some ways than reality *du jour*.

My life today has become a cartoon in so many ways, a Wayback Machine, but the early years give me ballast.

Way back, my late maternal grandmother, Brooklyn-born Loretta Sinnott Brown, called me "snippy snooper" as a young boy because I was always "snooping around," asking too many questions, forever wanting to know the minutiae of life. She and my maternal grandfather, George Walter Brown—born in Manhattan, an earnest man who had owned several Upper East Side brownstones and munificently forgave missed rents during the Depression with a heart the size of SoHo—lived on Rye Beach Avenue in Rye, New York, in a classic red brick two-story home, a short walk from Rye Beach on Long Island Sound at the mouth of New York Harbor. My grandparents had grown up in the city, worked there, then made their way north, as with all my relatives, maternal and paternal, since kin began arriving generations ago from the old sod, from places like Dublin, Wexford, County Clare, and Belfast.

My grandfather, whom we affectionately called "Daddy George," had close ties to Magherafelt, Ireland, in the Northern Ireland County of Derry where family members were baptized and married in the Little Chapel of Woods, which still stands today, framed by a family burial marker.

Once or twice a week, my mother used to take me and two of my sisters, Maureen and Lauren, to see my grandmother and Daddy George. Grandma was petite, short, and thin, a woman of incalculable resolve—perseverance that she clearly passed down to my mother. Daddy George was handsome, gentle, and erudite, an intellectual in his day—small in stature, large in bounty. He didn't talk much, as we observed as kids; Grandma did all the chatting, distracting us with sandwiches and desserts, piping hot chocolate in winter in a tall steaming glass, and in summer, fresh lemonade and blackberries from the backyard. I spent much time with her in the kitchen, snooping around and playing with her dog, a Mexican Chihuahua named Poncho, appropriate in dimension for the household. Mom, meanwhile, sat on the couch visiting with her dad, trying to make conversation. The moment seemed awkward.

In time, I began to realize that something was terribly wrong with my grandfather. His sentences were becoming shorter as his voice trailed off. He didn't recognize us on occasion, and he stared a lot in withdrawal. Often, he just shook his head in an acknowledgment when asked a question. I thought he was hard of hearing.

There were times, my mother told me later, when Daddy George in great confusion would walk to the Rye train station without telling anyone, taking an express to Grand Central so he could stroll the streets of the Upper East Side—a place that made him feel whole. He was trying to go home to his office on 28th Street. The local New York cops knew him and would phone my grandmother, then make sure he returned safely. No one seemed to grasp what was happening.

Daddy George, doctors said, had "hardening of the arteries," the cipher in those days for dementia. "Your grandfather is very sick," Mom would tell us.

I'll never forget the day we came for a visit, and all the dining room furniture, including the mahogany table on which I had done my grammar school homework, was gone—replaced with a stark hospital bed. Daddy George could no longer walk up the steep oak stairs and was confined to the bed.

The deterioration had a solemn impact on me. My grandfather, who had been slowly waning before us, was now in a deep slide—in the rear-view mirror of Grandma, who cared for him like a trained nurse; my mother, who adored him for all he was; and my siblings and me, who felt the pull of a family tree. We loved him. A photograph of Daddy George, sepia in tone, in a suit and tie in his professional Manhattan days, hangs in my office today; it's the same photograph that I hung on a wall at the foot of my mom's bed at EPOCH Senior Living in Brewster months before she succumbed to Alzheimer's. The night before she passed away, I pointed at the photo, and my mother recognized him. With his wire-rimmed glasses and the shape of his face, I look a bit like him.

Weeks before my grandfather died, Grandma on her loving rounds was stunned one day to see Daddy George sitting up in bed. He spoke for the first time in months and said in muted tones that he was aware of all she had done for him; he thanked her and told her that he loved her. It was a last expression of love—testimony that those suffering from dementia and other mental handicaps still observe and can retain far more than one might imagine. My mom rushed over to the house to speak with her dad. Doctors counseled that the enlightenment was fleeting, a last flow of blood to the brain or a remnant brain cell flashing a final distress signal. Daddy George quickly fell back into the abyss.

I will never forget the day he died. Still haunts me. When I returned to the red brick house, the hospital bed was gone and the dining room furniture was back in place, as if nothing had happened, yet I knew that nothing would ever be the same.

Nothing ever is the same, beyond history that repeats itself. "No man ever steps in the same river twice," the Greek philosopher Heraclitus of Ephesus wrote in 500 BC, "for it's not the same river, and he's not the same man. Other waters are forever flowing on to you."

In Alzheimer's, the currents of the disease rise slowly. Those with early-onset, with an acuity of what's to come, hold a collective breath, awaiting progressions of the loss. "Oh waste of loss," Thomas Wolfe, one of my favorite writers, observed in his 1929 novel, *Look Homeward Angel*. "Remembering speechlessly we seek the great forgotten language, the lost lane into Heaven, a stone, a leaf, a door. Where? When?"

The where and when is always front of mind with me. When my grandfather chased the forgotten language in Alzheimer's, he was lost cerebrally in a back alley; he never found it. Grandfather was never the same again, yet my mother rarely spoke of his illness, other than to say that he had suffered greatly, but with inspiring dignity. That's the way one should suffer, she told me. Always suffer with great dignity. Later, when my mother was diagnosed with Alzheimer's, family members were equally voiceless about the illness, in sync with denial, reacting to a stigma—a common antiphon to Alzheimer's and other life-changing diseases. Myself included.

"It's not denial," once observed cartoonist Bill Watterson, creator of the precocious, at times sardonic, comic strip *Calvin and Hobbes*. "I'm just selective about the reality I accept."

Aren't we all . . .

More than one in three today (far more in years to come) are touched in some way by the disease—either fighting it, or knowing a family member, colleague, or friend with Alzheimer's—and yet, the disease rarely gets attention in an obituary or in a death certificate. Family members often decline even to acknowledge Alzheimer's, or call it by name. This collective denial has been the subject of scores of newspaper, magazine, and medical journal commentaries. "Scientists say that when they try to trace the inheritance of Alzheimer's disease in family members, or to learn the age of onset, they come up against family members who will not admit that a parent or close relative had anything seriously wrong with them," noted *The New York Times* years ago in a report. "Adult children frequently try to protect their parents by not telling them that they have Alzheimer's disease, a situation reminiscent of the days when no one would tell cancer patients that they had cancer. The stigma, experts say, is because of the disturbing symptoms and the fears of family members that they could inherit a gene that will give them the disease." And so, family members across the board often reach, explicably, for a shallow, "drive-by" diagnosis after a brief encounter or a hasty phone conversation. It's fully human to deny what we find unpleasant or chilling, but when the drive-by precludes one from the facts, from facing real-life implications, then it's wholly unproductive, a dead end.

Such observations are akin to saying to one who cannot hear: "But you don't look like you're deaf."

You can't hear much on Pluto. It's a dark icy place, dense with denial, isolated to the point of impenetrable peace.

In 1930, Walt Disney introduced an obtuse canine companion for Mickey Mouse named Pluto, an apparent callout to a planet with a thin atmosphere of nitrogen, methane, and carbon monoxide gases, the kind of place in deep space of suspended animation where not much cohesive thought occurs. Beyond Pluto, three times farther from Earth and 900 times Earth's distance from the Sun, is Sedna, a surface composition of sixty percent of methane ice and seventy percent of water ice; it is capable of supporting a subsurface ocean of liquid water, scientists say. This dwarf planet will become closer and brighter over the next seventy-two years before it begins its 10,500-year trip to the far reaches of the solar system and back again, making it much easier for some to hop on a ride from Pluto, a sling shot. You can hear God from here.

The trip to Pluto, a metaphor of survival instinct for my flight from reality, can be a comfort, a release from the angst, fear, sadness, and rage—a surrender to numbness, those unfathomable blank stares, to feel peaceful again, avoid the pain of losing control. Daily, I fight against the impulse to let go, a welcome release, even just for minutes. There are days I have to prompt myself to come back. Often, my wife, children, or friends summon me with a snap of a finger.

The drifting is similar to sailing in a slack wind. In Alzheimer's, one doesn't move fast, but the journey is soporific—respite from the interruptions of a brain gone awry, a flickering light whose plug is loose in the socket. On Pluto, the mind and body are at peace, no longer on high alert. The metaphoric gravitational pull of Pluto, for me and others with the disease, draws deep. It's soothing at this stage just to let go. At some point, the light goes dark forever.

Often, I look, with soulful flashlight in hand, for my mother on Pluto, but I know she's not there. She's with God. Many months ago, one evening when I couldn't sleep, typical of my journey, I was lying late at night on the couch in the family room, watching reruns of *Planet Earth*. I sensed a woman sitting next to me. I wasn't sure if I had drifted off, was in-between sleep, or was just dreaming. Still not sure. At first, I thought it was my wife, Mary Catherine; her back was to me. Then the woman turned and looked at me. It was my mother. She stared straight at me.

"Mom," I said. "I can't sleep!"

"It's ok. I can't sleep either," she replied in a calming tone.

From what I recall from the encounter, she then rubbed the back of my head, and within seconds, I fell into a deep slumber. It was the most restful, peaceful sleep of a lifetime.

My mother in time would make her presence known elsewhere, once in the form, I suspect, of a flowering hibiscus. My sister Lauren had received a hibiscus from a friend, but the plant would only flower on rare occasions, remarkably rare occurrences and in yellow: on my mom's birthday and when family gathered at Lauren's outside Boston. As if to reinforce like the elementary teacher she was, my mother's presence was felt again. Driving down to the Cape on a summer day shortly after my mom's death, Lauren spotted a yellow jeep as she queued up for gas along Pilgrims Highway. Her attention was fixed on the license plate, surrounded by a sea of yellow. It read: "RIP Mom."

Rest in peace, always.

These types of happenstance are daring to attest; one opens themselves up to all sorts of second-guessing. I get that. So analyze away.

Yet, on a cold January night a year later, I was sleeping on the couch again, my wife was in the throes of a horrific sinus infection. I got up, as I do every two hours, just to walk around the house, often aimlessly. This time, I had to take another pee, and on the way back to the couch, I checked the digital clock on the stove. It was 4:12 a.m., still dark, black as night. As I walked to the couch, I noticed something moving slowly to port side of the wood stove where embers were alight. It was an image of sorts, but instinctively, I was serene with it. At first, I thought it was just another visual misperception, or as we scribes might correctly call it, another hallucination. I was wide awake at the time, focusing intensely on the image. I saw the outline of a woman. She had blonde hair, dressed in clothing familiar to me. The image moved slowly toward me, then backward, then toward me again. The woman was beckoning me with her right hand to follow. She kept summoning. I realized then it was my mother, or a likeness of her. The shadows of a man stood behind. Slowly, she summoned to him, as she had with me, to move forward. I wondered if it was my father. The image in the shadow hesitated, and I thought in the moment that if any of this were real, my father was probably saying to Mom, "Ginny, let's not scare the shit out of Greg!"

I was at peace, but it wasn't my time to move forward. So, I turned on a light. Saw nothing. I turned it off. Saw nothing. Then I went back to bed in great calm, intuitively feeling that I wasn't alone. I told my wife about the experience the following day. I joked with her that my mother was looking for one of her recipes. I want to believe it was my mother, but what if it wasn't? What terrifies me is yet another manifestation of this disease.

7

Smart Pills

Sleep is good for the soul, but waking hours are when work gets done, with the brain in the "on" position. Whatever one's aspiration in life, an engaged brain is fully focused with vigorous mentoring. Among great tutors in my life, I had exceptional coaches in high school at Archbishop Stepinac High School (class of 1968) on Mamaroneck Avenue in White Plains, five exits up Route 95 from the Bronx. I had a passion for sports, but enjoyed the expression of theater and turned to the stage. Drama coaches Father James Cashman and Father Bernie McMahon were particularly inspiring, instructing to express, yet stay within, to never show fear, to ad lib in a manner that always built confidence. They were lifelong teachers. Two of their prized students went on to far greater successes—Academy Award-winning actor Jon Voight, class of 1956, and Alan Alda, class of 1952, of *MASH* fame and other generational movies. But the actor I seem to emulate most these days is the late Lenny Montana, who played Luca Brasi, the dim hitman in *The Godfather*. My favorite scene is Luca Brasi's reprised, slow slur, preparing himself for a wedding salutation to Don Corleone, just to get it right.

"Don Corleone, I am honored and grateful that you have invited me to your home on the wedding day of your daughter. And may their first child be a masculine child," Brasi kept practicing in a slow, deliberate, and discomfited pace.

Before business meetings these days, before every family gathering, every outreach, every salutation, I rehearse my lines, just to get them straight. I prep for the quips, the thoughtful commentaries, and salutations. I study the lines. Sometimes, I keep crib notes. Nothing is ever left to chance these days. Then, it's showtime! I'm pretty good at it; damn good, in fact. Fathers Cashman and McMahon taught me well—teachers who trained me with great insight, humility, and faith in one's ability to row harder.

You have to row harder with dementia, or you drift. In the sport of crew, with roots dating back to ancient Egyptian times, you must work as a team, propelling the racing shell through churning waters. But in Alzheimer's, one must pull an oar with the strength of a strokeman, only there is no one else in the shell for the "catch" and "recovery." At the catch, a rower's hips are aligned with the oarlock for maximum thrust of the blade in the water. The rower then applies pressure to the oar by pushing the seat toward the bow by extension of the legs. As the legs approach a full extension, the rower pivots the torso toward the bow, and then finally pulls the arms toward the chest. The hands meet the chest right above the diaphragm, and then drop enough to take the blade out of the water. At the very end of the stroke, with the blade still in the water, the hands drop slightly to unload the oar so that spring energy stored in the bend of the oar gets transferred to the boat. This eases removing the oar from the water and minimizes energy wasted on lifting water above the surface in splashing.

The recovery phase follows the drive—removing the oar from the water and coordinating the body movement to move the oar to the catch again.

And so it is with Alzheimer's—a catch and recovery to engage a brain on its way to deluge.

Sure, there are many who encourage from the shoreline: family, friends, doctors, and colleagues, many of them not fully understanding why they are waving. In Alzheimer's, one is in the boat alone. So, you row a little harder!

Dementia today comes in many flavors, a cornucopia of medical terms. Old-style labels like "hardening of the arteries" have given way to a more technical lexicon. Now there are more than eighty types of dementias identified. Alzheimer's is the most prevalent; others include: Lewy body dementia, Creutzfeldt-Jakob disease, Huntington disease, frontal or temporal lobe dementias (including Pick's disease and Primary progressive aphasia), HIV-associated dementia, dementia pugilistica (Boxer's Syndrome), corticobasal degeneration, and other genetically related dementias.

The progression of Alzheimer's can be slowed, to some extent, with state-of-the art prescriptions used to diffuse symptoms, producing "decoy" chemicals that trick enzymes that break down the transmitter chemical (acetylcholine), allowing it to perform as well as it can. I take a daily cocktail of drugs. The combination dosage helps slow the rate of decline on good days. The Aricept (donepezil) works to improve the function of the nerve cells by slowing a breakdown of the transmitter chemical acetylcholine. Namenda (memantine hcl) assists in blocking transmission of chemicals in the brain that kills nerve cells.

Close friends call them my "smart pills!"

Consider the 1982 movie *Tron* in which a computer programmer is transported inside the software world of a computer mainframe and engages terrifying sequencers in an effort to get back. That's my world today, and the destiny of millions of others, unless something is done to subdue the insidious intruder.

Mornings for me are always the same. In disarray. At first light, I must focus on the five W's: the who, what, where, when, why, and how of life, as if rebooting my faithful MacBook Pro before tossing the covers and organizing the scattered files of my mind. I do it out of instinct, but there's always the depression, fear, and angst to walk through, and that's just on the way to the bathroom where, on doctors' advice, I've begun labeling the toothpaste, liquid soap, and rubbing alcohol. I have attempted often to brush my teeth with liquid soap, and on two occasions gargled briefly with rubbing alcohol. Scope is far better!

Then, I go deep into my lists—notes for everything, printed and on my iPhone calendar with repeat advisories. My life has become a strategy. I have a playbook, a script, backup for everything. Sometimes, the stratagem is just showing up, other times it's deflection; more often, it's an ongoing quest for excellence, understanding as best as possible the new boundaries. I have a formidable enemy—my mind. It used to be my best friend. I don't see any chance now for reconciliation. *Illegitimi non carborundum*, as I say: don't let the bastards grind you down. Cartoonist Gary Larson always got right to the point. A classic 1986 image underscores a debate over whether the brain can expand. In Larson's illustration, a student with a bulky frame and a particularly tiny head, raises his left hand in a crowded classroom. The clock on the back wall reads 10 a.m. "Mr. Osborne," the caption reads, "may I be excused? My brain is full."

Clinically, our brains are never full, but there are days when I feel that mine is empty. The eerie image of novelist Jack Torrance in the Stanley Kubrick chiller, *The Shining*, haunts me—Torrance, played by a young Jack Nicholson, working his manuscript to the point of madness in a whiteout of a blizzard at the deserted Overlook Hotel, drafting horrifying pages and pages: "All work and no play makes Jack a dull boy."

The play for me is a daily exercise of body and mind to engage the brain, as if pulling the chord to a cold chainsaw. You gotta rip at it, attempting at least to understand how the brain works. Some say the brain acts as a computer; others suggest it's a symphony orchestra. The brain is probably a little of both, perhaps more of an orchestra with various sections that must execute on cue for bravado of a performance. Hence tune-ups of mind, body, and spirit are critical to the process.

So at twilight, I'm back on the mat with the monster. That's why I run several miles each night to increase the cerebral flow as the sun sets, and more confusion takes over; I run until my legs give out. Due to my recent diagnosis and pain of acute spinal stenosis and scoliosis, I'm unable to run as I did, so now I crank the treadmill at the gym each night to an elevation of fifteen at a speed of up to 6.2, and race walk four to five miles. The pain is still present, though there is less pounding on the spinal cord. My daily physical routine helps reduce end-of-day confusion and restlessness, common in dementia patients and known as "sundowning," caused as light fades to black. This can be a time of greater rage, agitation, and mood swings, much like dandelions that behave differently at night; their heads close up tightly as the sun goes down.

On doctors' orders, I try vigorously to exercise my body and mind every night. After the gym, I usually write for two hours. Medical experts encourage those with Alzheimer's and other forms of dementia to pursue the creative arts, particularly writers, musicians, and artists with the disease. The writing makes me feel whole again— until the confusion takes over.

In Alzheimer's, mental and physical fatigue increases, and the restlessness can lead to pacing or wandering because an individual can't sleep. Theorists say that with the development of plaques and tangles in the brain related to Alzheimer's, there may be a disruption at sunset in what doctors term the "suprachiasmatic nucleus," associated with sleep patterns and changes in lighting—bringing on a sundowning effect.

With this disease, the sun rises and sets on a foggy bottom, a haze at times that precludes one, among other things, from recognizing familiar faces; or worse yet, the disease transposes a face, like the 1997 action thriller, *Face/Off*, starring Nicolas Cage and John Travolta. My life now, it seems, is a series of anecdotes. In Alzheimer's, there are times when one sees and experiences things that are not real, and times when one can't distinguish people and places that are.

There have been mornings when I haven't recognized my wife lying next to me. I knew I was supposed to be in the bed with this attractive woman, but I wasn't sure who she was. She looked familiar, but I had no understanding for several minutes of my relationship with the woman I have slept with for nearly four decades. It is disturbing; I never let on to her about the shame of it. She was asleep, so I just let it go.

And then there was the time at Kennedy Airport in New York in November 2010, awaiting my brother-in-law, Carl Maresca, and two of my brothers, Tim and Andy, for a flight to Shannon on an annual visit to Ireland, a place that restores the thinker and writer in me.

We were flying into Shannon to tour again the bucolic West Coast, a place that has attracted writers and artists for centuries, from Dingle to Donegal with its tiered cliffs, surging green pastures framed with moss-covered stonewalls, and snug, mottled villages that inspire poetry. From there, we were to hop a train cross-island to Dublin to take in this magnificent ancient city at the confluence of the River Liffey and the Irish Sea, a city that traces its beginnings back to 140 AD and claims among its sons James Joyce, William Butler Yates, and Samuel Beckett.

Sitting at the gate at Kennedy, I thought in long-term memory about walks through Trinity College, founded in 1592, along O'Connell Street, the site of the 1916 Easter Rising, the War of Irish Independence, and the Temple Bar, *Barra an Teampaill* in Gaelic, an area on the south bank of the Liffey. This cultural, and yes, pub district, likely received its name from the Temple family, who lived here in the seventeenth century; Sir William Temple was provost of Trinity College in 1609. In the core of the Temple Bar is Fishamble Street— the site of the first performance of Handel's *Messiah* on April 12, 1742; the annual performance of the *Messiah* is held on the same date at the same location. At a nearby tavern on Eustace Street in 1791, the republican revolutionary group, the Society of the United Irishmen, was formed. The group launched the Irish Rebellion of 1798 in an effort to end British rule over Ireland and to create an independent Irish Republic. In a maze of narrow, cobblestone streets, the Temple Bar captures the spirit of Dublin.

I'd rather muse on history than reality—the past is more redeeming to me than the future. It is a place of peace. My daze, call it reverie, was interrupted by a tap on the back.

"Hey, Lunchie!"

I earned the moniker "free lunch" years ago from my father because of my penchant for a free lunch, handouts from the nuns, and anyone with a basket.

"Hey, Lunchie!" the man called out again.

I stared at him intently, and didn't know him. I was getting pissed that this man in his sixties was calling me "Lunchie." New Yorkers are always in your face.

"You ok?" the stranger inquired.

Do I know you from Pluto? I wondered.

I stared at him again, carefully studying his expression, then began to connect the dots. The mosaic slowly resonated with familiarity. I focused in again. It was my brother-in-law Carl—a first-generation Italian American with Solarino roots. I've known him from the second grade; we attended Resurrection Catholic School together. He has always been an older brother to me, and always has my back.

"I'm your legal guardian on this trip," he said with a smile. "So shape up! We're going to make you wear a sandwich board with a phone number on the back of it; if you get lost, people will know who to call."

It was the last trip I took to Ireland with my surrogate older brother Carl, my "guardian" who had accompanied me on annual trips to Éire. Not long ago, shortly before his retirement, Carl, an avid athlete and outdoorsman fell from high in a tree cutting a branch and died instantly.

‎—⟋*⟍—

Not far beyond the bend of Doanes Creek in Harwich on the Cape, back on the lip of Nantucket Sound at the mouth of stately Wychmere

Harbor—a full circle of geologic perfection—is the confluence of all that is Cape Cod.

At the entrance to the harbor, marked by a sturdy stone jetty, is a graceful wide swath of sandy beach, one of the few accreting beaches on the Cape and growing at a rate of up to seven feet a year, given the steady ebb and flow of littoral currents.

Inside the harbor to the north is a row of sleek sailboards and pleasure craft in summer, guarding like sentinels on watch the comings and goings of the channel and overlooking the site of the legendary Thompson's Clam Bar, once one of the largest seasonal seafood restaurants east of the Mississippi. It served some of the finest clams known to man. Patrons would wait up to an hour and a half for a table in the 450-seat water-view restaurant, turning out more than 2,000 seafood dinners on a hot July night. The venerable structure is now the cornerstone of the exclusive Wychmere Beach Club in Harwich Port, a luxury private club.

On cue the afternoon of Sunday, June 19, 2011, the beach club's opening, the sun was glistening high above Nantucket Sound. My job as a media consultant was to lure the press and work the crowd over pricey chardonnay and cabernet and an assortment of fresh seafood and a raw bar that you would find at the finest New York and Boston bistros. I do nice work, arriving fashionably late, but on cue, and dressed in Tommy Bahama chinos, saddle shoes, and a shirt I bought in Dublin that looked like it was right off the deck of the Titanic. No assembly instructions required on this assignment, I assumed. Everything was perfect. Even my good buddy John Piekarski was there, standing by the pool with a handful of oysters and chatting up the elite. John hadn't told me he was coming.

I interrupted his conversation with a definitive pat on the back. "This guy boring you?" I asked.

The cold stares, even from John, could have frozen my retinas, only it wasn't John. It was a high roller from the city, not the kind of guy who appreciated a slap on the back and a stab in the shoulder from a less-than-perfect stranger. I finally realized all this after standing inelegantly next to the man for about a minute. With dots in the brain reconnecting, it wasn't even close. This guy didn't even look like John now.

So, I did my best Roseanne Roseannadanna of *SNL* fame, the character perfected by Gilda Radner: "Well, never mind."

"My mistake," I apologized. "Sorry!"

I walked away, feeling a pulse in my throbbing head.

It was the first time I had such an extraterrestrial experience. I have known John Piekarski for thirty years. I immediately thought of my mother and the times she had such disconnects. The realization was deadening. I moved on. All was good now, so I thought. When you fall off a horse you get right back on. Time to start up another conversation, I reasoned.

"You probably don't know me," I said minutes later to another gentleman standing near a walkway that led to the beach.

I reached out my hand. He shook it, and laughed. "Funny!" the guy said, shaking his head.

How did I go from being an idiot to a funny man in the space of a few minutes, I wondered?

I looked at him closely, stared intently. No recognition. "Sorry I didn't get right back to you after our meeting the other day," the man apologized.

The deadness was upon me again. Like the dutiful student, I started asking questions, trying to fill in the blanks, stitching together a story. Something. A clue that would give me direction, edification. Nothing. The mind was blank.

I pursued a line of conversation and questioning, with a reporter's instinct—small talk about sports and the summer ahead. Don't panic, stay in the moment, never let on. As Roman emperor and stoic philosopher Marcus Aurelius advised in the first century, "Confine yourself to the present." I've employed this strategy for years; it's a wait-and-see approach until I can either make a connection or exit the conversation gracefully.

"Greg, I want you to meet a friend," he said of the man to his left. "I think you can help him in his business."

Both had their business cards out on a table. Finally, a clue. *Shit.* I realized then that I was in conversation with a close client I had known for years and whose wife is a friend of mine.

Coming full circle, I suppose the silver lining in Alzheimer's, if you're good on your feet, and even if you're not, is you get to meet new friends daily.

I would have that chance to meet new friends again months later at a consultant meeting at Gillette Stadium in Foxboro where I've been a consultant to the Kraft Group for years, working in areas of community outreach and communications strategies. I arrived early for a meeting with Scott Farmelant, a friend and fellow consultant, a principal of the Boston communication firm Mills Public Relations. Months earlier, I had confided in him about my Alzheimer's diagnosis, as doctors had suggested with close clients and consultants. We discussed future projects and Scott's willingness to help fill in the blanks outside of my protected box of writing and communication skills. It was a business arrangement, born out of friendship and Scott's empathy for the progressive disease.

I was a bit out of sorts that day, but covering myself in the best reportorial spin. Some of the dots, as they often do unannounced, weren't connecting. I had been off my medication for a day or two— simply forgot to take it. But I was determined to fight through the haze on this brilliant sunny January day.

As I entered the room, I didn't recognize anyone; they looked vaguely familiar, but assumed a new crew of campaign workers had moved in. A guy to my left, a friendly, enthusiastic individual, started chatting me up about the campaign.

We talked about project benefits, opposition issues, media, and messaging. He clearly knew me, but I was embarrassed to ask who he was.

"Let's go grab some coffee," he said after some chat. "That's good with me," I said, "but I'm waiting for Scott Farmelant, then we can all go." There was silence.

The guy put his arm around me and whispered into my ear, "Greg, I'm Scott!"

Altogether mortified, but not off my humor game, I replied, "Well then, that's good, Scott. Now we don't have to wait for you."

We walked out of the room for coffee on a one-two count, and never spoke about the disconnect again. Scott's a good friend.

8

Rocks in My Head

Dr. Seuss once advised, "You've got brains in your head. You have feet in your shoes. You can steer yourself in any direction you choose."

Not if you have rocks in your head.

Since I was a boy, my mother said I had rocks in my head; now after decades, they are literally calcifying, obstructing signals to the brain. Early-onset Alzheimer's will do that.

I've always been a good rainmaker, the art of inducing precipitation, in this case, generating puddles for the family to pay bills, but of late, the signals are crossing. While I was never an exemplary steward, I'm spending money today in odd ways, at times like a drunken sailor. At doctors' directive, I've turned all my credit cards over to my wife, who along with my faithful sister Lauren, an accountant-type, views all my online bank and debit-card statements daily to make sure nothing is awry. Surprises were occurring regularly, until I was forced to hand over a hidden American Express card I had kept to maintain a sense of self.

The final straw was Christmas 2011. I'm a Clark Griswold, "Sparky" dad; each Christmas Eve after church service, the family has an intimate dinner at the Chatham Bars Inn, overlooking Chatham's inner harbor, then we ceremoniously watch Chevy Chase's *Christmas*

Vacation. We still laugh so hard we cry—aping all the iconic lines seconds before they are delivered.

I usually go overboard for Christmas, akin to Evil Knievel attempting to jump the Grand Canyon on a revved-up motorcycle. This particular Christmas was no exception in holiday largesse, but early that Christmas Eve was a moment of unusual stillness for me, the cerebral kind. Listening to *Silent Night* on a speaker outsider a retail store at noon, I was flush suddenly with the fear that I had no gifts, that everyone else in the family had gone Christmas shopping but me. I began to panic. So, I whipped out the American Express Gold, and within fifteen minutes bought close to a thousand dollars of stuff that I had no recollection of buying—the kind of crap nobody wants: shot glasses with Boston Celtic logos, paper plates and plastic forks, a doormat. I wrapped the "presents" like a good elf, placed them under the tree, and awaited Christmas morning.

To my horror, on Christmas morning, I realized that I had bought the mother lode weeks earlier, nice presents actually, and when it came time to open my inane offerings of late, I first got stares from my wife and kids, some humiliating laughs, a few loving cautions, and then a big hand from son Brendan—asking for the American Express card so that everything could be returned for a credit.

Talk about pissing your money away. I hope you kids see what a silly waste of resources this was, my wife must have thought in her best impersonation of Clark's mother-in-law after he had placed 250 strands of lights with 100 bulbs on each strand for a total of 25,000 light bulbs on the house, and none of them worked.

If I woke up tomorrow with my head sewn to the carpet, I wouldn't be more surprised, I thought.

Like the Griswold house, the lights in my head blink; they are full on, off, back on, then off again, on again. Sometimes, I can sense it coming; other times, I can't—the disconnects, dropped calls, mental pocket dials, short-term memory losses, and the tingling of the mind, which starts like an ocean swell in the forehead and works its way cresting in intensity over the top and sides of my head, then down the neck, rolling into my shoulders in anesthetizing sensation. I can feel the pressure. At first, I panicked; tried to stop it, but I couldn't. So, I tried to learn to dance with it. But I suck at dancing. On a good day, the rhythm is smooth, though out of step in places. On a bad day, the beat is off—stumbling with two left cerebral feet over time, place, and person.

But I now have a repertoire of banter always at the ready on sports, politics, and religion for those who want to go deep. It's a defense mechanism, while I try to find my bearings. I play a game with myself, upping the stakes every day—how long can I pull this off without someone noticing? There are times when the conversation drifts to a disparate subject with no grounding, and a friend or colleague will ask politely, "You with us?" And there have been times when I have emailed a client a newspaper piece on a story pitch, carefully checking the story for date and subject matter, only to find out later that the clip was several years old and had nothing to do with the story at hand. I lost a $5,000 monthly retainer that way. I don't blame the client; I blame myself. I blame the disease.

Such mental collapses are motivation to dig deeper into the cognitive reserve, knowing in the moment that I can't go to the tank forever. The process of fighting off symptoms is exhausting, and yet exhilarating when one succeeds. It is a forceful fight for clarity, one that I win more than I lose now. For me, it's akin to the olfactory phenomenon displayed in Atlantic herring, alewives, as they make their annual migration at the strike of spring—just down the street through the ancient Brewster Herring Run, thousands of them fighting, like salmon, against a flush of water, as the alewives rush in gut instinct up the slick, steep water stone ladders of the run from Cape Cod Bay to the Upper Mill Pond to spawn in fresh water kettle ponds where they were born. The fish repeatedly are flushed back by cascading water, hitting fish heads on rocks, yet instinctively climb the ladder again.

Cognitive reserve in primal nature! Late mentor John Hay wrote about the Brewster marvel in his inspiring book, *The Run*, connecting dots to the survival instinct in all of us. "The fish kept moving up," he observed. "I watched the swinging back and forth with the current, great-eyed, sinewy, probing, weaving, their dorsal fins cutting the surface, their ventral fins fanning, their tails flipping and sculling. In the thick, interbalanced crowd there would suddenly be a scattered dashing, coming up as quickly as cats'-paws flicking the summer seas. They have moved by 'reflex' rather than conscious thought."

Conscious thought is survival; loss of reason is demise. In Alzheimer's, one fights against the drifts, those vacant staring moments when the mind floats, and you can't control it. And then there are the visual misperceptions—the polite phrase for hallucinations. They started several years ago. One night watching ESPN's *Sports Center*, after nothing stronger than coffee with milk, I noticed some insect-like creatures, with stringy, hairy legs crawling along the top of the ceiling toward me. It wasn't the sports scores. I watched in horror as they inched closer. It was like the bar scene in *Star Wars*; they crept from wall to wall, then began to float toward me in packs. I remembered my mother telling me about them. So, I brushed them away. They vanished, though I was in a cold sweat. They kept returning at different times of day, about once every few weeks. They still come. Sometimes in packs, sometimes alone, often appearing as a spider or some other distorted vision. Sometimes they come in an army, like the time I was in Phoenix two years ago at the house of my old friend, Ray Artigue, a communications analyst and former vice president with the Phoenix Suns. I was awake in a guest room at about 8 a.m., and a phalanx of the imagined approached me. I swiped at them; they disappeared.

The hallucinations don't frighten me anymore; Mom taught me that they will come, and they will go. An artist herself, she often counseled about fear: turn the tapestry over. Don't look at the threads beneath it, just look at the art, and don't be afraid to move on.

So I do, and keep evoking an anecdote of the great Protestant reformer Martin Luther, a man of incredible faith, who in the early 1500s was frequently terrorized by his personal demons. One morning, as the anecdote goes, Luther awoke to Satan in full horror sitting at the bottom of his bed. Luther, at first, was terrified, then realized he had the faith to press on.

"Oh, it's just you again," he said to the apparition. Then he turned over and went back to sleep, like a rock.

Rocks have always held my attention, ever since I was a kid vacationing on Cape Cod. Leaving the Cape at the end of summer was always a sad experience for me. I can remember the empty feelings as I filled my duffel bag—the sneakers with the holes in the tips, my jeans with sand in the pockets, a surfing jam bleached by the sun, my wrinkled baseball cap—and carted it out to the station wagon. It always seemed to rain that day.

About a half hour before the family was ready to leave, all ten of us, I would take one final walk from the cottage off Herring Brook Road in Eastham to nearby Thumpertown Beach on Cape Cod Bay. Along the way, I'd relive the summer—days fishing on Salt Pond, the time we hiked to the old Coast Guard station, the bicycle rides along the back roads to Orleans, the soothing pounding of the ocean, the sweet smell of beach plums. Each memory was precious as time was slipping away.

When I reached the bluffs of the beach, I paused for one last look with the hope that I could freeze the moment in my mind. I then walked down the wooden steps to the beach—each of the thirty-two planks creaking from summer wear and tear; the gray paint peeling back; many of the nails rusted from the sea air. I could see the charred remains of Labor Day campfires that had blazed the night before. Once on the beach, I ceremoniously walked, as I did each year, to the surf.

There is something about a Cape Cod summer that no other summer place can match: The sky is brighter, the sun more radiant, the sand softer, the air more pure, the mood more peaceful. Like many before me, I sought some tangible connection to this fragile, narrow sliver of land—something, a part of me, which I could leave behind. And so, each year at this time, I would walk the beach looking for a special rock, a memory to file deep within. It had to be perfect in every detail— symmetric, polished, and about the size of my fist. It had to have just the right feel. It had to feel a part of me.

I usually picked up about three dozen rocks until I found the right one—my selected memory of that Cape Cod summer. The rejects were tossed into the bay for more polishing. I then walked back to the staircase and buried my treasure about twelve inches from the foot of the stairs.

All winter long in New York, I'd think of my rock; the summer memories it conjured helped me through the dreary days.

Then, each summer when we returned to the Cape, the first thing I'd do, after unpacking the duffel bag, was to race to the beach to retrieve the rock. I always found it, of course. I had convinced myself—and tried to persuade my mother—that any rock of similar size was the one I had stored. I collected these rocks in the back yard of the cottage we always rented, walking over them barefoot, at times, like a cobblestone path to a paradise.

I'd like to think they're still there.

9

American Pie

Westchester County was "American Pie" in the 1960s. You could drink whiskey in Rye when I was young. Growing up here, just four exits up Route 95 from the Bronx, yet time zones away in culture, one could order the best brand of Bushmills on an eighteenth birthday. I did, and paid the price at the Five Points on Midland Avenue, now Kelly's Sea Level bar, owned today by a childhood buddy, Jerry Maguire, and his family—hardly the alter ego of Tom Cruise.

By all measure, Rye is more than a bar stop. It's a storied place on Long Island Sound at the mouth of New York Harbor, the locus of Rye Beach and Playland where movie scenes from *Fatal Attraction* with Glenn Close and *Big* with Tom Hanks were filmed. I will always remember the scene in *Big* with Zoltar the Magnificent, the fortune-telling machine that transported a young Hanks, the character of Josh Baskin, from childhood to adulthood and back. Where is Zoltar when I need him?

Rye is a place of long-term memories for me, a shoring up of a past that can never be forgotten—memories that offer great solace at tangents of a change in life. The long-term memories sustain me; the short-term is a thin reed. In Alzheimer's, brain cells in charge of short-term memory are losing the war. But long-term memory is still safely tucked away in a relatively peaceful neighborhood. Those memories are like a loyal, trustworthy friend, an ally to spend time with, at least for now. The significance and yet illusiveness of memory for those with Alzheimer's is edifying. We all need memories; they define us. Saul Bellow, the Pulitzer and Nobel Prize winner, once observed, "They keep the wolf of insignificance from the door."

Rye, in so many ways, defines my mother and me, and a legion of ethnic transplants, in its simplicity, idealism, and in the everyday ordinary that delineated a time and space, silhouetted by the demographics of a generation—long-term memories to hold tight. Rye was everyone's town. In the 1950s and '60s, it was a Norman Rockwell community from central casting, a mix of Stockbridge and *Mayberry R.F.D.*—bleached, white picket fences, flannel shirts and faded jeans, Oxford button downs from the Prep Shop on Purchase Street, and some Sax Fifth Avenue suits for the city folk.

I've never left my childhood; I exist there today, to every extent possible, moments frozen in time of great joy, peace, security, immaturity, and potty talk at times. On some days, it's the only peace I know. Alzheimer's brings one home to long-term memory—in my case, to a time when doctors made house calls, nuns wore black sweaty wool nineteenth century habits, baseball was king, and a McDonald's hamburger, fries, and a Coke cost just twenty-five cents. The memories keep me whole, and serve to stitch a patchwork quilt of experiences that leave indelible images of a life that cannot be forgotten.

Rye was the quintessence of "American Pie." The Big Bopper, Buddy Holly, and Ritchie Valens were icons in my town, and the night a single engine Beechcraft Bonanza, model 35, serial #D-1019, wing number N3794N, crashed in a Clear Lake, Iowa, cornfield on February 3, 1959 was the day the music died here. I was in the third grade when the plane went down, and even Sister Timothy, a plump, stern, but benevolent Sister of Charity, took note of the loss. We called her the "Big Bopper."

The day the music died was the first communal tragedy Boomers experienced, a shared loss of innocence to be followed in four years by the assassination of John F. Kennedy, and three decades later by the death of Mickey Mantle, the "last boy." No doubt, the Father,

Son, and Holy Ghost of a generation took the last train to the coast. But we Baby Boomers survived, a bit tougher, more cerebral, and always idealistic. Perhaps we should have seen a flood of disasters and dementias coming, like the rise of high tide on a foggy Long Island Sound. But instead, we chose to clip priceless Joe DiMaggio, Mickey Mantle, Roger Maris, and Willie Mays baseball cards with wooden clothespins to the spokes of our bicycles to mimic the roar of a motorcycle. Made us feel childishly reckless. In street value today, we shredded the collective investment of college tuitions and retirement. And we think we're so smart.

Rye—a place where George Washington slept, Ogden Nash and Amelia Earhart lived, and once the seaside retreat of the Manhattan elite—was inhabited decades ago by ethnic, first-generation working stiffs. Today, some of the wealthiest, most successful in the nation live here. But to me, Rye simply is home, a place to remember, a patchwork quilt of hometowns across the country. Everyone needs a memory of home, real or imagined; mine is more real than imagined. Innocence, as it was elsewhere, was the coin of Rye in the '50s and '60s—a town where first-, second-, and third-generation Irish and Italian Americans bonded with Jews, connecting on ball fields and sandlots here and in neighboring Port Chester. Young Italians from "the Port," as we called it in button-down Rye, often cruised Milton Road on Friday nights, beating the shit out of us Irish guys in madras shorts, pink shirts, and deck shoes. I don't blame them now. I grew up with an ethnic mix in Rye and Port Chester, regular guys like Tommy Casey, Jimmy Fitzpatrick, Vinny Dempsey, Jimmy Dianni, Billy St. John, Tony Keating, Ritchie O'Connell, Al Wilson, Brian Keefe, Chuck Drago, Dino Garr, Carlo Castallano, Rocco LaFaro, Tancredi Abnavoli, Dante Salvate, Ronald Carducci, Ritchie Breese, Micky DiCarlo, and yes, Ricky Blank, one of the most gifted Jewish shortstops I've ever known.

Many of us played organized baseball on the same teams together after we realized that an infield rundown was more fun than a slap down—later communally on a hold-your-breath, mix-and-match Rye/Port Chester All-Star Team that twice won the New York State

Senior Babe Ruth League Championship with two trips to the Senior Babe Ruth League World Series regional tournament—a non sequitur of young jocks if there ever was one. In time, we all became best of friends. Six of our starters signed major league contracts. I was among those who didn't, but as a catcher, faithfully wore the tools of ignorance, first presented in the third grade at a Pony League practice.

Rye was a melting pot, boiled to perfection by the nuns. The town was predominately WASP—a hornet's nest, in fact, with three Presbyterian churches and one Catholic church, as well as a synagogue. But you could have fooled us fraternal Catholics, who reproduced like rabbits. We were tokens, often looked down upon in social circles, at the country clubs, and in line for groceries at the A&P, but we thought we owned the damn place. And in spirit, we did.

At Resurrection Grammar School, sandwiched between Milton Road and the Boston Post Road, and in the shadows of the Church of the Resurrection, a Gothic stone cathedral, one hardly messed with the nuns whose names sounded like the guest list of first-century saints in Jerusalem. Sisters Timothy, Syra, Turibius, Aloysius, Monica, and Joseph, along with a convent full of accomplices had your back, your front, your top, and your bottom. But don't screw with them. You moved only on command. Our parents exceedingly impressed this dictum on us. It seems so wildly anachronistic, looking back. My parents, as most of the day, sung in this choir of didactic discipline. Church was second to family, first at times. Discipline was the order of the day. My dad, with oak-like roots in County Clare, was the first-born son of Edmund and Helen (Clancy) O'Brien. He was raised with his brother Larry by his mother's sister, Annette, and her husband, Bob O'Dell (who never missed one of my baseball games), on gritty Sedgwick Avenue in the Bronx in the shadows of the "House That Ruth Built," where he played his sandlot baseball on a diamond whose pitcher's mound today is second base in the new Yankee Stadium. His parents died of tuberculosis, the quick consumption, when he was a young boy. My father was schooled at St. Nicholas of Tolentine and Fordham University. He was one of the youngest Naval LST captains in World War II. A cerebral type, he read four newspapers a day in his professional years for a balance of news and opinion: *The New York Times, Wall Street Journal, New York Daily News,* and the *New York Post.*

He was a "layman reader" at Resurrection, one of the first ever in the church when Mass in 1969, at the decree of Pope Paul VI, was transformed from Latin to the vernacular. When Dad, an everlasting Yankee fan, was named to head up this new order of laymen, we in the family thought of him as Moses with hair dye. In a papal order from Rome, *"Ad Déum qui laetíficat juventútem méam,"* was rendered "to God who giveth joy to my youth." Not the same ring of high-church elegance to it, and besides, the English translation extended the length of a Mass. One could always burble through the Latin: *Mea Culpa, Mea Culpa, Mea Maxima Culpa!* Our pastor, Monsignor John D. McGowan, an arthritic pastor in his eighties, still holds the record for saying Mass from start to finish in twelve minutes, including the homily. As a plebe altar boy, I served Mass that day and clocked him, as fellow altar boys looked on with pride. The aging McGowan genuflected as quickly as a wideout making a cut for the end zone.

I couldn't wait to race home to tell my mother, a beautiful woman, barely five-feet tall and a hundred pounds with platinum blond hair. "A lean horse for a long race," my dad would always say. Mom was all about the church and was impressed with such records. Raised in the shadows of the American Museum of Natural History and Hayden Planetarium in New York, she played hopscotch on the sidewalk at a time when milk was delivered in a horse-drawn carriage. Mom was educated at a French convent school and later at the College of New Rochelle in the Ursuline tradition, the first Catholic college for women in New York. Few women in the day went to college; most stayed home to have babies. A teacher later in life, she first worked as a banker, far ahead of a long-awaited shattering of the glass ceiling for women, and then she became a devoted mother, deeply involved in Resurrection as a Cub Scout and Brownie leader. Life for us at the time was the epitome of the '50s sitcom *Leave It to Beaver,* exemplifying the idealized suburban family of the mid-twentieth century. My mother—God bless you, Eddie Haskell—frequently wore a lovely red dress.

Both parents, respectively, were members in good standing of the parish Mothers' and Fathers' Clubs. They also taught CCD, "The Confraternity of Christian Doctrine," established in Rome in 1562 for the purpose of giving religious education to the heathens. In later days, the nuns defined heathens as the children of Catholic parents who weren't sent to Catholic School. Faithful parishioners taught CCD on Wednesday nights; the nuns instructed the heathens on Thursdays at 1:30 pm, as if caring for lepers. We were dismissed early on those days. Officially, it was called "Released Time," and we were told to clear the playground as quickly as possible. The collective body language suggested that we scatter swiftly from the heathens and Huns. *Run home to the bosom of your mothers,* the nuns admonished us!

And God help us, Jesus, if we ever looked at a Protestant! We were warned never to gape at the spiral of the nearby Gothic Rye Presbyterian Church, designed in the 1860s by Richard Upjohn, the renowned church architect who built Trinity Church on Wall Street. If we even stared at this magnificent edifice, we feared, it would be akin to looking back at Sodom. We'd be turned to pillars of salt.

Pass me the salt shaker. Every Thursday, sometimes on Fridays, the nuns queued us up to "confess" our weekly sins to the priests in confessionals—dark, dank places, the darkness of which struck me as the gateway to hell, rather than a trap door to enlightenment.

Some of us innocent types (we were the brown-nosers) felt we had to manufacture our sins, presuming that if we were not in the confessional long enough, the nuns would assume we weren't coming clean. Beyond all priests, we all feared Father O'Brien, no relation; he was a former U.S. Marine chaplain who wouldn't put up with any crap. Later he arose to the rank of monsignor. I've always assumed that on Judgment Day, he'll be the henchmen in Heaven, tossing the miscreants into the ring of fire.

At the confessional, by dumb luck, I often landed in Father O'Brien's court. I spilled my guts in the usual manner. Then in the sixth grade behind a dark screen that silhouetted a ghostly figure, Father O'Brien, apparently tired of my manufactured sins, commanded, "What more have you done, son; what more?" I panicked, so I told him that I often had "impure thoughts, bless me, Father, for I have sinned."

"YOU WHAT?" he shouted so everyone in line could hear. "YOU WHAT?"

The words echoed throughout the cathedral, like a pipe organ in *Phantom of the Opera*.

On the way out of the confessional, the girls wouldn't even sneak a peek at me, like I was a leper; the boys all gave me eye contact, the equivalent then of a High Five.

My penance was to say three Hail Marys, two Our Fathers and a Glory Be. I've often wondered if the "Glory Be" was a signal to me from Father O'Brien: "About time, son…"

The mile walk from pastoral Brookdale Place to Resurrection was problematic for me. I had to pass the towers of Babel, careful not to glance up, just look down at my scuffed Buster Browns. My sisters, brothers, and I walked to school every day—the girls were dressed in the uniform of plaid skirts, white blouses, blue jackets, and black patent leather shoes; the boys were required to wear a white-collared dress shirt with a blue tie, gray flannel pants, a blue blazer, and dark socks; we all looked like *Encyclopedia Britannica* salesmen. The only exception to the socks rule was gym day. On gym days, guys wore white socks with running shorts underneath their trousers for a quick change in the basement for a stinging game of dodgeball or stickball in the playground. To this day, one can detect someone who was educated in the metropolitan New York Catholic school system; they will quip at work to a friend or colleague wearing white socks: "Got gym today?"

Once at school, regardless of the temperature, five below or pushing ninety, we gathered in the playground behind the red brick schoolhouse before the start of class. We were sorted in grades by cracks in the pavement. It was a blueprint to avoid chaos, the equivalent today of those invisible electronic dog fences. If you crossed the line, you'd be zapped by the nuns, unless you were queued up at the convent steps to carry the bags—the nuns' briefcases, not the old battle-axes themselves. "Brown nosers" like me waited as hungry puppy dogs outside the convent to carry a black bag; I often wondered later if they contained the nuclear code in case Khrushchev stepped out of line. At the back door of the school about 200 feet away, the exchange was made: a pat on the head, a passing of the bag, a return to the playground. We then waited within our assigned cracks, engaged in kickball, punchball, flipping cards, or just yapping. Minutes later with great thunder, an oversized glass window in the principal's office opened—an ancient kind that moved on string cords, not tracks, and made a noise like the trumpeting of angels in the Book of Revelation. The hairy, muscular arm of the Mother Superior then reached out with a cowbell the size of a boxcar. She flushed three times:

DA-DING, DA-DING, DA-DING.

The first ding ordered us to stop in motion. Instantly. Didn't matter if you were in the air, mid-sentence, or taking a pee in the hedges: you held the position. The second ding was a call to line up in silence like prisoners of war; the third ding heralded our entrance to the cellblock, err, school. All in stillness, mind you, looking straight ahead. The nuns excoriated the boys that there was to be no staring down at the shiny patent leather shoes of coeds to see their undergarments in reflection. Of course, none of us had ever thought that was possible, but what a great freakin' idea.

In class, we had thirty to forty kids packed to a room, and hardly anyone stepped out of line. There were always exceptions. The nuns, with cold stares, would burn your retinas with a force that would frost a lawn. In the first grade, Sister Syra took no prisoners. If you were out of line, you were hung out to dry in the "clothes cupboard." Literally. In those days, the blue blazers had collar loops made of tin, and if you acted out, Sister Syra hung you on a cupboard hook like a piece of meat until your mom claimed you at the end of school, or if you happened to have a more modern blazer, the ones with a cloth loop, you were relegated to a crouch position under her desk. The discipline, while clearly over the top and flirting with abuse, had a stinging influence on me. I was afraid to go to class and skipped school one day in the first grade, hiding out in a side altar of church, one designated for Our Lady of Perpetual Help. The nuns, realizing I was AWOL, went nuts. My mom was called, and the boy hunt was on. Mom ultimately determined that I was probably hiding in a pew. In short order, I was returned to class.

Second grade with amicable Sister Monica was a slide, but third grade and beyond was a call to arms. Sister Timothy would slap you silly in the mind; Sister Anthony in the fourth grade sported a moustache, and I thought I saw her once on a black-and-white television heavyweight wrestling match against champion Bruno Sammartino from Abruzzi, Italy; and Sister Joseph in the eighth grade, a long, thin women who looked remarkably like the Wicked Witch of the East, could cut right to the heart!

"I'll get you, my little pretties, and your little dogs, too!"

I still recoil at the thought of what seemed like a long, bony index finger, the length of a tractor trailer in my young imagination, reaching down a row of desks to pluck by the chin an insubordinate and carry them, on the sheer strength of hand ligaments, all the way to the front of the class for a holy thrashing, then a trip to the principal's office for yet another ceremonial kick in the ass.

Our classroom was a cattle call with the likes of incorrigible Jimmy Dianni, my alter ego in some ways, a guy who rose later in life to the position of lieutenant and chief fire inspector in the Rye Fire Department.

Dianni's foil was a classically awkward, blameless kid of the day; let's call him Liam Kelley, to protect the innocent. Kelley likely now heads up a Fortune 500 company, but Mom always felt sorry for him; she had a heart for the muddled and affronted. We've all had them in class, and many of us will do hard time in Purgatory for not coming to their relief. But as Divine or dumb luck would have it, the nuns always found a way to fuse the two—Dianni and Kelley, repelling magnets. I looked on as a voyeur just for the mere fascination of it.

Serendipity, possibly, but it all started in the fourth grade when Dianni, a freckled-faced, slightly chubby boy, hurled, for some enigmatic reason, his tattered brown book bag, the kind with silver metal corners at the bottom, into a crowded playground. Perhaps he was just mad at his mother. But who did it hit right in the squash? Kelley! Was it by design? Maybe just dumb freakin' luck? But, game on!

Halloween, no doubt, was in the air late on a Friday afternoon in October in the early 1960s. Dead, fallen oak leafs were swept by a coastal wind across the asphalt parking lot at Resurrection, like screaming pucks at a hockey practice, as the nuns herded us from the bulky red brick school building to Resurrection Church for weekly hymn practice for the obligatory 10 a.m. Sunday Mass, which students and families were all expected to attend; the nuns took names at the church door. At this particular Friday practice, Sister Aloysius was orchestrating like Leonard Bernstein—spine upright, arms pumping in baton-like fashion, thick white-matted hair beneath her black bonnet. We filed into the church like lambs to a slaughter; no one was allowed to speak; we were entering "Oz" after all. We were warned: Nobody talks to the Wizard. God has the whole world in his hands, and frankly, there's no room for you. So, buck up, just sit in silence, pray the Rosary, hope you're not struck by lightning, and listen up for further orders. I got it, but Jimmy missed it.

For some delightful reason, maybe the sheer pleasure of it, the nuns positioned Dianni in a pew next to Kelley, who sat unaffected up against a granite pillar that rose from the floor to the roof of the church that seemed to us the height of the Empire State Building. On this particular Friday, I was sitting to the left of Dianni; Kelley was to the right of him, plumb against a cold stone pillar with enough room between the pew and pillar for a small pumpkin. We were rehearsing the hymn *Army of God* in full, uplifted voice:

And I hear the sound of the coming rain, As we sing the praise to the Great I Am

And the sick are healed, and the dead will rise And your church is the army that was prophesied

As the chorus reached its holy peak, and the Lord's grace was raining down on us, we could hear a piercing cry from the back of the church.

"Get my head out! Get my head out!"

Kelley had dropped his hymnal between the pew and the pillar, and Dianni obliged on cue by wedging Kelley's head between them.

"Get my head out!" Kelley yelled in a voice that overpowered the saints.

"Dianni, you fuck, get my head out!"

The sisters were apoplectic. They raced to the back of the church as if someone had just burned down a convent full of nuns. At the scene of the crime, a decision was made to call in church sexton, John Quinn—a gnarly man with a brogue as thick as Guinness and looking a bit like Bilbo Baggins in *Lord of the Rings*. He was asked to pry the swelled head loose. With the sturdy hands of an apostle rebuking the devil himself, Quinn safely extracted the head intact.

"It's free, it's free!" he declared, having snatched Kelley's head from what all had feared were the jaws of death.

With baton still in hand, and looking as if she had just witnessed a vomit scene from *The Exorcist*, Sister Aloysius tersely dismissed hymn practice. "I think we've sung enough today!" she said, the pleats of her habit swaying with a shake of her knees.

The imbroglio ensued, and I looked on in awe of Jimmy, yet with a guilt of Jesuit proportions, but I knew that Kelley would have his day. Witnessing the conflict refined me in calculation of character, moments in long-term memory that I can never forget. It is reassuring for me.

Months later, with thirty-eight students sandwiched in math class, authoritarian Sister Joseph ended the session with a repressive homework assignment from our *Progress in Arithmetic* textbook. The room groaned as if crushed by a school bus. Dianni, sitting again next to Kelley, goaded him to protest, and Sister Joseph became enraged at the class defiance.

"Add to your assignment," she ordered, "the worksheet at the end of chapter two!" she ordered.

The moans continued with Kelley leading the charge.

"And just for that, copy all the times tables in the back of the book, three times!" Sister Joseph declared, as if challenged by the underworld.

The wailing subsided, although some laments could still be heard. Dianni prodded Kelley again for a response. Kelley was waiting to pounce.

"Fine," Sister Joseph screamed, the veins in her neck popping, that long index finger poised. "We're gonna have a test tomorrow on the first four chapters!"

There was a frightening silence. Sister Joseph had prevailed. Not so quick. Dianni looked at Kelley, Kelley looked at Dianni, and then Kelley cried out, *"Ah, shit!"*

The words echoed throughout the classroom. Sinewy Sister Joseph sprinted to the back of the room and pounced like a linebacker. What was left of Kelley seconds later was sent to the principal's office.

But God is good, justice is certain, and in Dublin, one never gets mad, right? Kelley retaliated in time.

It is important these days to keep exercising long-term memory—that loyal, trustworthy friend.

A rite of passage at Resurrection in the seventh grade was the day students moved up from writing in lead pencil to fountain pen, filled to the brim of the cartridge with blue India ink. A successor of the dip-pen that Ben Franklin once used to sign the Declaration of Independence, the fountain pen had a stainless steel or gold nib that washed a wave of ink onto a page. You had to write fast, or the ink flooded; a practical reality that may have taught us Baby Boomers to think quicker when writing.

A bottle of precious blue India ink rested on the oak eraser ledge below the blackboard, and one approached the ledge for refilling the fountain pen with all the reverence of standing before the Holy Grail.

The nuns had taught us that it was a mystical privilege to write in blue ink. One day in the seventh grade, I saw Kelley in line for ink; he had the look of a gunman, as the rest of the class sat passively in their seats, blue jackets off, white shirts exposed. Kelley filled the cartridge slowly and deliberately, getting every ounce possible into the reservoir. He turned with intent, walked down the middle aisle toward Dianni's desk, his eyes affixed to the back of the room so as not to draw attention. Passing Dianni, still in stride, he waved his pen in a fierce jerky motion in front of Dianni's new clean white shirt, the one his mother had warned him not to soil. In an instant, a large "Z," the size of the Mark of Zorro, was indelibly imprinted on Dianni's shirt. Kelley, in the role of the swashbuckling Don Diego de la Vega, a.k.a. Zorro, had left his mark on Dianni, now the dupe, and relegated to the role of Sergeant Demetrio López García.

Nobody messes with Zorro. Class dismissed.

Seasoned altar boys, Jimmy (in his makeshift pinstripe shirt) and I immediately fled for the sanctuary of the church—not for the confessional, but to light up incense in a closet of a room off the sanctuary. The Catholic Church interprets the burning of incense as a symbol of the Prayer of the Faithful, rising to Heaven, a purification process. The incense is burned in a metal container called a thurible, to be dispensed in three ritual swings for the Trinity. The imagery is recorded in Psalm 141:2, "Let my prayer be directed as incense in thy sight: the lifting up of my hands, as evening sacrifice."

But Jimmy and I weren't there for the prayer. We just liked the smell of the stuff. Besides, as captain of the school safety patrol and altar boy Master of Ceremonies, a position in the church pecking order akin to Michael the Archangel, I had access to the room. Keys to the Kingdom. It pleased my mother; she was also proud of the way we held sway with the nuns at Mass. Jimmy taught me to hold the gold-plated altar communion plate just above the Adam's apple of nuns queued up for communion. When the sisters lined up, we would press the plate gently against their throats, just to let them know we were there. A presence almost as good as a supernatural power.

Jimmy always has been a presence with me. Fifty years later, when he learned that I had been diagnosed with Alzheimer's, he called to express his love and support; he promised me that he wasn't going to treat me any differently. It was music to my ears. He ended the conversation with a play on Alzheimer's: "Remember, buddy, you still owe me a hundred bucks!" I've passed the exchange along to other friends, who have responded in kind, "You owe me a hundred bucks, too! And don't forget it."

Bada-bing, bada-boom.

The boom came in October 1962 with the Cuban missile crisis of the Cold War, a 13-day war of words between the U.S., the Soviet Union, and its ally Cuba—a Russian roulette among titans of the day—Soviet Premier Nikita Khrushchev, Cuban Prime Minister Fidel Castro, and John F. Kennedy. No one was ready to blink.

Two months earlier, after unsuccessful covert U.S. operations to overthrow Castro through a failed Bay of Pigs invasion and Operation Mongoose, the Cubans and Soviets secretly began constructing medium-range and intermediate-range ballistic nuclear missile bases with the ability to strike most of the continental U.S. Photo reconnaissance captured proof. It is generally regarded as the moment the world came closest to nuclear holocaust. After rejecting tactics of attacking Cuba by air and sea, the Kennedy brain trust opted for a naval blockade of Cuba—no Soviet ship would be allowed to enter Cuban waters. In a letter to Kennedy, Khrushchev called the blockage "an act of aggression, propelling humankind into the abyss of a world nuclear-missile war."

"Ah, shit!" as Kelley would say.

On October 25, 1962, the Soviet ships were steaming just off Cuba, and the U.S. was not standing down. We were on the edge of extinction, we thought. The nuns were abuzz with images of Armageddon, and tuned-in transistor AM radios throughout Resurrection for the holy unwashed to hear. Last call for us, and no one had passed the height line yet at the Five Points. After wet-your-pants radio reports and a mock class exercise of duck and cover under our desks in the event of a nuclear attack (as if to vaporize us in a position of kissing our asses goodbye), the bell rang to end school, and we all spilled out of the building like flushing tap water, down the second floor stairs, to the first floor, heading to the back door. Billy St. John and I then hung a quick right to the basement.

"Where are you guys going?" cautioned Tony Keating, a life-long friend, who walked home with us every day. "Keats, we're going to the basement to get ready for the boys' basketball team tryouts," replied Billy.

Few seventh graders had ever made the eighth-grade team, and Billy and I were on the precipice of greatness, hoping Coach Pete McHugh would tap us.

Keating stopped us in our tracks. "Where do you want to be when the bomb drops? On the basketball court with Mr. McHugh, or home with your parents where you belong?"

The logic was unassailable. And so, like lemmings, we followed Keating down Milton Road to safe haven. When I got home, I hugged my mom, and then went to my room to pray.

"Dear God, not now, please not now!"

Prayers were answered. The next day, no bomb. Kennedy and Khrushchev had agreed in back-channel negotiations that the Soviets would dismantle offensive weapons in Cuba, and the U.S., in return, would agree not to invade Cuba and dismantle missiles in Turkey and Italy. Still, Billy and I were cut from the eighth-grade team for missing practice and racing home to pray. A small price, I suppose, for saving the world.

Prayer was always a part of the daily routine at Resurrection, drilled into our thick "cabezas" through all the smoke and mirrors of *Mad Magazine* and *Playboy* centerfolds. Every May, we had special devotions to the Blessed Virgin Mary, honoring the mother of Christ as the "Queen of May," a ritual that dated back to the sixteenth century. We were all schooled in the virginity of Mary, and many of us, at the direction of the priests, nuns, and our parents, wore scapulars—the Blue Scapular of the Immaculate Conception, scratchy cloth images of the Blessed Virgin that were suspended over the chest and the back by thin twine. While often causing a rash, the scapular came with a sacred promise, known as the Sabbatine Privilege, that the Blessed Virgin, through special intercession on the Saturday after the death of a devotee, would personally liberate and deliver the soul from Limbo.

I was all over that.

On May Day, the nuns instructed us to write private letters to the Blessed Virgin, our personal prayer requests, nothing to be held back. It was to be a solemn exercise. We were then assembled, as if awaiting the Rapture, at the rear of the parking lot behind the church in front of a tall granite statue of the Blessed Virgin. At the base of the statue was a large wire bin into which we tossed our prayers to Mary. Then, Sexton Quinn, on orders, lit the prayers on fire, and we all watched our words drift up to Heaven in the smoke. I could see them.

Still can.

Each year, I had the same prayer: that my mom and dad would live forever.

10

Forget-Me-Nots

In the spring on Brookdale Place, the forget-me-nots bloomed like a botanical garden, a sea of soothing pastels that kindle the memory. The Greeks called the flower Myosotis, translated "mouse's ear," an allusion to the shape of its leaf. Who could ever forget a patch of ensuring forget-me-nots, delicate five-lobed blue, pink, or white flowers with yellow centers? German folklore says the Almighty once overlooked the petite plant in naming all the other flowers. Legend suggests that one of the tiny lobes cried out, "Forget-me-not, Oh Lord." To which God replied, "That shall be your name."

Often in life, we remember the diminutive. Henry David Thoreau wrote of forget-me-nots, "It is the more beautiful for being small and unpretending; even flowers must be modest."

I grew up in a modest neighborhood where memories last forever. Forever is a long time, yet in a long-term memory, it's a place of persistent peace, a steadfast mooring when the swift high tides of life pull one to treacherous waters where memory implores the brain: forget me not.

It took forever in Rye for our stickball games to end on Brookdale Place. Used to drive my mother nuts, as she tried diligently to prepare dinner in two shifts for ten. Most of the time was taken up trying to find the errant ball in Phil Clancy's shrubs or Mr. Androtti's ivy, or secure another broom handle for a bat when we had exhausted our stash. I used to sneak broom handles out of the rectory at Resurrection Church, telling Bridie, the matronly Irish woman who cared for the priests, that I needed another broom to sweep the sidewalks for Monsignor McGowan.

Bridie was a tough Gaelic doyenne; it was difficult to discern her age from the deep crevices in her face and her youthful voice. She was always accommodating, but she intuitively knew that I was up to something, yet seemed to enjoy the repartee. After securing another boom, I always tried to do something helpful on my way out of the rectory, like putting a plate away in the kitchen or a glass back on another shelf, usually a spot where Bridie had just baked a stack of chocolate chip cookies.

"Anything else I can do for you?" I would ask with a handful of plunder in one palm, the prospective stickball bat in the other. "Yeah," she always replied, "stick that broom up your ass and sweep the floor!"

When Bridie's stock ran out, we looked to Jim O'Rourke, the guy from Killarney that looked two decades beyond his age; the priests had hired him to cut the lawn. Jim loved to drink, and usually began about 10 a.m., walking down to McGuire's Market, owned by Jerry's dad, for a morning Bud, while most in the store were looking for the cream. By noon, O'Rourke was usually sleeping it off in the janitor's room; so we'd sneak in and steal a broom. He lost a lot of brooms on the job.

But we never lost the bases on Brookdale Place. We didn't need to take them home at night. The field was the street, long and narrow like the fairways at St. Andrew's. First base was the birch tree on the curb lip in front of Pappy Langeloh's house; second base was the large, sweeping oak in front of Lou Kelly's home; and third base was the blunt edge of Ronnie Buckie's driveway. Home plate was chalked in the middle of the street, batter's box and all.

As often as we could, we'd have Hungarian-born Zena Kelly, Lou's trophy wife, throw out the first ball for special effects. She was Zsa Zsa Gabor incarnate to us kids. She had some big *casabas*, knew it, and always obliged us. Al Wilson frequently dropped the ball when handing it to her for the opening toss. I don't know if he was just nervous like Hermie in the *Summer of '42*, or he was just looking for Zena to pick it up. Al was no fool. Mom often watched from the kitchen window, her fixed position over time, as she gazed out, taking it all in, sorting out what it all meant or what she thought it to be, as she often talked to herself or to an imaginary friend. The conversations continued. Over the years, the neighborhood stickball players came and went, depending on age. If you could swing a bat and stood taller than a tricycle, you could play.

The regulars included my brothers Paul, Tim, and Andy, and my tomboy sister, Lauren, a pretty good hitter, also played from time to time. My sister Maureen, a "Hot Lips" Houlihan-type, frequently watched from the sidewalk, as did sisters Justine and Bernadette from their scooters.

Stickball, a variation of a Northeast inner city game invented in the 1750s, takes ample coordination, but if you hit the sweet spot of the broom handle, you could drive the pink Spalding high-bounce ball, the Spaldeen, almost to Monument Park in Yankee Stadium. The crowd always cheered as the ball lifted, like a Project Mercury rocket, above the canopy of trees—prompted by a din from deep inside the throat of the slugger, as he mimicked the roar of a standing ovation, pushing gusts of air up the esophagus, then instinctively limping into a Mickey Mantle trot, aping the weak knees of "The Mick," head cocked to the left for balance.

"Holy cow! Did you see that?" we mocked in our best Phil Rizzuto.

We commonly ran out of digits counting the scores. Games were often called on account of the bell, not a lost ball, weather, or darkness, but the bell.

We all lived by bells; I often felt like a cow. On the back porch at 25 Brookdale, Mom would ring a cowbell the size of a grapefruit with a long cord that my dad had hung from the porch ceiling. The knell was a summons for all the O'Briens, no exceptions, to head home. Game over!

Da-ding, Da-ding, Da-ding!

The clangor was a directive for the other kids to go home as well, a dictate from my mother that neighborhood parents relied on to gather their flocks. Brookdale Place was an extended family. Mom was the bell ringer, the arm of authority on a dead-end street with a tidal brook at the end that meandered to Long Island Sound. We never had to worry about speeding cars, other than some of the relatives after too many whiskey sours over the holidays. Brookdale parents watched out for every kid. We had group cookouts, block parties, and in the summer time, the neighborhood kids roamed freely through backyards playing flashlight tag or catching fireflies. Bernadette Burgess, who lived across the street, had the best swarm of fireflies.

There were few organized sports in those days; pickup was the rule: stickball, Wiffle ball, stoop ball, basketball, and of course, slow-motion tackle football in the fall and winter after Pappy Langeloh had cut down his corn stocks in the field next to us. The most fun was plowing through the snowdrifts of December on fourth down and short yardage, and giving the ball on a fullback drive to four-year-olds, bloated in their puffy snowsuits like the Pillsbury Doughboy.

With the largest family on the block, my folks ruled the neighborhood. There were a lot of big Irish families in Rye then. Birth control in the Catholic Church was anathema. Judging from the size of families in Rye the "rhythm method" of birth control was working about as well in New York as Casey Stengel's curve ball. Priests and nuns, presumably most of whom never had sex, instructed mothers of the parish to recognize the days of a fertile womb and avoid intercourse—a game plan gone with the wind after a few martinis. "I got rhythm," as the Gershwin song goes.

Then bango, bingo! The wives got pregnant again. My mother gave birth to ten children and had five miscarriages— fifteen pregnancies in all. I've always considered younger brothers, Gerard and Martin, who died in infancy, part of the family, and always will. The miscarriages will remain nameless until Heaven. Large Catholic families were *de rigueur* in the day. The Caseys had eight, the Cunninghams seven, and my godmother Eileen Clavin had sixteen. Everyone used to call her, with Mother Goose distinction, the Old Woman in the Shoe: ... *She had so many children. She didn't know what to do. She gave them some broth. Without any bread; Then whipped them all soundly, And put them to bed.*

Not really. We never got whipped at home, nor did Eileen's kids; she was an angel of a godmother. But the thought of a thumping kept us on the straight and narrow, and it was just a train ride away. My father worked in Manhattan in the old Pan Am building above Grand Central as director of pensions, a twenty-five-minute ride on the express New Haven line. When I or one of my brothers or sisters stepped out of line, my mom threatened to place the call, and "The Belt" would be on its way. Infractions ranged from mouthing off, to failing to do chores, to bad grades, or in Lauren's case, one of her virtuoso "drop-dead" looks. Lauren, third in the pecking order, had perfected a look of contempt with trademark Irish diplomacy—the ability to tell someone to go to hell, in a way that they looked forward to the trip. I was always impressed, but Mom was on to it.

"Wait 'til your father gets home, and you're going to get the belt!"

The threat alone was sobering.

My mom, a Donna Reed mirror image, was petite but she had the will, when necessary, to inflict one badass guilt trip. Her nickname in later years was "Boomer," a moniker passed down from brother-in-law Carl, a reference to a hard-hitting Minnesota Vikings tailback named Bill "Boom Boom" Brown with a reckless, almost violent running style. Like the late '60s All-Pro tailback, Mom could bowl us over, knock us right off our feet, with the largesse of her great intellect, wisdom, and ceaseless love—good and tough, always justified and in abundant measure.

I never actually saw the belt, but envisioned it laid out on my parents' bed, stiff like a corpse in a casket. The "belt" I dreaded was a ten-foot-long, four-foot-wide strip of rawhide with sharp nails poking up and a belt buckle the size of a suitcase. But worse than the belt was my mom looking me squarely in the eye, cutting deep to the back of the brain stem, and declaring, "I'm disappointed in you. I thought you could do better."

Please, I'd rather the belt. Just give me the belt. A few swings and it will be over. The sting of disappointment lingered. *Ouch!*

My relationship with my mother came full circle. Growing up as the oldest boy, early on I received a disproportionate amount of attention from my father. I adored my dad; he was my exemplar, but I always looked to my mother for inner strength. She knew my heart and the souls of all her children. But I strayed in time, and being the "free lunch" of the family, a Prodigal Son in some ways, I disappointed her, pushing the boundaries selfishly in sophomoric ways, defiant of my parents' munificence and limited resources. Mom and I didn't have much of a relationship for a time; then we found each other in Alzheimer's. End of life has a way of doing that.

She was big on confession. You always had to come clean with her. Confession as a youth was a ritual in our house. On Thursdays at church, you were directed to the confessional box, sort of a spiritual "time out," for a weekly unloading of a bolus of sins, often defined as missing the mark. We sat inside a dark cubicle with a dividing wire screen and a phantom, ghostly figure behind it that had all the redemption of death row. Three Hail Marys, an Our Father, and a Glory Be, and you'd be on your way, off sinning again, constantly reminded to tow the line. Praise the Lord, and pass the *Playboys!*

My parents, greatly influenced by the Bible, frequently read passages to us, particularly when trying to make a point on Christmas Eve, Easter, or when the spirit moved. They gave us all strong biblical or Irish names: my brother Paul for Saul of Tarsus; Timothy and Andrew for the apostles; Gregory after the writer pope, Gregory the Great, who took office in 590 AD, although I never lived up to the name; Bernadette for the miller's daughter, born in 1844 in Lourdes, France, who asserted to have seen the Virgin Mary in a cave grotto; and so on. Sometimes, Dad would let us vote on the names of new arrivals in the family, a majority of one vote; however, we did nix my dad's choice of the name Thaddeus, a disciple and close friend of the Apostle Jude, not to be confused with Judas. Like an oversized diaper, the name was too much for an infant. My mom and the voting siblings were all in agreement on this. There was no division.

Division generally is the rule in a large family, which has become a dinosaur of our culture, a Tyrannosaurus of tradition. Either by birth order, intent, or a shuffling of the deck, or just dumb luck, my parents divided the brood into "the older kids" and the "younger kids," a classification that would appall most child psychologists today, but one that sticks, with some of the siblings retaining their birth-order roles, as do others in Boomer families. The older kids, by my parents' declaration, were consecrated to be: Maureen, me, and Lauren; the younger kids: Justine, Paul, Bernadette, Timothy, and Andy, the baby. Ironically, the baby, now an EMC Corporation executive in Manhattan, is the big breadwinner, probably making threefold the rest of us, with the exception of brother Paul, also an EMC honcho.

The family expanded exponentially over time to the point that my folks in the summer had to rent two cottages off Thumpertown Beach Road in Eastham on the Outer Cape. A colleague at Pan Am had introduced my dad to the Cape when he was in his early 30s. The older kids were dispatched to the snug, yellow cabin, next to the gray mothership of a cottage where the younger kids were kept near my parents. Maureen, Lauren, and I will never forget the night, in the early '60s in the early morning hours, when someone tried to break in the back door next to our bedroom. Looking back, I suspect it was my dad, just trying to make sure we didn't become too independent from the family. No chance of that! We all relied on one another. Maureen, a nurse to be, was the second mother, "Mother Superior," as we called her; Lauren took no prisoners in family disparities. I was initially relegated to lawn duties with a manual push mower, trimming the front hedge with sheers, and snow shoveling the driveway. The younger kids stepped up as we stepped away, in some instances, doing a far better job.

When I stepped away to pursue the low fruit of the world, no one seemed to notice.

My parents, for the most part, were exceedingly close, fully romantic in the early years, but with the heaviness of life, they became more distant, then intimate again in the final days. They were like blueberry bushes that seem to grow better in pairs. My parents were typically competitive, too, and instilled stiff competition among us, a rule of family law that kept us lean, mean, and hungry for our grades in school, and always competing for the cleanliness of the four-floor, six-bedroom stucco home we occupied. We all had Friday cleaning chores, from the finished basement to the attic. And when it came to our "marks" in school, my folks were cutthroat, particularly with the older kids. In grammar school, if we brought home a ninety percent over-all academic average on a report card, it simply wasn't enough.

"You can do better," Dad would say, holding out the prize of his affection for the highest grades.

And so we were pushed to bring home ninety-eights and ninety-nines, which we did, and then moved on to private Catholic high schools, most of us, where we studied logic, philosophy, and learned to translate from Latin Cicero's letters and Virgil's *Aeneid*, sometimes with the help of a black-market translator called a Trot.

The CliffsNotes of our family life read like Frank Capra's *It's a Wonderful Life*. My dad was indeed George Bailey; my mom in the role of Mary Hatch. In Rye, we had our various Uncle Billys, Ernie Bishops, and Bert the cop, even an Aunt Bee and Roger the Dellwood milkman, who delivered three times a week twelve to fourteen glass bottles of milk to our house and stacked them in our refrigerator. And we were surrounded by guardian angels; Clarence Odbody, I swear, lived down the street.

⚹

My mother was a living angel; she loved the primary color yellow. Yellow angel rays, we were taught, represent the enlightenment that the Lord's wisdom brings to the soul. Social in every respect, my mother attended all the gatherings of the day. She met my father at a college dance in New Rochelle. He was a Fordham University student at the time and a Naval officer candidate. Dad was the rudder of the family; Mom was the main-sail, and stood out among the Greatest Generation of women of her day—wives and mothers who helped shape and define their spouses and children in diverse ways, both in what they were in life and are today in memories. These women gave selflessly in child-rearing years, then later as caregivers for their war-hero husbands, never receiving a medal for it.

And in the end, the Greatest Generation of men, independent conquerors of world evil, clung to their spouses in old age; survivors still do. This generation of women has never received the accolades it deserves.

My dad needed mollycoddling. Losing his parents to tuberculosis as a young boy, he never fully recovered from the loss. An athlete, thinker, a man of letters, and a Roosevelt Democrat, my father found comfort in excelling beyond his means with a Gaelic will to succeed and sustain his passions. He was once asked at a Fordham University oral theology exam, seated before a table of schooled clerics in the shadows of high Gothic walls that seemed to reach to the Heavens, to prove there was a God. He answered with great clarity, faith, and Jesuit logic, pointing to the world around him. And today, he has the irrefutable evidence.

Holding court with us one day on the beach, he reflected on the imperfections of life, likely quoting another academic. "Life is like a river," he intoned, "You need to study it as it goes by, then decide the right time to put your feet in the water." Dad was a man who got right to the point. He once told one of my brothers: "Don't get me wrong, Greg's a nice guy, but he's like medicine; you have to take him in small doses." Yet Dad was loving, like my mom, in what one might call marital photosynthesis: they emitted love and life to each other.

Still they were strict, always pursuing the narrow road. At times, they lost their way; as years passed, my mom, given her Alzheimer's, more so than my dad. We began to notice over the years wholesale lapses in memory and continued engagement in conversations with people and objects that weren't real. At first, we ignored it: phones left off the hook because she couldn't figure out how to end a call; wearing shoes that didn't match; those distant, vacant stares; and, at times, an out-of-body persona, a mix of aberrant rage and adolescent fancy. Still, the distractions of a large family, all the school, sporting, and church events camouflaged her illness, as well as the routine of teaching duties at parochial Most Holy Trinity in nearby Mamaroneck and St. Gregory the Great in Harrison.

In time, the symptoms worsened, more so after my parents retired to the Outer Cape in 1998, a place of further isolation in winter, a precursor to Pluto, a venue where she went from clothes shopping at Bergdorf Goodman in Manhattan to Brown's Superette for baloney in Eastham.

Mom departed from Rye reluctantly, following my dad as she had done instinctively from the day they met. She brought with her a quilt of long-term memories to last a lifetime that was now measured in short years, not decades.

I couldn't imagine until now the isolation she must have felt. Mom left a dead-end street for a dead end in her life. As peaceful and bucolic as the Cape was, the lights were growing dimmer.

Da-ding, Da-ding, Da-ding!

Bye-bye, Miss American Pie, on to a dead-end street. Forget me not.

11

Dead-End Street

Cestaro Way in North Eastham is hardly a proper name and easy to remember for a narrow lane on Cape Cod, lined with dense patches of scrub oak and scrub pine on the fringe of the Cape Cod National Seashore, about two miles from the frothing Atlantic. It's a dead-end choice, on a dead-end street. But developer Arty Cestaro wouldn't have it any other way after he bulldozed a swath of sandy forest off School House Road in the late 1960s, sold my parents two lots for a summer house, then dug a drinking well down "sixty tree" feet.

A burly, stubby Italian with a touch of Genoa in his voice, Arty was a man for all seasons on Cape Cod, all three of them. Spring arrives for a day in June.

Since the Pilgrims first arrived in these parts, year-round survival on this narrow land has required a range of cunning and skill. Depending on the time of year, Arty—who sported a face of peppered stub—cleared lots, built homes, fished for bass and blues, and baked a cloistered family recipe of thick lasagna and crusty Italian bread to sell to the tourists—all under the banner of Cestaro.

So, why not Cestaro Way?

The street was a mirror image of Arty, as it was for my family: course, bumpy, potholed, with thin strands of oak attempting to reclaim the road. It was perfect in an old Cape Cod way, just perfect.

Ours was the first house built on Cestaro Way. It was a two-bedroom cottage with an unfinished attic that served as a sleeping porch for most of the kids; we camped out on molded mattresses or in sleeping bags, some with a slight hint of urine, depending on a Friday night out. The attic had a natural alarm system for wake-up calls. On hot summer days, the sun baked the framing beams and sandy plywood floors to the point of driving a deep sweat. My dad had the house built as a family retreat and for retirement. Mom, abidingly along for the ride, enjoyed the view on Cestaro, particularly from the back deck that overlooked the dense scrub pines—a place, she often said, where she could lose herself. And ultimately did.

After a decade of summers renting a nearby Thumpertown Beach cottage complex, having a place now to call home on the Cape was like pouring Super Glue over the family. We all stuck together—sand, gravel, pine needles, sweat, and all. Mom and the siblings stayed for the summer, as was the custom for summer people, and Dad flew up weekends between vacation times. My parents were immensely proud of their Cestaro Way anchor, testament to family values they wanted to share: *Mi casa es su casa!* My father covertly, yet with benevolence, hid a spare key on a rusted nail under the back porch, then proceeded to tell Arty Cestaro, the North Eastham postmaster, everyone at Betty's Beach Box and Brown's Superette, vagrants at the laundromat, all those in line for coffee at Fleming's Donut Shack, the fishermen at Goose Hummock in Orleans, and just about everybody he met on the Cape, Manhattan, Westchester County, and all along the way. Thank God Al Gore hadn't invented the Internet yet.

Trust was a maxim of the day. Life on the Outer Cape in the '50s, '60s, and early '70s was simple and quiet, like my mother, in a Norman Rockwell way. Creation of the Cape Cod National Seashore, signed into legislation in 1961 by John F. Kennedy, who summered in Hyannisport, saw to it that some of Henry David Thoreau's pristine vistas, 43,500 acres in all, remained undisturbed. The Cape was uncomplicated then. When Jack Kennedy, for example, stopped receiving his weekly edition of *The Cape Codder* delivered to the White House, the president phoned his good friend, Malcolm Hobbs, the paper's publisher, to inquire about his favorite local read.

"Let me check on that, Jack," Malcolm said from the newsroom.

There was a pause on the phone, while Malcolm made his way back to the subscription office.

"Hey, Jack," Malcolm replied minutes later, "your subscription has run out! Send a check, and we'll send you the paper."

Kennedy laughed, fully relishing the moment amidst world convolutions. A check was dispatched, and Kennedy never missed an issue of *The Cape Codder* again.

That simple, that direct, an exchange that wholly defined the Cape decades ago, a far different place than today. The beaches were wider, ample room for the wooden playpens, sticky from apple juice, that the fathers of large families schlepped down a steep flight of wooden steps from the top of the bluff. Surfers and surf casters on the beach were as plentiful as shorebirds; beach bonfires were the proxy of a summer night on the town. We bathed with soap and shampoo in clear freshwater kettle ponds where you could see bottom fifty feet from shore; and on Saturdays just before sunset, we all raced to the sea to watch a squadron of Navy planes from Otis Air Force Base line up in a mock carpet-bombing mission to drop live, pulsating ammunition on the "Target Ship," the 417-foot U.S.S. *James Longstreet,* a decommissioned World War II Liberty Ship named after a Confederate general. It had been towed to a site in Cape Cod Bay a few miles offshore. The final run of the night was greeted with applause up and down the beach, as if Ted Williams had just hit another dinger. The *Longstreet,* rusted to submission, now lies in a shallow grave below the surface.

My mother felt safe in Eastham. We all did. The place felt to her like Rye in the '60s. There wasn't much crime on the Outer Cape: a few fisticuffs here and there and a botched drug drop or two. Nearby, Wellfleet and Truro police cruisers in those days often marked time by playing tag with spotlights in the woods; a Wellfleet police officer once had to pedal his bike to work after receiving a DWI; selectmen fought in bars after disagreeing over town business; and the kindly Wellfleet watchman, always willing to offer a helping hand, once unwittingly assisted drug smugglers unloading bulky burlap bags of marijuana off a sailboat, named *Mischief*, moored in the harbor to a waiting truck in the parking lot for flight off-Cape. When the watchman finally discerned the nature of the cargo, he called the Wellfleet police, who came screaming down to the harbor with sirens on full alert from miles away to avoid a possible gunfight. The smugglers fled; nothing was ever found, other than an embarrassed watchman. I covered the scene as a cub reporter for *The Cape Codder*. Alec Wilkinson—a gifted writer for *The New Yorker*, a successful author, and a Wellfleet summer cop in his youth—chronicled the antics, and more, in a remarkable book: *Midnights: A Year with the Wellfleet Police.*

The Outer Cape, over the years, has always attracted its share of eccentrics, and square foot by square foot, some of the finest intellectual, artistic, and writing talent in the world, who shaped the culture of a generation. Among them, writers like Eugene O'Neill, Tennessee Williams, Sinclair Lewis, Norman Mailer, Mary Oliver, Poet Laureate Stanley Kunitz, Arthur Schlesinger, Jr., Annie Dillard, and Marge Piercy, to name a few, along with some of the most notable artists and therapists of the last century, not to mention the sweet oysters here. It's still said that you can't find a shrink in Manhattan in August because they are all vacationing on the Cape.

Hidden deep in the Wellfleet-Truro woods, not far from the Great Outer Beach, is one of Cape Cod's best kept secrets— remnants of a summer colony that once housed some of these gifted architects, diplomats, and critical thinkers from the 1930s. These homes on stilts—designed by the brightest and most inventive modernist architects in Europe and America—were functional, yet radical; sort of floating boxes, oriented to capture views and breezes, perching lightly on the land with flat roofs that often rise to gradual pitches. The buildings are as significant to the region's built environment as any antique Cape or saltbox, all part of the allure of isolation in the Outer Cape woods, a place of intense privacy for creative inspiration and low-impact buildings that were "green" long before there was such an environmental color.

And then there was intriguing Charles Flato, a hunch-backed intellectual writer who had suffered from polio as a child, worked later as an investigator reporter for the civil liberties subcommittee of the Senate Labor Committee, served under Nelson Rockefeller in the Latin American division of the Board of Economic Warfare during World War II, lived in retirement in the Wellfleet woods, and oh, yes, was a Russian spy. Flato was outed when KGB files were opened to researchers after the Soviet Union collapsed. His codename in the Gorsky memo, written by Anatoly Gorsky, then chief of Soviet intelligence, was "Bob" and in another Verona transcript, cryptanalysis of Soviet intelligence dispatches, Flato is believed to have the codename of "Char."

I thought of him as Charlie, and he was always willing to talk. He was a good local source in my early reporting days. My mother liked him as well. Charlie and I shared a plantation of coffee beans over the years on his back deck. I just thought he was a guy with a brain and a cane.

"I couldn't think of a better place to get lost," Charlie once told me.

The isolation, stark natural beauty, and anonymity of the Outer Cape drew many—the famous, infamous, and regular people, like my folks—to dead-end streets, and held them captive here.

The early retirement days for my parents were blissful, but the isolation finally resonated with my mother about three weeks into her first winter here, as the reality of year-round residency on this patch of sand, jutting sixty miles into the tempestuous North Atlantic, settled in with the starkness of a whiteout in a coastal storm, a place where the major highway, Route 6, resembled a walking trail in February. It never snows on the Cape, the locals promote, and you can play golf here year-round. But grab the Dramamine and check the map. "The bared and bended arm of Cape Cod," Thoreau wrote, is where "a man can stand there and put all of America behind him." The remoteness in winter on the Outer Cape, while inspiring and cerebral, is no place for someone who is losing their place. My mother never got the memo.

Neither did the Pilgrims, who never "landed" in Plymouth in the strict definition of the term. They anchored instead off Provincetown on the Cape's tip on November 11, 1620, where William Bradford, the first Plymouth Colony governor, Myles Standish, and thirty-nine other passengers commissioned the Mayflower Compact, the first governing document in the New World. They then explored the back shore from Truro to Eastham before moving on to Plymouth Harbor for greater shelter. Plymouth Rock is merely an invention of the Chamber of Commerce. In fact, there is no official reference to the Pilgrims landing on a rock at Plymouth; it is not mentioned in Edward Winslow's eminent *Mourt's Relation*, written in 1622, nor in Bradford's historic journal *Of Plymouth Plantation*, published twenty years later. The first recorded reference to the Pilgrims landing on a rock in Plymouth, in fact, came 121 years later.

What is an undeniable fact of history, however, is that my mother's favorite Eastham beach, First Encounter on Cape Cod Bay, is where Pilgrims first encountered Native Americans in the New World in a hostile introduction. Arrows flew, shots were fired, and all safely scattered. Historians speculate that the Native Americans might have been responding to the starving Pilgrims' discovery a month earlier in Truro of a lifesaving cache of buried corn.

"And sure it was God's good providence that we found this corn for else we know not how we should have done," Bradford wrote in his journal.

My mother loved First Encounter, a place of retreat, a refuge to gather her thoughts or watch a blazing red sun at dusk dip into the bay to be extinguished like a candle. She equally savored Coast Guard Beach in Eastham, my favorite ocean retreat—site of the old Life Saving Station whose courageous crews patrolled the stormy shoreline in the 1800s in search of shipwrecked sailors. Since the wreck of the *Sparrow-Hawk* in 1626, more than 3,000 ships have run aground in the treacherous shoals of the Great Outer Beach. The

Pilgrims were a near miss here. On November 9, 1620, the *Mayflower*, sixty-five days out from Plymouth, England, made landfall off Coast Guard Beach, caught on the shifting shoals. Far off course from its intended destination of what is now Northern Virginia, a miraculous change in wind freed the *Mayflower* to sail north to Provincetown.

History abounds off Coast Guard Beach.

At my mother's bearing, during the spring, summer, and fall of the early '70s, often after an ocean storm, I walked south along Coast Guard Beach about two miles to a snug, wind-blown twenty-one-by-sixteen, two-room beach shack with a frugal wooden writing desk overlooking the surf. It was called the "Outermost House" venerated in the classic Henry Beston nature book of that name, chronicling a lone year on the Great Outer Beach. A Harvard-educated writer and naturalist, Beston built the cottage in 1925 mostly from scrap driftwood, dubbing it the "Fo'castle," given its ten windows and commanding presence atop a high dune overlooking the open Atlantic that offered the sense of being aboard a ship. In 1964, the cottage was preserved as a national literary landmark "wherein he [Beston] sought the great truth and found it in the nature of man." My mother, after reading the *Outermost House*, first took me there. I was possessed, and returned alone often to peer inside at the crude, wooden writing desk, and to sit on the outside porch and contemplate the isolated nature around me. It was here that I decided to pursue a life of writing. My mom, as she had many times before and would again, led me to a solitary place in life.

You can hear the sound of the sea in Beston's writing. "Listen to the surf. Really lend it your ears, and you will hear in it a world of sounds: hollow boomings and heavy roarings, great watery tumblings and tramplings, long hissing seethes, sharp rifle-shot reports, splashes, whispers, the grinding undertone of stones, and sometimes vocal sounds that might be the half-heard talk of people in the sea," he penned.

Like my mother, I felt at peace here, a calm shattered by the Great Storm of February 1978 with sustained winds of close to 100 miles an hour and an overwash of nearly fifteen feet that swept the Fo'castle out to sea. The loss was devastating, but a fitting burial for a place that had brought us closer together.

Our relationship wasn't always that way. I was close to my mother growing up, but distant over time. She clearly saw a lot of my father in me, and often channeled her angst toward him through me, more as years progressed; then it turned to rage. Perhaps she felt comfortable directing it at me. In some ways, I was the embodiment of my father: male, selfish, and clueless. I was an easy mark.

By the 1990s, there had been a tidal surge in our relationship, as my mom's shifting moods were vented more and more in my direction. Looking back, I know now that she was reaching out in fear and anger over what was happening to her, and yet I was pulling away, never grasping the moment.

"I'm your mother!" she would scream at me repeatedly, as if to convince herself. I thought at the time she was pulling rank, but she was just seeking reinforcement. I never saw it coming. We had chilling moments of conflicts, both of us pushing back at one another with the force of a wave crashing a sturdy bluff. Neither of us moved.

My fortieth birthday was a ceasefire, a surprise for which everyone dressed as a person of history. My mom came as Rose Kennedy, attired in a dark wig with all the graciousness of a Kennedy; it was an appropriate rendering, given their collective love and respect for family. Wrote Kennedy in her 1974 autobiography, *Times to Remember*: "I looked on child rearing not only as a work of love and a duty, but as a profession that was fully as interesting and challenging as any honorable profession in the world, and one that demanded the best I could bring to it." My dad, in contrast, came as Panama's Manuel Noriega, the Latin strongman accused of drug trafficking, racketeering, and money laundering. Dad had filled condoms with sugar looking like hanging bags of cocaine tied to the buttons of his shirt. It was an unforgettable night of family and friends laughing, drinking, and dancing. It was one of the last times that I remember my mother fully articulate and bountifully engaged. She wrote candidly in a birthday scrapbook of recollections, a testament that defined our relationship:

I remember when Greg in the Third Grade served his first Sunday Mass as an altar boy. He was with a more experienced altar boy, and somehow got confused and ended up on the side of the altar with the bells. In those days, bells were a big thing at Mass. Greg was terrified. At the time of the consecration of the host, no bells rang. Greg froze! The other altar boy kept telling Greg to ring the bells. Still no bells. Repeating this several times had little effect, except Greg did pick up the bells; he just couldn't ring them. He froze again. No bells. Finally, the exacerbated priest, host in hand, turned and yelled at Greg, "Ring the God damn bells!" At that point, Greg started ringing like St. Patrick's Cathedral, and didn't stop until the priest turned around once more and said, "Greg, stop the bells!" The nuns were all laughing, the congregation was laughing. I was crying.

We had each other's back; we just didn't know it at the time. Mom reminded me that night of the time I was asked to read a scripture verse at my brother Paul's wedding. Typically, I lost my place in the reading, but instead of panicking, I relied on my altar boy training and earlier counsel from her to ad lib when your back is against the wall. So, I *ad libitum* the balance of the passage—tossing in a few "thou(s)" and some fire and brimstone. No one caught on, but my mom. When I returned to the pew, she patted me on the knee and said, "Nice work: Matthew, Mark, Luke, and John would be some proud!"

Ad lib was to become a cornerstone in our lives; in the months and years to come, it would become more apparent, as I began experiencing similar moments of confusion, recurrent memory loss, trouble at times finding the right words, problems with balance and problem solving, and a pendulum of emotions that I couldn't manage.

We talked about it; the symptoms wouldn't wane for either of us. Following my mother's example, I just ignored the signs, focusing instead on work, my spouse, children, and friends—a focus, however, that fades as the disease evolves and one is wedged in isolation.

As a caregiver for my mother and breadwinner of the family, I found it difficult to ask for help. My role had been on the giving, not receiving, end, and to reverse roles was an admission of failure. I preferred, like my mother, to keep to familiar patterns of behavior, the routine, rather than concede the awful changes in play. I was trying desperately to hold on to who I was for as long as possible, knowing the disease ultimately would rob that from me. We were both feeling terrible isolation. My mother had only two good friends on the Cape, my father notwithstanding—Tom and Mary Collins, an affable retired couple, who lived directly across the street on Cestaro Way. Mom spent much time with them. They didn't seem to mind her quirkiness. They met for lunch, for talk, for end of the day cocktails on occasion. One afternoon about ten years ago in early fall, Tom came over to the house to chat with my mom. My dad had gone for the New York papers. Tom and my mother talked about family, politics, sports, and anything else you could squeeze into a half-hour visit. When the conversation ended, he turned to my mother as he walked out the door.

"You know, Ginny, I've lived a good, full life," he observed. "As far as I'm concerned, if the Lord wants to take me, He can have me any time He wants!"

Tom gently hugged my mom. She waved to him as he walked across Cestaro in his characteristic enthusiastic gait. He opened his front door, stepped across the threshold, then dropped dead instantly. Bang. Massive heart attack. The Lord often takes us at our word.

Mom was devastated. She was never the same. She let go a bit that day. Within a few months, Mary had moved back to Connecticut, and Mom was alone again. I noticed a softening in our relationship. Beyond my father, absorbed in his own medical issues, she now had no friends on the Cape, and thus turned to me, emotionally and for chores around the house, as she faced down her demons.

I always had thought of myself as Mr. Green Jeans, the genial sidekick to Captain Kangaroo. Mr. Green Jeans always performed ably with hand puppets, talked to Grandfather Clock, introduced live animals, taught little children to care for the Earth, but he couldn't fix squat. Neither could I. Accepting of this, my mom kept it simple, just asking me in late spring to install the bulky window air conditioner in the living room, replace screens with storm windows in the fall, paint the outside trim, clean the gutters, and wrap the hoses for storage. I think she just wanted me around the house to talk. She was lonely, and when she wasn't talking, she just stared out of the window. Blank stares, as if she were on Pluto.

On a late Sunday afternoon in October 2000, I finally started to get it. Mom asked me to take her to the bank; I wasn't sure why. She said she needed to use the ATM. A banker earlier in life and one who had used a cash card often, she told me she was having difficulty with the machine. She couldn't figure out how to use it; tried several times. She was completely out of sorts.

"Greg, I'm scared," she told me in the bank parking lot. "I can't do this anymore. I get confused all the time. I need someone to talk to. Will you help me? Please don't tell your father!"

I will never forget that day. The sky was gray, the wind was blowing on shore, and there was a penetrating chill in the air.

"Sure, Mom," I said, beginning to realize her inner fear of losing control. "We're good now. We're just good, Mom."

I never looked back on the relationship, my anger over her rants at me; I only looked forward now. I was Mr. Green Jeans, wholly useless, yet destined to be a caregiver. Hand me the Phillips screwdriver! Just tell me which end is up.

Confusion in time gave way to chaos. Mom began putting garbage in the trunk of the car—forgetting to take it to the dump, opting to horde. The maggots and stench were revolting, yet my siblings and I were reticent to deal head-on with it. Mom began hiding money in the house from my father, wads of it; she slept in her clothes; made up words for lack of recall; often refused to shower; and grabbed for liquid soap at times to brush her teeth. Then there were the "menu issues." Dad in his wheelchair would ask for ice cream for dessert, and she'd serve him eggs, sunny-side up. The behavior upset me and equally distressed my father, who observed it nightly. At first, we collectively passed it off as a change-of-life transition, but the shift intensified.

After all the anguish in our relationship, my mother and I were on parallel tracks. She was years ahead of me, but I could see her in the distance, not sure where she was headed. Yet, I followed. Then one day, my ticket to Pluto arrived by way of a blissful bicycle ride from Brewster. On a postcard-perfect day, I had taken my son Conor and his friend, Ryan White, both about twelve at the time, on a trek along the Cape Cod Rail Trail to Eastham, about a fifteen-mile ride, to visit my mother—a pastoral passage beside sparkling cranberry bogs, lush meadows, saltwater marshes, and fresh water ponds. In all ways, it was a cleansing, majestic Cape Cod day. Mom, however, was more muddled than usual. With the temperature inching toward eighty, she scolded all of us for not wearing winter coats. To take the "chill" off, she insisted the boys don these heavy, oversized sweatshirts from a spare bedroom closet, largesse from winters past. They balked at first, but sensing her resolve, I instructed them to oblige.

"Mom's right," I summoned. "It's cold out."

Conor, having witnessed corresponding episodes in the past, concurred, and Ryan graciously consented. The second we peddled out of the driveway, turning left on Cestaro Way toward the bike trail, the boys ripped off the sweatshirts and tossed them at me.

"No way, we're not wearing these things!" Conor declared.

I thanked the boys for being good sports, and draped the heavy sweatshirts across the handlebars of my bike as we headed back to

Brewster, taking in a panorama of primal nature. I was euphoric, in the Zen, incredibly at peace. I felt like a kid again, and plied the trail in full speed far ahead of Conor and Ryan. Faster, faster! The wind was soothing. In the moment, I recalled that, as a youth, I had prided myself on riding a red, three-speed Schwinn racer, no handed! And like a child, I wasn't wearing a helmet that day. For thirty seconds, I peddled back in time, a kaleidoscope of images from youth: Rye Beach, the ball field at Disbrow Park, town marina, and out to the American Yacht Club where you could see the Manhattan skyline and Twin Towers in the distance. Then, as abrupt as a clap of thunder, the imagery shifted. I sensed something awry. In horrifying slow motion, what seemed like frame-by-frame, I witnessed the sweatshirts on the handlebars slip slowly into the spokes. My bike, at full gallop, stopped on a dime, and I was hurled headfirst over the handlebars fifteen feet into the air, but with the presence of mind at least to shield my left hand over my forehead before impact. I hit the tarmac with the force, it seemed, of a .45 caliber bullet, the impact cutting deep into my knuckles right through to the bone. On the second bounce, my face hit the pavement in a pool of blood. I was numb, out of body, yet felt something cold pouring down my face.

As I finally stood up, I must have looked like the lead role in a Bela Lugosi movie; in pure fright, Conor and Ryan sprinted off into the woods. Two Samaritans sitting on a nearby back deck came to my aid, and collected the kids. The rest is fleeting; a half hour later I was rushed to Cape Cod Hospital in an ambulance, sirens ablaze. After multiple stitches to the head and left hand, I was discharged.

Little did I know that I had unleashed a monster.

12

Passing the Baton

The legendary track star Jesse Owens faced a monster. In the summer of 1936, just years before the start of World War II, demon Adolf Hitler and his Nazi faithful were goose-stepping across Eastern Europe. At the Berlin Olympics, Hitler sought to showcase purported Aryan superiority and chastised the U.S. for engaging gifted African-Americans, whom he termed "sub-humans," to compete against his Aryan Nation. Owens stared the demons down, winning four gold medals: 100 meters, 200 meters, long jump, and 4x100 meter relay, the final affront to Hitler, making Owens the most decorated athlete of the 1936 Olympics. Owens ran the first leg of the relay in a record 39.8 seconds, picking up a two-meter lead, and resolutely passing the baton to Ralph Metcalfe, an African-American who was the fastest human from 1932 to 1934, and later served in the U.S. Congress. A purposeful passing, at this critical moment in time, propelled Metcalfe to a four-meter lead, the measure of success. Foy Draper, who ran the third leg, maintained the lead, and 100-meter world record holder Frank Wykoff, with baton firmly in stride, lengthened the winning margin to fifteen meters, beating his Italian counterpart, Tullio Gonnelli.

An efficacious passing of the baton in a relay race is as elemental as lacing up a pair of running shoes, and has relevance in the race against Alzheimer's. Timing is critical. When a runner hits a mark on the track, usually a small triangle, the awaiting runner—on cue and face forward—opens a backward hand, and after a few strides, the lead runner has caught up and exchanges the baton. Often, the lead runner will shout "*stick!*" several times as a signal for the awaiting runner, glancing behind, to put out a hand. Passing the baton has significance on many fronts—on a track, at home, at work, in disease, and into eternity. In the relay race of life, one can't run alone. You sprint your leg as best as possible, then hand off with precision, letting others carry you as they can. Looking back, I realize now that my mother, in trying to outrun Alzheimer's, was yelling at me, "*Stick ... stick ... stick!*"

You can see eternity from Eastham and elsewhere. Ever look between two facing mirrors, at home, in a barbershop or a beauty salon? You face a seemingly endless line of images fading into the distance. In principle, it's called "looking into infinity." Each mirror reflects the image into the other mirror, bouncing these reflections back and forth into infinity—gateways, some speculate, to parallel universes. If you squint, you might see Pluto and beyond.

My mom was a mirror, preparing me as only a mother could to see through her lens into infinity and pass the baton. The day after I was released from Cape Cod Hospital after the bike accident, she arrived early in the morning at my house in Brewster with bandages and rubbing alcohol in hand. In her altered state, she was rushing over to stop the bleeding. I was covered in hospital bandages with more than twenty stitches to the face and hands, all washed up, and yet, she insisted on cleaning the wounds. Her signals were confused. She was still my mother, knew it, and proceeded to clean the bandages with rubbing alcohol. I let her, realizing she was living in the moment, and at that moment, so was I. She was my mother, even in her Alzheimer's, and I desperately wanted to be her son.

I hope my children, as this disease progresses, will allow me to be their father. It is vital for those with Alzheimer's to connect with the past, the long-term memories and relationships. The short-term is a flash.

Parallel universes between my mother and me collided after my accident. We were over the handlebars, and together could see into infinity.

But one must squint to see into infinity, stretching the mind. The word, with mathematical definition, has derivation in the Latin word *infinitas,* meaning "unbounded," a noun with roots in the ancient Greek word *apeiros*, which translates to endless. In my mother's final years, I had endless conversations with her, including regular Sunday night *tête-à-têtes* at the dinner table with my folks in Eastham beside a large picture window overlooking a patch of scrub oak and pine, bent from winter winds into forms that stretch the imagination. The curved oak table with sturdy legs and high-back Queen Anne chairs forced one to sit upright. Bought at a discount home improvement center, it still had the emotive feel of a medieval round table, not because it resembled an antique, but because a Prodigal Son now had occasion for final wisdom from his parents. I cherish those moments, some of them painful, all of them imbedded in my soul.

Dad, as usual, drove the conversation with pounding, penetrating queries, challenging me on politics, sports, religion, sibling rivalries, and just about any other subject one is not supposed to talk about in public. Mom was quick, as she could, on rebuttal. It kept her mind challenged and active. She deflected my dad's barbs like a veteran hockey goalie, which were meant more to make her think than overreact.

My cerebral training early on was served up in Rye at the family dinner table, a relic today. All of us were seated on Brookdale Place on Sundays around that thick plank of mahogany. We were akin to knights in shining armor; only our swords were stainless steel, barely sharp enough to cut the overcooked beef, and our breastplates were paper napkins slung from the collar. Still, we were a force. My folks would query us, like a pop quiz, about our lives, our friends, attitudes, beliefs, and trouble on the horizon, just to get inside our pointy little heads. I thought of the exercise, at the time, as a holy inquest, but as I grew older, I enjoyed the banter. It brought us all together. But there were exceptions. Like the time when my older sister Maureen called me out in high school, lobbed a grenade under the table, for my dating on the sly a well-endowed, exceptionally attractive coed several years older than I was.

"So, Greg, why don't you tell us about it?" said Maureen, the self-appointed "Mother Superior" of the family.

Dad dropped his fork. Mom glowered at me. And I stared intently at Maureen in an attempt to burn her retinas, but they were blocks of ice.

"So, what's this all about?" Dad asked.

The sizzling meatloaf before me that I had so coveted had all the appeal now of a pair of worn sneakers after a sweaty basketball drill.

"Oh," I said lamely, "We just went to the movies together. I think it was the *Ten Commandments*."

"Yeah," Maureen interjected between mouthfuls of mashed potatoes, "Thou shalt not sin!"

"That's enough," Dad declared, shutting down the discourse. I wasn't sure if he was disgusted or proud of me.

Mom nodded in a way that said firmly: *Greg, you can do better.*

The look alone served to bring me up short, but those words have become a mantra throughout my life. I still envision my mother urging me on. In the moment, the exchange that day was discomforting, yet enlightening. Looking back, such wordplay reinforces the family dinner table as a forum for in-your-face instruction, edification, and for unforgettable family bonding.

Such illumination continued decades later at the more intimate dinner table on the Cape. Observing my mom's frontal assault on

Alzheimer's, the wisdom was abundantly enriching. Perspective has a way of cutting through a disease. Every Sunday at twilight after leaving Willy's Gym in Orleans, I drove alone to Eastham for introspection with my parents. The drive was a timeline of sorts, passing Town Cove to the starboard where schooners once delivered their consignment from the Old World; Salt Pond, a brackish estuary, rich with shellfish, that empties into the Atlantic; Evergreen Cemetery, where the markers date back to the time of the Pilgrims, and where my parents eventually would rest; and across from the cemetery, Arnold's Lobster and Clam Bar, a family favorite where the sweet, salty aroma of fresh seafood off the dock wafts across the tombstones. Arnold's, formerly Betty's Beach Box, is run by a childhood friend and Pilgrim descendent, Nate Nickerson, a.k.a. Nathan Atwood Nickerson III, whose *Mayflower* forbearers settled the Cape. Arnold's was my mother's favorite eating hole; she always enjoyed talking with Nicky. Since birth, he has known the difference between a steamer and a quahog, and probably could pronounce the word *in utero.*

Such distinction was lost in time on my mother. A quahog, to her, could have been a kitchen utensil—a knife or something sharp to stick into an electrical socket, as she often tried. We had to hide the knives. One day, she noticed the kitchen paper towel rack was empty; staring at the exposed cardboard tube, she knew it should be covered with something white, so she laid pieces of bread over the tube as if hanging out clothes to dry. The slide continued with both parents. The dinner table reinforced their decline. At times, my mother served my dad coffee grinds on toast. He never let on in front of me, nor did he want to embrace the stony reality. That bothered me and my siblings terribly. In retrospect, I believe he was trying to protect my mother from reality, as he began his own fearful, slow slide into dementia himself, complicated by the throes of circulation disease and prostate cancer. It was a shit show.

At first, none of us saw the warning signs of Alzheimer's. We were all numb to it: my mother's memory loss, challenges in planning and with problem solving, difficulty completing familiar tasks, confusion with time and place, trouble understanding visual images, problems finding the right words, inability to retrace steps, poor judgment, withdrawal, swings in mood and personality, and finally, intense rage.

In the fall of 2007, reality was sinking in. At the dinner table, my parents and I talked more intensely about family, politics, and life; we talked about religion, eschatology, about God, a genderless definition of all-love, and about facing the Almighty one day. I told them several times that something wasn't right in my head. Dad dismissed it, but Mom always tried to instill courage in me.

"You must have courage," she counseled. "Never give in!"

In the final months, our dinner table discussions centered around topics we had never entertained before. End-of-life stuff. My father, now in a wheelchair with little use of his legs, waxed on about the genius of Roosevelt Democrats, the need to care for the disadvantaged, the moral obligation to pursue a passion in life that made the world just a bit better, and he probed knotty questions about what happens to you when you die. A rock-ribbed Catholic who had lost both his parents in childhood, he feared death, and like many of us, wasn't quite sure of what awaited him on the other side. He was deathly afraid.

Mom seemed to embrace it.

Many years ago, I had a dream about death, one of what was to be several. In the dream, my father had passed away. He was in Heaven. No longer confined to a wheelchair, he was sprinting like a high school tailback, with jet-black hair combed straight back. I told my parents about it over the dinner table on September 16, 2007. I remember the day.

"Was I running to Mom?" Dad asked.

"No," I said. "You were running to your parents." He paused.

"Was Mom there?" he asked.

"No," I said, knowing the implications of the response. "She hadn't left yet."

"Not my time!" Mom evoked with confidence.

And it wasn't. My father was to die first on January 5, 2008, my brother Tim's birthday. Mom died four months later on May 21; she was buried on my sister Lauren's birthday. So much for birthdays.

In that moment, collectively, we were well into the stages of grief: shock; denial and isolation; anger; bargaining; depression; testing; acceptance; and hope. We hadn't turned the corner yet on hope.

The dictionary defines hope as desire with anticipation; scripture describes it as faith in a seed form. All of us were in need of watering. Mom knew her time, but always held her tongue. Liberal in some ways, conservative in others, walking lockstep with traditional spiritual values, she often said she regretted not speaking her mind on more occasions. It was a sad commentary, given her diminishing state of intellect. Sadly, women a generation ago were to be seen, but not heard. They carried babies, cared for children, and were the fabric that held families together like glue. Imagine what we all could have learned had we listened more.

I listened too late, learning far more from my mother's assail on death than from her wisdom and duty to family. I whiffed at that. In contrast to the culture today of self-indulgence, the mothers in the Greatest Generation were selfless in devotion, not out of diffidence, but in maternal instinct—a promise of love, beyond the capacity of most men. Even in Alzheimer's, the love persisted.

My mother in her bruising fifteen- to twenty-year progression of Alzheimer's, refused to lie down. She carried us at times like a soldier in Patton's army, when she wasn't quite sure what planet she was on. I watched in awe, as did my sisters and brothers. Mom's role had changed, and would change again. Yet, none of us wanted to concede the obvious: our mother was slowly sliding off the face of the Earth, pulled into the metaphorical orbits of Pluto and Sedna.

The nursing of my father took its toll on Mom's health. Her memory continued to fade, like cedar shingles bleached by the sun; her rage intensified; she didn't recognize family members and friends at times; she wandered and drifted; she was scared. But she cared as best she could for my father and for the rest of us. The ancient Greeks called it *Agape*, the purest form of unconditional love, far purer than *Eros* (physical passion), *Philia* (brotherly love), and *Storge* (affection). Mom wanted to hold to her role as wife and mother, but roles were changing. She was fighting demons, forever pushing back against monsters in the shadows.

In 2007, Dad was back in Cape Cod Hospital for a second, life-threatening circulation bypass surgery and she stood with him again against all odds. It was her final stand. She was about done. Over lunch at a restaurant on Hyannis Harbor, walking distance from the hospital, she took my wife, Mary Catherine, aside in an emotional breakdown, and within my earshot, she growled with venom, *"I hate him. I hate him. I hate him. I just haaaaate him!"*

She wasn't referring to my father, but venting rage against me, perceived in the moment as the surrogate husband. She was reluctant to confront my father in his suffering, dutiful to the end. The elephant was under the tent. It consumed the space, and it just blew me away.

The tent flaps opened wide and led to EPOCH nursing home in Brewster where Dad was sent for rehabilitation, and Mom followed because she could no longer safely be alone and because she wanted to be with him. They were side-by-side in separate beds in an antiseptic, sterile first-floor room. It was difficult to tell which one was the patient. Mom was somnolent, and when she spoke, made little sense—a chilling contrast of a little child, then a raging adult. The brain simply wasn't firing. Signals were crossed. The scene was an awakening, a cold shower, for the siblings who had visited; they were appalled at Mom's plummet. For his part, Dad was ever distrustful, fearing in his advancing paranoia that we were attempting to commit him to the nursing home. The irony was that Mom needed to be cared for far more than he; she was out of sorts to the point of insentience, yet laser sharp with long-term memory about the particulars of her life and family. The following day when the devoted EPOCH staff took her by the hand to the library filled with four walls of books, they asked her what she wanted to read. The nurses told me later that she scanned the shelves for fifteen minutes, and then quietly, emotionlessly pulled out two books.

"I think I'll read these," she finally said, not grasping the title or author.

The books she chose were *Secrets in the Sand* and *A Guide to Nature on Cape Cod and the Islands*—two books of mine published many years ago, and books that she had kept in her living room in Eastham.

"They just felt comfortable in her hands," the nurse told me later.

At EPOCH, it was clear to presiding physician Dr. Robert Harmon that my mother was on tilt, moving from mid-stage Alzheimer's to end-stage; still she wanted to be the wife and mother. Dr. Harmon called for family intervention, a conference at EPOCH that looped in siblings over the phone who could not attend. It was a disaster of a family conference, as it might be with other large families. Many of the siblings, in this College of Cardinals, were at different end points—from positions of denial, to circumspection, to anger, as Dr. Robert Harmon sought to bring us to a place of irrefutable reality: Alzheimer's was consuming Virginia Brown O'Brien, and there was nothing that any of us could do about it. Nothing.

In the weeks to come, I sought, as my parents' designated Power of Attorney and Healthcare Proxy—a position of impotence in a large family—to find common ground among the siblings, something similar to striking peace on the Gaza Strip. The warring factions, with all good intentions, were split. The girls justifiably wanted Mom protected in a nursing home, and the boys sought to keep my parents together at home. We were split in a moment of crisis, and the crevasse was widening. Deep into confusion myself and privately questioning my logic, I cast the defining vote. Mom and Dad would stay at home, here on Cestaro Way, the dead-end street.

My parents returned to Eastham the following week with the commander-in-chief, holding tight to the concept of hunkering down in the cottage below the tracer bullets. Dad's survival instinct, motivated by fear, was to ride out the storm with my mother. And so, at his unrelenting direction, we hired 24/7 in-home healthcare to be paid out of his Pan Am pension fund at a nosebleed rate of $25,000-a-month for both parents. These were well-meaning, dedicated professional caregivers, but do the math.

It was a free fall, medically and financially. "Only the dead have seen the end of war," Plato once said, a declaration that opened Ridley Scott's classic 2001 movie, *Black Hawk Down*. We all sat back in horror, as if observing in slow motion a horrific airshow crash—my father in a wheelchair, with internal bleeding and no use of his legs; Mom in short circuit, with little use of her intellect. Regularly, I called them at night, just to check in, and when no one answered, I would race in a fire drill to Eastham, sometimes at 11 p.m., thinking I would find them dead, only to realize my mom forgot to hang up the phone.

The reality was debilitating for my brothers and sisters who lived off-Cape, as it would be for any family with such a commute. Over time, Mom's rage and Dad's incessant crusade for survival accelerated, for various and incongruous reasons. I tried to underscore the point one night over the Sunday dinner table, but Dad wasn't getting the fact that his wife of sixty years was slowly drifting out, that I was drifting as well, and both of us were getting angry.

Regrettably, my father, once my hero, never read Ernest Hemingway's *The Sun Also Rises*: "You can't get away from yourself by moving from one place to another." The trip from EPOCH back to Eastham changed nothing. The thoughts of collateral damage stunned me, as I confronted my own demons. I started shifting fidelities. I had no choice. Mom was alone and vulnerable.

October is a special time on Cape Cod and the Islands. The sun rises later in the morning and sets lower on the horizon, yet high enough to light up the emerald salt-marsh grass. Indian summer is in play, a period of unseasonably warm, dry weather, a bonus for the locals. The Cape in fall is heated by the warmth of water surrounding this narrow spit of sand; consequently, summer is longer here, and spring generally arrives for a day in early June.

As the sun set over Cape Cod Bay on Sunday, October 14, 2007, Columbus Day weekend, I headed to Eastham after restarting my brain at the gym. I was in full flush on the way to Eastham, reflecting on my parents, their fading health, and my conflicting instinct about keeping them together at the cottage, for better or for worse.

My father—months from dying and he knew it—was particularly prickly that night with incessant pain, internal bleeding, and a continued breakdown of the body and mind. Dad clearly was on tilt; my mom couldn't think at all; and the professional caregiver at the house, God bless him, had trouble with the English language. Mom, that night, had served pickles sprinkled on Cheerios for dinner; last time I had that was in college after smoking some recreational dope. All the ingredients were in place for a blow-up of denial when I arrived. My father, fully paranoid, had assumed I had come to take him and my mother to a nursing home. He was itching for a fight. We were at the anger and bargaining stage of grief.

"*Tell your brothers and sisters that we're doing fine here, and that we don't need your damn help!*" he bellowed. "*You can leave now, son! We don't need you!*"

"Dad, I'm just here to see Mom," I said quietly.

"*Well, your mother doesn't want to see you either.*"

Immediately, my mother moved to a seat next to me, putting her right arm over my shoulders. She never said a word. Perhaps a sign she was switching allegiances.

My dad persisted. "*The bodies are still warm here, Greg. Go home. You haven't done a damn thing for us. So, just go away, go A-W-A-Y!*"

"Dad," I said. "I get it; you're scared of dying; I get that, but Mom is very sick, and she needs our help."

"*You've done nothing for us, Greg. Ever! Nothing!*"

The words cut to my heart. They were delivered in my father's fear, but I was done with it.

"*Dad,*" I screamed in a spray of expletives. "*Do you think you're the first person in the world to die? Dying sucks, Dad. I imagine, it freakin' sucks, but we all die someday.*"

I paused for a second, which seemed like minutes, fully aware of what I was about to shout: "*SO WHY DON'T YOU TRY NOW*

TO DIE WITH SOME DIGNITY, DAD, AND TAKE CARE OF MOM ALONG THE WAY!"

There was deafening silence; you could count heartbeats. We were all crying, and the elephant in the room had consumed the oxygen. We were emotionally gasping. Gabriel, my parent's faithful caregiver, intervened as a messenger angel. He stepped in and separated me from my father, directing me to a back room. Still traumatized by what I had just said, I followed Gabriel, and Mom followed me. The torch had been passed. Gabriel brought me a glass of water, an act of kindness still imbedded in my memory. He made no judgments, and then returned to my father, as any caregiver should.

Mom and I then sat quietly in the back room, surrounded by family photographs—her mother growing up on a horse farm in Brooklyn, my dad as a handsome Navy lieutenant, her children as young kids on Nauset Beach. She was still crying.

"I'm scared," she said. "What's happening to me?"

"Mom," I said, looking into her eyes. "I know the pain. I feel some of it. You're not alone. We are all here for you."

I pointed with my right index finger to her forehead. "Do you remember that little girl who grew up on the West Side of Manhattan, do you remember the little girl who went to the French convent school, then grew up, got married, and had ten children?"

"Yes," she said, intently staring at me.

"Well that little girl, Mom, that wonderful mother, hasn't left yet; she's still inside you. Believe that!"

"*REALLY?*" she asked drawing out the word, sobbing now, perhaps the first time she admitted she was lost in space and not coming back.

"Yes," I affirmed. "And that little girl will never leave you as long as you fight until you can't fight anymore. You understand that, Mom? Do you understand that?"

"I do," she said definitively. That's all I needed to hear.

We walked back hand-in-hand into the living room. Dad had calmed down, and Gabriel was hovering next to him.

"I love you, Dad," I said as I walked out the door. "But you really pissed me off tonight. You're better than that! Much better than that."

The following day at 7 a.m., Dad called me.

"I'm sorry," he said. The contrition was short, to the point, deeply sincere, and duly noted.

It was behind us now. Finally, we were all on the same page. The roles clearly had changed, but it was a downhill slope, reminding me of the Outer Limits run at Killington, Vermont. I was hitting red marker poles along the way, collectively in the depression, reflection, and the loneliness of grief, a changing of the guard for a fate that lay ahead. I never confided in Mary Catherine about this; wasn't sure she could or would go there. Still not sure. And who would blame her? I was looking inward, trying to protect what I could, a matter of duty as a husband and father for as long as I could.

13

Angels Unawares

M y mother loved yellow, the color of the mind and the intellect, the third chakra of the solar plexus, representing personal power and spark. Yellow is the hue, most visible of all, of memory, hope, happiness, and enlightenment. Yellow inspires the dreamer; encourages the seeker. My mom's rapture with yellow was an upward, heavenly turn in the stages of grief.

Yellow is a color of angels, and in the Bible it symbolizes a change for the better. Mom believed in angels. So do I. The word, derived from the ancient Latin *"Angelus,"* translated "messenger" or "envoys," resonates with peace. And in the throes of Alzheimer's, that's pure gold; if you scratch below the surface of life, messengers may abound, as Hebrews 13:2 counsels: "Be not forgetful to entertain strangers for thereby some have entertained angels unawares."

My mother, I believe, entertained angels unawares. Seven months before her death, in late fall 2007, she became obsessed with yellow. She saw the color everywhere, mostly on cars. All she talked about was yellow. I dismissed the thought outright. Weeks later, driving my mother to Brown's Superette, across from the Eastham Windmill, the oldest working gristmill on the Cape, she exclaimed, "Greg, do you see that yellow car? Look, there's another one, *and another one!"*

Holy schnikes, I was seeing yellow now, myself. In time, so was my brother Tim, who lives in Guilford, Connecticut, and faithfully visited my parents frequently. So, Tim opted to buy a yellow Jeep Wrangler. My mother was thrilled every time he drove into the driveway, somewhat of a second coming. Taking a cue from my younger brother, I also bought a yellow Jeep. We were Heaven on wheels—Mom's angels-at-arms. She loved driving in our Jeeps, like a kid on an amusement ride at Playland in Rye. My brother still has his yellow Jeep. So do I. And I'm taking mine to the grave.

As a New England November gave way to December, the days were tersely shorter—a sundowner effect for all. The sun, lower in the sky at the vernal equinox, now dipped into Cape Cod Bay at 4:09 p.m., as the hourglass sand of my parents' lives was slipping through our fingers. Alzheimer's was bearing down on my mother in the final stage of the disease; Dad was succumbing to his circulation disorders, the progressing effects of prostate cancer, and advancing dementia; and I was adrift on days, off my mooring, tethered to a lifeline, a loving family. We were all living on the edge of faith, with a bit of attitude from Alfred E. Neuman, the red-headed urchin of iconic *Mad Magazine;* the kid with the blissful grin: *"What, me worry?"*

My mother was worried, but endured the disease resolutely as it moved to full bout. The progression was much like watching paint dry on a moist day, ever steady and slow, but the results were unassailable. Still, she functioned as a dutiful military nurse, endeavoring to care for her husband, as other wives of this generation had selflessly done with spouses. Somehow, these women were lost in the headlines. They prevailed against all odds. But where were the medals and headlines for them?

There were yet more crisis runs to Cape Cod Hospital in December. Responding to my father's critical internal bleeding and the unrelenting strain of holding a thought wore my mother to a nub. I followed in tow. We were at the tipping point—an irreversible moment in time, like a glass of fine bordeaux cabernet sauvignon spilling over onto a white linen table cloth. Standing up the glass will not retrieve the wine, nor will it remove the crimson stain. My mom was packing for Pluto, and Dad, forever the Navy man, was setting up deck chairs on his *Titanic*, awaiting a rescue that would never come. The siblings were apoplectic.

My father, meanwhile, kept his humor. After one of his many Lazarus-like resurrections, he barked when the phone rang at home, *"If that's Nickerson Funeral Home, tell them I'm not ready yet!"*

Mom was ready, but didn't know it. Rudderless and adrift, she fought alongside my father—perhaps fearing being left behind, maybe out of instinct. Dad was her rock; we were her kids. She wanted it that way, never ignoring the chain of command. While Alzheimer's can ravage a mind, it cannot erase instinct, the capacity to acquire knowledge without interference or reason. Instinct has history in the Latin verb *intueri*, "to look inside." My mother taught me to look inside, to turn over the rocks, particularly when one cannot fathom the reality, the certainty, of what is happening on the surface.

Certainty was served up bedside to my parents at Cape Cod Hospital on November 11, 2007, a month before my father's eighty-fifth birthday and about eight weeks before his death. Dr. Alice Daley, a skilled internist and compassionate woman who had closely studied my parents' medical records, discerned that it was time for a come-to-Jesus talk. Damn the denial, Dr. Daley knew life was short for both. With Dad in the prone position, Mom seated by his side and insisting she stay, anticipating the worst, and me, a stunned observer, at the foot of the bed feeling like a voyeur, Dr. Daley gently asked the patient if he was prolonging life or death: "If life is a desire to live in some quality, real or imagined, then one is prolonging life," she said. "But if life is fear of death, then one is prolonging death."

Dad, deep in the throes of his own dementia, was prolonging his death. So was my mom.

Dr. Daley, in one of the most remarkable, powerful exchanges I've ever witnessed, then asked both of my parents to give each other permission to die—the "working through" stage of grief.

"Virginia," she began softly, "how do you feel about Frank dying?"

In instinct, Mom rose to the occasion.

"I will miss him terribly," she said. "And that frightens me." Sensing the moment, fully aware of my mom's state of mind, yet knowing that she might later regret a moment lost, Dr. Daley asked her point blank, "Do you give your husband permission to die?"

The words pounded through my brain.

There was a pause, as affected as I've ever witnessed.

"Yes, I do," Mom said, tears welling up. She knew where life and death was heading for the both of them.

"Did you hear that, Frank?" Dr. Daley asked.

"I do," he replied.

"How do you feel about dying first?"

"I want to die first," Dad said quietly. "I don't want to be alone. I don't want to live without Virginia. I can't handle it."

Mom reached for his hand.

Denial in the moment had given way to soul-searching truth.

Another baton had been passed in the resurrection of their relationship.

"Do Not Resuscitate," the forbidding acronym, DNR, is the kiss of death. We were all raised to cherish life, and this core belief was now being called into question. A DNR was in play for both parents, a "no code," as nurses call it, a signed affidavit to respect the wishes of a natural death. And I, the Prodigal Son, "Lunchie," the guy growing up who often was missing in action, was to make the final call. Not good. It wasn't the position I had anticipated earlier in life; as a young man, I had squandered my parents' moderate means on travel, good wine, and trying in vain to sway women far above my station in life. The DNR weighed heavily on me.

The fire drills continued. After Christmas, my sister Lauren, who lives north of Boston, came for a visit one afternoon and found my parents home alone. A substitute caregiver had run to the store to pick up *The New York Times* and *Daily News* for my dad. When my sister arrived at the cottage, my father was sitting in his wheelchair facing the wall. A horrific chain smoker, he was puffing a cigarette queued up to his oxygen tank, behavior as rash as lighting a match in a nitroglycerin factory. My mother was wandering the house, insisting no one was home. KaBOOM! We were, as a family, at ground zero, a place many Boomers have been with parents, as their own children one day will be with them.

New Year's 2008, I had hoped, would bring new promise, but faith was not of this world. My dad had made it clear to me that more ambulance runs to Cape Cod Hospital were *verboten*. He was done, and I instructed the caregivers as such. But on January 4, with Archangel Gabriel off duty, a replacement caregiver in a medical crunch freaked, and rushed Dad to the hospital in an ambulance. A half hour later, Dr. Daley summoned me from a meeting in Boston. I flew down Route 3 to the Sagamore Bridge, like a seagull chasing an offshore dragger so laden with fish that the scuppers were taking on water.

Walking down the corridor of the intensive care unit, I immediately instructed the medical staff that my father was going home the next day. *Got it, tomorrow!* There would be no question about it. I then went to his room. In full horror as I walked through the door, he was even more a skeleton of himself, withered in days.

"Greg," he demanded, "What the hell's going on? I don't want to be here. I told you that! I want to be home with Mom."

"I know, Dad," I apologized. "You're going home tomorrow. I have spoken with the doctors, and you're going home."

"Good!" he said.

"And you're never coming back, Dad."

"Good..."

"And you're *never* coming back again."

"Good."

"Dad, you're *NEVER* coming back here ever again!"

In one of my father's last rational moments, he pulled his scrawny frame upright to a sitting position and addressed me as only a father could lecture a son who wasn't getting it. His body language told me to stand the freak down.

"I get it," he said as if addressing a third grader. *"I … GET … IT!"*

The exclamation point was a hand gesture, cupping his fingers at the middle of his breastplate, then ever so slowly, for emphasis, drawing his hand to the extremes of his shoulders.

I got it, too. They were the last words my father ever spoke to me.

The hospital dispatched my father to hospice care at home the following day. My mom, I believe, knew in her heart that we were on final watch; still not sure of time and place, frozen in the moment, but knowing the moment was at hand.

The doctors prescribed morphine for Dad's intense pain to allow him to let go, and die with some dignity, free of his fears. I was asked to pick up his final orders at the pharmacy and bring the morphine up to the nurses in Eastham that night. The reality was chilling. I was bringing home my father's death sentence.

The drive to Eastham was disorienting, unlike the Sunday rides from Willy's Gym. Random images of my folks, childhood, my brothers and sisters, flashed through my head as I pondered the past, the present, and future. Only the past held hope for us that evening, and that was now on the brink.

Entering the house through the back door, fumbling with the screen that I had never fixed properly, the cottage felt as though it had the life sucked out of it. The quiet of imminent death filled my parents' bedroom. Dad was lying motionlessly in bed, eyes open, unable to talk, still resisting. Mom, steadfast as ever in Alzheimer's, was sitting by his side, not quite sure what was about to happen, but dreading horrific change in the air.

I gave the morphine to the nurse, the mother of my daughter Colleen's close high school friend. I felt as though I was wearing the mask of an executioner.

"You need to say goodbye to your father," the nurse counseled.

"What do you mean?"

"It's time, Greg."

"Time? Time for what?" I said anxiously, "I have to call my brothers and sisters; I need to get them here."

My head was throbbing.

"There is no time left. You need to say goodbye. Your dad is ready to go home."

She stared intently at me, like the Sisters of Charity at Resurrection.

Instincts locked in. I grabbed Dad's hand. Mom, without prompting from me, put her hand gently on top of mine. It just seemed, for her, the right thing to do.

There is no training, no manual, for this.

"Dad," I said looking closely into his dim brown eyes. "Shake your head if you can hear me."

He nodded his head.

"I want you to know, Dad, that we will take care of Mom, all of us. I promise!"

He shook his head.

"Dad, you are very sick, and it's time to go home."

He shook his head.

"Can you see a light, Dad, a peaceful light?"

He shook his head.

"Dad, move to the light. Embrace it. We will take care of Mom. I promise you!"

He shook his head.

"Dad," I then said, "I love you, and it's been an honor to serve you."

He shook his head.

Tears were slipping down his narrow, ashen face. Together, we were at the door of acceptance and hope, looking to infinity—my dad, my mom, and me—through facing mirrors of reality. I felt as though I was gazing through a kaleidoscope, a tunnel of reflected light and colors in patterns that both comfort and confuse. It brought me back to the innocence of childhood when all seemed right. But it wasn't tonight.

Moments later my father closed his eyes. He never opened them again.

The following morning, Dad was pronounced dead. He passed in peace at home just where he wanted to be, lying in his bed and shielded by the unremitting love of my mother, who lay next to him, with her arms instinctively across his chest, unsure of her reality, frightened to be left alone, but dutiful to the end. I got the call from caregivers at 6 a.m. and raced to the cottage. When I arrived, my mom was sitting alone at the dining room table, staring blankly out into the scrub oak forest behind the house. A cold, piercing drizzle pelted the picture window; it might as well have been a rabbit hole into the fantasy world of the Queen of Hearts and the Mad Hatter, images she had faced before and would again, months later, in the nursing home. Mom was terrified. I took her by the hand to the bedroom for final valediction. Dad was still—resting in his peace. Always the wife and mother, she sat next to him and brushed his hair back, as if preparing him for an appointment. "Mom, Dad's dead," I said.

"I know," she replied. "I'm alone. I don't know how much longer I want to be here."

Minutes later, the crew from Nickerson Funeral Home arrived. In a small Cape Cod town, everyone knows one another, and today was no exception. The crew expressed regrets, and then carefully wrapped Dad's body in a white bed linen, placing him in a long black plastic bag with a zipper. As the attendant slowly zipped the bag shut, I was overcome with the certainty of death. So was my mom. In the moment, yet knowing better, I zipped down the bag so Dad could breathe. I thought Mom would want that. All in the room seemed to understand. I then instructed the funeral home crew that I would walk my father out to the hearse in the stretcher. It seemed like the right thing to do.

"Mom, don't worry," I said. "Dad's not leaving here alone!"

Putting the stretcher, feet first, into the back of the hearse, I reached down and kissed him on the forehead. I zipped up the bag. Dad was safely home now.

Mom was left behind and lost in the crushing wake of his death. My father was waked days later at the Nickerson Funeral Home in the center of the snug fishing village of Wellfleet where my parents, years ago, had walked hand-in-hand at the harbor. He would have been pleased, knowing that he lay in state wearing his Yankees cap, an act of respect, thanks to my brother Andy. Mom just kept staring all night, the vacant gaze of Alzheimer's. Her children and grandchildren were consoling, but her spirit was far away; she was preparing for a trip to Pluto and beyond.

On the day of Dad's funeral, the January weather was howling, emblematic of my parents' blustery fight for survival. The shrill wailing of the Irish bagpipes split the stillness of St. Joan of Arc Church in Orleans and resonated the isolation of County Clare. In my eulogy, I quoted Shakespeare, a depiction in *Hamlet* that captured my father in a universal way: "He was a man. Take him for all in all. We shall not look upon his like again."

At Evergreen Cemetery in Eastham, he was buried with military honors, as Mom slipped deeper into an abyss. She never left the car, just stared out the window at us. In the weeks and months to come her plummet was precipitous. Confusion intensified, the filter was shot, the rage intensified, and more and more she was seeing and hearing things imagined. The hallucinations in her final stage of Alzheimer's increased far beyond the crawling spider and insect-like creatures I've witnessed; demonic figures were reaching up at her from the floor, as if to pull her to Hell.

"They are scaring me!" she often cried.

We tried to calm her. All siblings stepped up. Some of us already knew, then, about the importance and power of long-term memory for those with Alzheimer's. My brother Paul in California called regularly to talk to her about the early years, the memories of a long life. Tim, Maureen, Lauren, Justine, Bernadette, and Andy visited as often as possible. Deceased brothers Gerard and Martin, I had imagined, were preparing a mansion for Mom in Heaven. And my dad, I had assumed, was stocking the celestial pantry, making sure there was a Black Dog chardonnay on ice for her, and a six pack of Heineken and a bottle of J&B scotch for himself.

The disease marched on—a steady, almost methodical gait from the time my mother let go, finally acknowledging she was terribly sick. That's the curse of Alzheimer's in concession; no redemption from here. The terror of reality: once you know you have something, a friend once told me, you have to live up to it. It was a teaching moment. In months to come, there were many alarming incidents with my mother. My sister Bernadette was horrified on a visit in the spring of 2008 to witness Mom brushing her teeth with tanning lotion. Lauren earlier had given the lotion to her because she had remarked that my sister's legs looked so tan. Mom's teeth were gritty brown after brushing with Coppertone. Bernadette gently told her to stop it.

"But the instructions say it's for fair-skinned people," Mom replied.

The disconnects worsened; my mother wasn't recognizing her children. I was braced one Saturday night with the dread of the disease. Walking into the living room, she screamed as if I were an interloper: *"Who are you? Who... are... you? Get out of my house!"* Her voice rose with each syllable.

"Mom, it's me."

"Get out of my house. GET OUT OF MY HOUSE!"

I was in shock and went immediately to the back deck to calm down, then returned minutes later to reassure her. She understood—realization in Alzheimer's that perception is ever-shifting. She hugged me. I let it go.

The following week, Bernadette visited again and asked Mom if she'd like to go to the cemetery to visit my father's burial plot. Mom was reluctant at first, conflicted over Dad's innate fear of death, then she finally gave in.

"Ok, I'll go," she told Bernadette in the haze, *"but please don't tell Dad!"*

No one did.

A cemetery is the dividing line between life and death. And like my mother, I also had been putting off a visit, having difficulty confronting the reality of end of life. I awoke that Easter Sunday to a glorious early spring day, determined that I would make the trip. I stopped off first in Eastham to visit Mom. We had a good talk on the couch, an Easter blessing for me. Minutes later, my brother Andy called, and caregiver Gabriel gave the phone to Mom. They talked for a few minutes; Mom was general and rambling, but I could tell Andy was feeling pretty good about the conversation. Then Mom, without notice, asked him point blank: "Do you want to talk to Dad?"

There was a nervous pause. Mom handed me the phone; she had been calling me "Frank" and "Dad" on occasion for some time.

"You sound pretty good for a dead guy," Andy told me. "Andrew," I replied, "today is the day of the resurrection!"

Cemeteries are spooky places. I hate them. But Easter seemed to take the edge off. The sky was deep blue, and a gentle breeze drifted in from the Atlantic. Salt was in the air. I had much to tell my father, regrettably things I never took the opportunity to say. I always thought there would be another day. Today was the day.

The unmarked gravesite was barren, no headstone yet, and the plot was still dirt. I was alone, so I got down on my hands and knees and started running my fingers through the dirt, deeper and deeper, from finger tips up to the wrists. I let my heart out, telling my father how much I missed him, that we were taking good care of Mom, that I was scared, and that I never had any sense of the finality of death until now. I was sobbing.

But I didn't feel the love. Something was radically wrong.

I reached for my cell phone to call Tim.

"Where's Dad buried?" I asked.

"Next to a guy named O'Rourke," Tim said. "Right next to him?" I replied. "Sure?" "Yeah, why do you ask?"

"Just wanted to know."

I had forgotten the location of Dad's gravesite. Slowly, I stood up, brushed the dirt off my hands and knees, and moved tentatively one step to the left, to my father's proper grave.

"Dad, as I was saying," I began.

I can imagine my father and O'Rourke belly laughing up in Heaven watching the fiasco, my dad telling O'Rourke, "That's my dumbass son. He doesn't even know where I'm buried. He's blubbering over some dead guy that he doesn't even know."

Death has a way of swaying truth from secular life. The truth is found in a soft, honest voice inside all of us, if only we listened more. "Death, where is thy sting," to quote Apostle Paul. But close to the end of my mother's life, I lost my inner ear, and began listening to others, like a wave tossed by the sea. Mom finally set me dead straight.

The siblings were at odds over whether she should stay at home in Eastham or move to a nursing home, a similar wrangle in scores of families. My sisters, yet again, wanted Mom in a nursing home, and the boys were pushing to keep her at the cottage with full-time caregiving. A nursing home, the boys felt, was a place to die. In retrospect, perhaps my sisters were right. Maureen, Lauren, Justine, and Bernadette advocated strongly for Mom to be placed in a Greenwich, Connecticut, facility, not far from Rye. I was finally listening and agreed to visit the facility in late April of 2008. It was a nice place, as nursing homes go— friendly, well-kept, and professional. Greenwich is a fine stately town for a woman raised on Manhattan's elite side.

"Mom would be safe here," I thought, still feeling in my gut that it wasn't right, but emotionally spent and wanting to accommodate my sisters. I was emptied of emotion, and giving in, verified that Mom was heading to Greenwich.

After I returned from Connecticut, my wife and I went to the cottage to visit my mother. Again, she was in a haze for most of the time, just gazing out the window into a dense patch of scrub oak and pine. I spoke with Mary Catherine within earshot of my mother about plans to relocate her to the nursing home. I was still ambivalent about it, searching for the courage to pull the cord. I was speaking as if my mother wasn't in the room; I had assumed she was on Pluto. We talked on.

"Greg," my mother interrupted, breaking fifteen minutes of staring silence. "*GREG*," she shouted. "*THAT'S NOT A GOOD IDEA. IT'S JUST NOT A GOOD IDEA!*"

She looked straight at me like a mother disciplining a son.

I signed on.

Mary Catherine was stunned. I was dumbfounded. But I had my answer. There would be no trip to Greenwich. Mom had spoken from deep within her soul, as those with Alzheimer's often can, if we would listen to them. She had set me straight and I was following orders from my mother.

Whether with Alzheimer's, other forms of dementia, autism, or some other brain default, the inner spirit, I believe, communicates at some level. I saw it with my mom and I saw it in my grandfather. Today, I see it with my nephew, Kenny McGeorge, a 24-year-old in Scottsdale, Arizona, who battles severe autism, with the help of selfless, loving parents, Tom and Barb. Kenny never gives up and always looks for the upside in life. Kenny and I text all the time, as he does with others, sometimes in the middle of the night. Often, I get a text from Kenny when I can't sleep and feel isolated. I realize then that I'm not alone. Kenny gets it. He's one of my best friends. He is not stupid either; he just has a disease. Brain defect and disease is not a mark of intellectual bankruptcy, but often a marker for courage and perseverance. Kenny is all of that; so was my mother.

But reality has its day and it was clear to me, over time, that my mother could no longer stay in the cottage. *Alea iacta est.* A die had been cast.

A compromise family decision was made—Mom would go to EPOCH in Brewster, a caring nursing home about two miles from my house. My brother Tim was on hand for the move. But I had to deliver the news first—a one-on-one discussion with my mother, who had fought her disease to the point of submission. The exchange between us was wrenching, immediate. When I arrived at the cottage, Mom was at her usual post—sitting at the dining room table, staring deep into the woods. I've had to deliver bad news many times in my life, all of which paled in comparison to this discussion.

"Mom," I began. "Today is the day you have to leave. We're going to a new home in Brewster," I said.

She didn't budge. She was shaking. Violently. And turned away.

"Mom, do you hear me?" I said, reconnecting eye to eye. "I'm going to take you to a place closer to me. Dad wants you there. I want you there. All the kids want you there."

She kept shaking.

"Mom, look at me, please look at me." Slowly, she turned her eyes toward me.

"Mom, I would never do anything to hurt you. I know this is difficult. We love you, but this is best for you. I promise."

She turned away.

"Mom, look at me. Do you love me? Do you trust me?" She sighed, exhaled as if letting the air out of a balloon, releasing emotion in an exhale that seemed like an eternity. "Yes," she said. "Yes."

She stopped shaking.

Minutes later, as I was in the backyard, speaking on the cell phone with an old friend and colleague, Mike Saint, she walked out the back door and headed to my yellow Jeep. Gabriel, the caregiver, was behind her, signaling the moment at hand. She was ready to go. We left without her bags.

On the drive to EPOCH Mom noticed yellow cars in front of us and behind us.

"Look at that," she said. *"I can't believe it!"*

"Believe it, Mom," I blurted in faith.

I called Tim at the cottage; he had been gathering Mom's things, given our hasty departure. "Tim, you're not going to believe this. There are two yellow cars in front of us and two behind us. Impressive, but freaking me out!"

Within a few miles, the yellow cars peeled off, only to be replaced shortly by another escort of yellow cars. The exchange occurred, on and off, all the way to EPOCH.

At the nursing home, Tim and I tried to make Mom's new room as homey as possible, hanging family photos on the walls, and bringing a few small furniture items that, hopefully, would jog her memory. We both felt sick that day, the kind of emotional pain that starts in the feet, hits the stomach in nausea, then races to the head. Purposefully, I hung a sepia tone photo of her father, "Daddy George," at the foot of her bed. He stared down in comfort right at her. The photo now hangs in my office today over my desk.

Tim's departure to Connecticut was particularly upsetting for me. My mother and I were now both alone. I returned to EPOCH with my son Conor to visit with Mom and brought along a glass of chardonnay for her and a beer for Conor and me. Within minutes, an elderly woman in a wheelchair, far into the depths of dementia, raced into the room, as if she had just jump-started a NASCAR race. I dubbed the woman "Mad Martha," and she was deep into Mom's personal space, and speaking nonsense. Mom, near her end, could still recognize nonsense when confronted with it.

"*Get out of my house*," she yelled at the woman. "*GET OUT OF MY HOUSE!*"

Martha departed in an instant.

"Dad," Conor said, "I think I'll have that beer now!"

Mom's stay at EPOCH was brief. She had gone there to die. Often, the two of us watched old black-and-white movies together in the facility's common room, filled with other men and women in late stages of dementia. The staff was incredibly caring, but the setting had all the ambiance of Ken Kesey's *One Flew Over the*

Cuckoo's Nest. I was getting a first-hand look at what lay ahead.

"That's right, Mr. Martini, there is an Easter Bunny," I recalled from the movie.

Sitting with my mother one day in the common room, watching black-and-white reruns of *It's a Wonderful Life*, I whispered to her that I had to visit the men's room.

"I'll be right back," I told her quietly, worried that she would wonder where I went. "I'll be right back."

"I CAN'T BELIEVE YOU JUST SAID THAT!" Mom replied in a loud, clear voice that resonated throughout the room, and reinforced in me that she was still my mother, I was still her son, and she was still in charge. But she was connecting dots that had no relevant tangent.

"I can't believe you just told the entire room that you had to pee!"

Her reprimand was greeted with universal applause—men and women in their eighties, all fighting Alzheimer's and all regaling in an opportunity to be in charge again. Dementia cannot rob an inner spirit. I was thankful to be part of this palace revolt, hearts crying out for relevance.

Weeks later, Mom was overcome with pneumonia and carted around an oxygen tank, as my father had before her. She was frightened; her frail body was breaking down. I told her not to worry, that we'd all stick by her side. She turned to me, looked me right in the eye, and said: "Like glue! We stick together like glue."

There would be no Easter Bunny today, Mr. Martini; the following morning when I arrived, I found Mom sitting at a table staring intently at a photo of her children, taken many years ago on the back deck of the Eastham cottage. She was about done at this point, I could tell.

"Mom," I said. "You don't have to stay here. You can go home."

She stared at me.

"You can go home to Dad, to your parents, and to sons Gerard and Martin. You can go home any time you want. You're the boss! You don't have to stay here and talk to knuckleheads like me!"

My brother Tim had delivered a similar message earlier.

Mom smiled, the forgotten glance of a young mother. She sighed again, closed her eyes, and slid wistfully back into her chair.

Later that week, I got the call about 10 p.m.

"You mother is not doing well," the nurse said. "She's scared. She needs you."

I raced to EPOCH, about a two-mile drive on a dirt road through the woods, hitting all the potholes left behind from the trotting of horses on this country road, rear wheels sliding left, then right as I pressed ahead. When I arrived minutes later, my mother was deep asleep. I woke her to let her know she was not alone.

"Mom, I'm here. Sorry to wake you up, but wanted you to know I'm here."

She smiled again. There was a countenance about her that said something was about to happen. She seemed more alert, more at peace. Her father, Daddy George, glancing down tenderly from the framed photo on a wall at the foot of her bed, was staring right at her. I felt his presence in the room.

I put my left hand over my mother's left hand as she lay in bed. She was so sweet at the end, much like a compliant grade-school child, like the ones she had taught in school. Slowly, she put her right hand on top of my hand, as she had done four months ago on my father's deathbed. We talked, as one can on the steps of death. I waited until she fell back to sleep, then kissed her on the forehead as I prepared to leave.

Her green eyes opened wide. "Greg, where are you going?" she said in a soft voice.

Knowing in my soul what was about to happen, I sat back down, held her hand, looked into her eyes, and said, "Mom, I'm not going anywhere. We're riding this one out together …"

The time was now. As I sat there, I recalled that she had told me just weeks earlier in what were to be her last instructions: "We all have a purpose in life. Go find it!"

I had trouble in the moment finding the purpose of death. But I stayed by her side until she fell back to sleep again. Then I kissed her on the forehead, knowing the long kiss goodbye was over.

She died hours later.

14

Groundhog Day

Death observed up close is a muscle memory that one never forgets. Memories of my mother and the reality that Alzheimer's had conquered once again washed over me, as we prepared at Nickerson Funeral Home for Mom's final trip to church. As the siblings queued up behind the black stretch limo, I told my brother Tim to pull his yellow Jeep in front of Mom's hearse, and that I'd pull my Jeep behind it.

"Mom's going to go home surrounded by angels," I said.

The funeral Mass was held at Our Lady of the Cape in Brewster on primal Stony Brook Road in the old historic district, a portion of which is listed on the National Register of Historic Places. Mom would have liked that. The church, with tongue-in-groove oak ceilings bowed like the hull of a boat, is an eight-minute jog from my house. The church was filled with extended family and friends. Older sister Maureen was the first to speak:

"How did Mom do it? She did it as many other women from her generation... with a great support system that they had among themselves. So, in the end, we thought she would stay with us a little longer, but she had other plans and kept to them. Mom, in all ways, was Dad's anchor. She was the glue that held him and us together through good and bad times ... What a job!"

And it was.

"But we have to stop meeting like this." I said from the pulpit. "Two lives. Two deaths. Two funerals. Four months."

My mom defined motherhood in an age when worldly accomplishment was all too often the mark of achievement. Ever petite, she could bowl the siblings over—knock us right off our feet like ten pins—with the largesse of her impressive intellect, wisdom, and ceaseless love. Good love and tough love, always justified and in abundant measure, as provided by most mothers of the Greatest Generation. She could burn our corneas with a polar stare, one that penetrated deep into the soul. There were many times I was convicted by her swift, rational judgments, but redemption is a wonderful thing. You have to give redemption to get it, and my mother had infinite capacity to forgive and to teach.

In death, she was still teaching.

My mother knew that I hated flying, primarily because the airlines always lost my bags. It was a regular occurrence. Two days after her death, I was in North Carolina for my daughter's graduation from Elon, flying back hastily for the funeral. Sure enough, one of my bags was missing at T.F. Green Airport in Providence upon arrival. After a computer check, US Airways determined that the bag, tagged under another name, had been sent to Akron, Ohio. Someone at the counter had put the wrong sticker on it.

So, I had to spring for a new suit for the funeral. Mom always liked picking out my clothes; apparently, nothing in my closet had suited her taste. Still, she was calling the shots. And she knew I liked a good ending to a story.

"Now wipe that smile off your face, Mom, and please find my bag!" I challenged her from the pulpit at the end of my eulogy, hoping she would engage St. Anthony, the patron saint of the lost and found. Apparently, she had.

Hours later, when I returned from the cemetery, there was something waiting at the front door—my bag with the mislabeled sticker.

The sticker read "Brown," my mother's maiden name.

My dad was home. My mom was now home. And I was starting to wonder when the hourglass would be drained for me. I can't get sick, I kept telling myself in Mom's mantra. I can't stop thinking, processing; I must stay wholly engaged; I can't let go. So, just look as good as possible, my mother had told me earlier, and don't let them see you sweat.

Letting go is surrender, Mom always said, yet freeing from the numbness of stress, fear, anxiety, and the fatigue of a fight. Pluto was looking pretty damn good to me now. But I knew better; at least I thought so. The progression of this disease is unnerving, cutting, and guileful. This monster will be slayed only when we collectively understand its extensive reach, not just at the end stage of the disease, but at the start of this chaos. As the sadistic Joker, Batman's supervillain archenemy—the archetype of Alzheimer's—observed in the 2008 movie, *The Dark Night*, "Introduce a little anarchy. Upset the established order, and everything becomes chaos. I'm an agent of chaos. Oh, and you know the thing about chaos? It's fair!"

No, it's not fair. No purpose in that. *C'est la vie.*

There is purpose in a driven life, but when the purpose ends, one must reset the timer. Death has a way of liberating one from duty. I had been honorably discharged. But, what now? When my folks passed away, my son Brendan—having witnessed the toll front-line caregiving had taken on me and the family—promptly declared, "Now we have our dad back!"

The toll had been extreme on Mary Catherine and the kids. I was missing in action as a husband and father, but saw no way around it. MC bountifully carried water for me as mother and surrogate father, buckets of it; still does, as she had for my mother. I felt conflicting obligation and guilt as resident family caregiver for my parents. I reasoned at the time that it's easier to ask for forgiveness than for permission. I asked for forgiveness.

I was back as a father, but would never be the same. I couldn't reset the timer. I couldn't even find the damn thing. The events of the past five years and a progression of symptoms had me several quarts down. I had been on high alert, and it wasn't until my discharge from service that I began to discern my present state of mind. I had awoken from a nightmare, only to find myself in the middle of one. Like wandering Pittsburgh TV weatherman Phil Connors, adeptly played by Bill Murray in *Groundhog Day*, I was in a Punxsutawney time loop, trying to get it just right, walking day in and day out in the footsteps of my mother, who had cut a trail for me. I began scribbling down more notes before the thoughts escaped, emailing and texting myself often thirty or forty times a day, as short-term memory began to disintegrate. One day after scribbling for hours in an Orleans coffee shop, a woman came up to me and asked if I was Stephen King; apparently she thought there was some resemblance.

"No," I replied, "but I'm writing about a horror story."

The plot unfolded weeks later in a car wash. My Jeep was awash in mud on a day when the neurons weren't firing properly.

Entering the automated car wash, those rubber slats slapping against the windshield became, in my mind, a platoon of horrifying creatures from the movie *Alien*. I panicked and drove off the guardrails, hanging up my yellow Jeep sideways inside the car wash rails. The attendants had to swing it around. I knew the manager, who quickly sized up the situation, accepting my loss of synapse. Redemption.

"Not a problem, Mr. O'Brien," he said quietly, with disquieting realization of what had just transpired.

Those with Alzheimer's need acceptance where they are, even in the flush of a car wash gone awry. So it is with cutting a lawn. I'm just a consummate lawn guy who enjoys riding my lawn tractor, as much as my Jeep. Weeks later, while on my lawn tractor when the synapse was failing again, I got this random idea as I began cutting my lawn—an acre of overgrown bluegrass and creeping red fescue: *Why not cut my neighbor's lawn*—Brewster's town administrator, Charlie Sumner, the "mayor" of the town—just across the street? Seemed like the right thing to do. As I headed down the steep hill on Stony Hill Road into heavy traffic on Stony Brook Road, whizzing by, often at close to 50 mph, something in the deep recesses of my brain told me this was a bad idea, a very bad idea. My attention was then drawn to a neighbor's lawn through the back woods behind our house where a delicate man in his seventies was placidly cutting with a push mower. The old way. Without rational thought, I took a hard right into the scrub pines, blades aglow, cutting through the underbrush—saplings of oaks, pine, and a few maple trees. The piercing grinding echoed throughout the neighborhood sounding like screams of mercy. My neighbor must have thought I was Freddy Krueger from Elm Street. I never made eye contact with him, just trimmed his lawn in perfect parallel lines, then sharply hung a left back through the woods, the grinding of the underbrush again intense. The poor man fled into his house, probably scared shitless. Four days later, he discretely delivered a hand-scribbled "thank you" letter to the house, presenting it to my son Conor; hopefully, not after seeing a shrink. Got a Christmas card from him that year, as well.

Long-time friend and watchful eye, Brewster Police Chief Dick Koch, a brother to me, commanded later that he never wanted to see me driving down Stony Brook Road on my lawn tractor. His boys would pull me over. Ultimatum accepted!

The nights were getting longer as 2008 faded to 2009. I couldn't sleep. More and more, I was seeing frightful images, knowing intuitively that they weren't real, yet terrifying. I chose not to discuss this, mostly out of embarrassment, for fear I was losing my mind. I didn't want Mary Catherine to worry; also didn't want—out of foolish Mick Irish pride—any pity, judgment, or sympathy. And the thought of telling my children about this was anathema. Try this one on: *"Hey kids, I'm losing my mind! But don't worry, your dad can still find the fly on his jeans when he goes to the bathroom."*

Such discussion in this earlier stage would have been demeaning for me and hurtful. I was beginning to comprehend how others with Alzheimer's cope, looking inward in loneliness, rather than seeking help from others. Who could ever understand? My self-esteem was, and is, at the low-water mark. More and more, I was not recognizing familiar faces, the rage was intensifying, short-term memory on the wane, judgment deteriorating further with an ever-slowing breakdown of mind and body, personal finances in greater disarray, and I now began engaging in random emailing, calling, and texting the wrong people in a breakdown of synapse. The experts call this "confabulation," a memory disturbance, defined as the production of fabricated, distorted, or misinterpreted memories about oneself or the world, without a conscious intention to deceive. I call it Alzheimer's, a place where the brain is searching for meaning with wrong data and randomly connecting dots.

My phone skills have become equally dyslexic. My iPhone is filled to the brim with numbers, scores of them. I see a name in my contact menu I'm supposed to call, only to find out, just like faces at times, that I have dialed the wrong person, convinced it was someone else. Such is the case with emails.

The disturbing confusion with time and place persists, along with great difficulty in determining spatial relationships; my Jeep has been dented front to back, although I destroyed the evidence with recent bodywork. The social withdrawal can be intense. I had once been a poster boy for the *Animal House* fraternity, Delta Tau Chi, and now all I want to do is be alone, not quite sure of whom I've become and where I'm headed.

The reality hit home years ago in a random Boston moment, a dyslexic day, lots of confusion and rage. I had just been given a new cell phone by a client, who wanted access at all times, with a specialized mobile radio band, keeping me on a short leash. After multiple cups of coffee and a queuing up in the men's room to take a leak, I forgot about the phone's then maverick technique. My client, on the two-way radio, began squawking, "O'Brien where are you? What the hell is going on?"

I thought I was hearing voices from my pants. The guy in the urinal next to me, apparently oblivious to the technology, was equally dazed.

Voices continued to rail. *"Godamnit, O'Brien, will you answer me!"*

Perplexed about what to say, I just shrugged it off, revealing: "Oh, that's just the little man who lives in my pocket!"

The fellow raced out of the men's room, dripping along the way.

On February 4, 2010, a cold, penetrating night in Boston, I was driving home from a meeting in nearby Somerville, just over the Leonard P. Zakim Bunker Hill Memorial Bridge, beyond the Thomas P. "Tip" O'Neill Jr. Tunnel that runs beneath the City of Boston. The bridge, at a distance, has the appearance of the masts of a schooner, and looking up at the guy-wires lighted in blue, it offered the lyrical essence that evening of Samuel Taylor Coleridge's "The Rime of the Ancient Mariner":

With sloping masts and dipping prow,
As who pursued with yell and blow
Still treads the shadow of his foe,
And forward bends his head,
The ship drove fast, loud roared the blast,
And southward aye we fled.

So south I fled with a dipping prow. A place as familiar to me as Nauset Marsh, not east toward the Cape, but southward aye. My brain directed me home to Rye on docile Brookdale Place, not to Brewster. Along the way on familiar highway road, the synapse misfired again; I just didn't know where I was. New territory. The lessons of my mother kicked in: don't panic, ride it out, and eventually it will come back.

Finally, it did. I was now outside Providence at 1:45 a.m., about an hour from Boston and an hour-and-a-half ride back to Cape Cod. I realized then that I was a bridge too far from Brewster and wanted, in my mind, to return to childhood, but instead I had to stay the course, living the nightmare. Pulling into my driveway at 3:15 a.m., ever so quietly, so as not to wake my wife, I exhaled—a deep protracted sigh that emptied the lungs, in much the same way my mother had respired months earlier during our dining room table talk after releasing her fear of yielding to Alzheimer's.

Exhalation is good for the soul; the movement of air from the bronchial tubes through the airways is soothing. The thoracic diaphragm relaxes when one exhales, ridding the body of carbon dioxide, a waste product of breathing. In short, it gets the crap out. We all need to get the crap out. Such expiration, as it's also called, links the mind, heart, and soul, staying grounded in the body. We are beings with parasympathetic and autonomic nervous systems, one purposeful, the other involuntary. In exhalation, the body does what the brain says—come down!

I find myself exhaling often these days, but on bad days, the confusion lingers, like the time when I felt compelled to join a long altar line at Our Lady of the Cape down the street. I was typically late that Sunday for Mass, and my family had gone ahead of me. As I walked into church, a line had queued to the altar. I saw my family sitting in a pew to the left; they were waving at me. I knew the consecration of the Mass hadn't begun, yet my brain told me to get in line. I could see Colleen, Brendan, and Conor in slow motion shaking their heads. My wife looked the other way. My brain told me to proceed. Others in the church whom I've known for decades were staring at me. I looked to the front of the line, and noticed that most were in their late eighties. My brain again told me to stay the course. As I got closer, I realized the call to worship was for the terminally sick. Now in a panic, I tried to discern an exit strategy. Everyone was staring at me. I stayed the course. When I reached the front of the line, two priests hovered over me in compassionate prayer. One asked gently, "Son, what's wrong?"

I searched for the right words, not knowing what to say. Still in denial about early symptoms of Alzheimer's, and months before a prostate diagnosis, I blurted out, for lack of a better thing to say: "Cancer!" It was a sobering declaration.

"Ireland sober is Ireland stiff," wrote the great James Joyce. My family toasted the Isle of Mists with throaty zest after the Shannon-bound Aer Lingus flight finally lifted off a rain-soaked JFK runway at 10:30 p.m. on Sunday, August 22, 2010 after a four-hour weather delay that featured boisterous thunder and angry bolts of lightning. It was an ill-omened start to a family pilgrimage to plumb the depths of our Irish ancestry and, in the process, rediscover one another and revel in the seven deadly sins. We skipped the wrath part: Mary Catherine with Dublin roots, and the kids—Brendan, named after the Irish abbot who, legend says, led a ragtag band of Irish monks in a leather-hulled currach across the Atlantic to present-day Newfoundland in search of land promised to the saints; Colleen, a diminutive of the Gaelic cailín, "girl from Old Irish"; and Conor, named after Conor Larkin, the chief protagonist from County Donegal in the classic Leon Uris novel *Trinity*. Larkin was an organizer in the late 1800s of the then fledgling Irish Republican Brotherhood in the struggle for an independent democratic republic. Conor is the namesake of the present head of the O'Brien clan, Sir Conor O'Brien, the Prince of Thomond, the 18th Baron Inchiquin, and a direct descendant of Brian Boru, the first and last king of Ireland. As for me, I have paternal and maternal roots in Dublin, Wexford, County Louth, and County Clare. I'm all over the place.

With high expectations, the Éire trip was the last time I felt in full command of fatherhood, teetering on an edge, perhaps the last time we felt fully whole as a family. In Alzheimer's, it is exhausting, grueling, trying to hold it together. I was on my "A" game, but got pulled in during the fourth inning.

The skies cleared as we landed in Shannon, crossing a cerulean blue River Shannon. The tarmac was still wet, but the heavens opened. My son Conor spotted a rainbow, a wondrous spectrum of red, orange, yellow, green, blue, indigo, and violet. "This trip is meant to be," he declared. Conor was on point. The week would bring the best swath of weather all season, as we plied the West Coast from Galway to the Ring of Kerry.

Driving was befuddling; we're a right-brain family, so maneuvering on the left side was vexing—given the distracting lush green countryside, the ancient stone walls that define centuries, the serpentine narrow roads, and wacky local driving habits. Evan McHugh was correct when he wrote in *Pint-Sized Ireland*, "When the Irish want to tempt fate, they play Irish roulette. No firearms involved—they just go for a drive."

Instinctively, I took to the wheel. Bad move. I have great difficulty now with directions, spatial measurements, and just plain driving, even when maneuvering roads I have known for decades. It didn't take long for Brendan to take over after I had wiped out a long row of orange traffic cones, brushing back one of the *Garda Síochána na hÉireann*, a.k.a. the local police.

"Get out of the car!" Brendan demanded, yet another passing of the baton in my progression. "You're not driving anymore."

Sheepishly, like a guilty young kid, I assumed the shotgun position. I didn't say a word. I knew the time was upon me. We talked about it.

"We've got your back, Dad," my daughter Colleen said from the back seat.

County Clare was a homecoming. We stayed at Dromoland Castle in Clare just outside Shannon for our last night. The castle grounds, the ancestral home of the O'Brien clan for 900 years, is now a luxury 375-acre estate. The Renaissance castle retains its old-world charm with splendid woodcarvings, stone statuaries, hand-carved paneling, brilliant oil paintings, antique furnishings, a championship golf course, and stately gardens. The reception area was majestic; the front desk had taken note of the reservation.

"Welcome home!" they greeted.

The rooms were noble, with sufficient space for a king's guard. But quickly, we were off to the bar that looked more like an ancient library than a tavern. Typically clumsy as an ox and not ready for regal prime time, I spilled a glass of good red wine in the bucolic gardens just outside, observing a turret with my daughter Colleen. Upon asking for a refill, I was told, "This one is on your ancestors!"

Later, over dinner, the family was observing the stoic floor-to-ceiling oil portraits of ancestors. "All O'Briens," our waiter told us, "are an ugly lot!" *What a dunce*, I thought. *Don't you think the castle is filled with O'Briens?*

Our final family fling was a night at Durty Nelly's in the shadows of nearby Bunratty Castle. There, we made good friends with the locals, likely for the draw of daughter Colleen. I made sure to stand close guard by her. In the meantime, Mary Catherine was having trouble finding the handle on her wine glass, dropping two of them on the ancient stone floor to raucous applause. The shattering echoed throughout. "My Gawd," one of the older locals exclaimed, "she's goin' for a foock'in hat trick!"

Saturday morning breakfast in the king's dining room before a flight home was a grounding for all of us. Seated in elegant high-back chairs at a white-linen table, in dignified style, I reached for the coffee and cream, then poured the cream all over my eggs, splashing the outer limits of the elegant white stoneware. It just seemed like the right thing to do. A pregnant moment had given birth to quintuplets. We all knew the drill.

That elephant in the room had reared its head again. Hard to deny the long tusk of reality. We talked briefly about the unmentionable, but the weight of a progressive disease can be heavy. Even in denial, on a trip to the homeland. My wife, ever stoic in protecting the kids, laughed as if to say: find the humor in this. The kids were starting to get it. The family pilgrimage to plumb the depths of our Irish ancestry just hit bedrock, hard, yet a solid foundation. That's the Irish way.

The Irish are often slow to embrace prickly realities below the surface. We can be an emotionally numb lot. Perhaps it's a survival instinct, dating back to the Viking invasion epochs ago. We generally don't talk about the ugly side of life. See no evil, hear no evil, speak no evil. We speak no evil when it comes to deeply personal, complicated matters, taking denial to soaring heights until the crash landing of a malevolent diagnosis. Still, many survivors don't want to engage. And so it is with my wife, a coping mechanism, not as evident in my children. We're all cut from different trees, more apparent to me than ever on this journey. Mary Catherine keeps me balanced in her rejection of harsh reality, often treating me, in her own fear, as if life goes on forever. It won't, but I am thankful at times for the delusion; at other times, more and more now, I prefer empathy and candid encouragement to press on. And so I checked what remained of my denial at the entrance to O'Brien castle.

We made our flight to Boston on time. As the boxy Aer Lingus craft lifted above Shannon, over the Cliffs of Moher, and headed out into the Atlantic, I kept looking back, feeling as though I had left a burden behind.

15

Out to the Kuiper Belt

The Kuiper Belt is an elliptical icy plane far outside the orbit of Neptune and billions of kilometers from the sun. It is a long way from Ireland's Ring of Kerry. The Kuiper Belt was formed from fragments of the Big Bang, spin-off from creation of the solar system, and is home to dwarf planets like Pluto, Haumea (named after the Hawaiian goddess of childbirth), Makemake (the god of fertility of the native people of Easter Island), trillions of anonymous objects, and the mysterious Oort Cloud, a suspected source of comets that flash about our sun. Here, deep into the cosmos, Sedna orbits—the first observed body belonging to the inner Oort Cloud. This remote expanse holds the answers to life.

Answers are impossible to discern in Alzheimer's but the metaphors abound. The asteroids, dwarf planets, and the Oort Cloud of this disease refract reality. One is left with random manifestations, successions of real-time, mind-bending warning ciphers that serve only to confuse, yet underscore the progression of a beast that attacks without forewarning.

I was seeking answers early in September 2010, on an out-of-body recce mission to the Kuiper Belt. There were none to be found among the cosmic dust. On this particularly dispiriting day, I resolved to take my life.

The drive back from New York after a client meeting on the campus of *Readers Digest* in Chappaqua was pensive, as I passed through pastoral Greenwich, Fairfield, then on to New Haven, Mystic Seaport, and points north. I was lost in thought, contemplating the vagaries of a new assignment, rewinding tranquil childhood memories in Westchester County, thinking about my family, pondering the aggregate symptoms of Alzheimer's, and brooding about a fourth prostate cancer biopsy scheduled that afternoon. Prostate biopsies are no fun; far less agonizing, to be sure, than childbirth, but stinging to the point of nausea. My imagination, maneuvering along Route 95 just outside Providence, was in overdrive. I had conjured up a beastly image of a ten-foot surgical needle with the doctor at the handle driving it to its intended delicate and private spot like a rip-roaring jackhammer. *Zap. Zap. Zap!*

I fought off the pain in past biopsies by associating the aching din with the sound of Red Sox icon David Ortiz, Big Papi, whacking a home run. The "zap, zap, zap" became a "whack, whack, whack." This was to be a championship season, I had hoped.

As I passed over the Braga Bridge where the Taunton River meets glorious Narragansett Bay, my attention was drawn east to the 11,248-foot Newport Bridge, a suspension work of art, and then on to the placid waters beyond. I felt in awe, at peace at first, followed by intimidation for what lay ahead. The scheduled biopsy was a transient distraction to escalating horrific memory loss, isolation, and loss of self. I was now deep into a pity party, questioning my future, my value, my essence.

Looking out over to the reflective beauty of Narragansett Bay, in an epiphany of conflict, I screamed out in my Jeep, "*Screw it! Just Screw it!*" I resolved to focus on my wife, kids, and work, and whatever else happens, it just happens. Screw it. I can't control the rest, I reasoned, nor could my mom. Gotta learn to walk in faith.

Moments later, I found myself smack behind a slow-moving yellow freight truck. Given an affinity for the color, I drew near, and was drawn to a large inscription on the back of the truck. It read: "You are NEEDED." Needed was in all caps, a sign perhaps of what was to come.

I felt the presence of God within. Call it what you will; perhaps it was my mother looking after me. Whatever, I felt on hallowed ground. I lingered behind for several minutes, absorbed with the message until I realized I had an appointment with a needle. So I passed the truck, and two miles up the highway, my attention was drawn to a digital sign loop at a local hotel, the kind of rotating message you often see off the highway. There was a message flashing. It read: "Thank you for all you can do!"

I was starting to get the point. About forty minutes up the highway, as I approached the Bourne Bridge, I was back in my pity party, fretting work, family, and life itself.

"This sucks," I thought.

A car passed me on the left. It had plates with the state logo: "Live Free or Die." The vanity plate read, "SECURE."

I felt as though the Lord had taken a two-by-four across my head as I pulled into the urologist's office. Immediately, I emailed my brother-in-law, Lou, in Phoenix, and a close Kansas City extended family member Jerry Riordan about it, both strong in faith, but I would need yet another wallop.

Whack, whack, whack. Big Papi had a banner afternoon. After the biopsy, I began bleeding from those secret places, front and back, a normal flow at first for the procedure, then the floodgates opened over several hours. I called the doctor twice and was told this would pass, but the only thing passing were pints of blood. I didn't call back again; my self-absorption with pity endured. I thought I had a way out. The discharge cycle, a hemorrhage now, went on for about twenty-four hours, a loss of an estimated six pints of blood; my exit strategy, I thought, without the guilt of a more hands-on suicide. I saw no upside in the direction of my life, and so chose not to tell anyone about the full extent of the hemorrhaging, not even my wife.

But "nothing in creation is hidden from God's sight," as Hebrews 4:13 notes. I should have remembered that New Testament verse drilled into my head as a youth.

I knew in my heart that if I fell asleep, I might never wake up, and that I didn't have the right to end it here. And so, with the family asleep and my blood count on empty, I drove myself, dizzy and disorientated, to Cape Cod Hospital about twenty miles away, testimony again to my diminished state of mind and to the grace of God. The emergency room nurse took one glance at my ashen face, sat my sorry ass into a wheelchair, and within seconds, whisked me to an emergency room cubicle.

I instructed the nurse not to call my wife. I wanted to ride this one out alone, particularly if I was heading to Pluto, as I had hoped, for the final trip. To my horror, I was directed to the same emergency cubicle where my father had been taken years ago with internal bleeding, and where my mother, tired of fighting, finally gave in to the demon Alzheimer's. In the cubicle, I bled out another two pints. The average person carries about eight to ten pints of blood; with a loss of four pints, time to call a priest, minister, or rabbi. Losing half your blood, medical experts agree, is a sure way to expire. I had lost an estimated eight pints of blood in all. I was on empty again.

"Do you know you're supposed to be dead?" a nurse asked me bluntly, trying to engage in conversation, keeping a solemn moment as light as possible, and yet discerning my motive. "Yeah, but no one had the courtesy to tell me," I replied. My mind was racing at the time. I thought of favorite writer Joseph Heller, author of *Catch 22*, who wrote, "He was going to live forever, or die in the attempt." I was trying to die in the attempt and was reaching for the stars, fully detached, and now fading in mind and body. Alone in my cubicle, as doctors tried to discern how to stop the bleeding, I had my come-to-Jesus moment. The light. I sensed a powerful, pure bright light at the end of a tunnel; I was at peace and hoped my mother, grandfather, dad, and brothers Gerard and Martin would be there to greet me, but in my gut, I knew this wasn't my time, not my call. I looked to the ground and saw the pool of blood on the floor, as I had witnessed years earlier with my father in a wheelchair. I cried out on the brink: "Lord, take me home, or bring me back, but please don't leave me in this place."

Within minutes, I was wheeled into a surgical unit, and doctors determined how to stop the bleeding. There would be no final trip to Pluto. The flight had been cancelled.

For all of us, there is a cycle of birth, life, and death. And there are second chances. The human body is intent on living, in spite of what happens in illness. Cells keep multiplying, breathing is involuntary; the brain, even when teetering, directs the intention to live and create. My second chance was reinforced with another encounter with Dr. Alice Daley, the physician on call, a caring individual who had presided over my parents' end-of-life conversation. Clearly, we were in an orbital path.

"I hope, Doctor, you're not going to give me the: 'it's-ok-to-die' speech today," I said as she entered the room.

Dr. Daley smiled in a way that said I had dodged a bullet, direct to the head.

"Go, and sin no more," the nurse on duty replied. It was a sobering directive.

Apoplectic over news of my hospital stay, my personal physician, Dr. Conant, was far more direct the following week regarding my failed attempt to bleed to death. He scribbled in my medical record after a follow-up visit: "Discussed ambivalent feelings, re: near miss with exsanguination. Very concerned about worsening memory; he has to use maps and tricks to function daily; long discussion regarding risk factors."

Dr. Conant then took a blank piece of paper and drew a bell curve, as if I were back in the sixth grade. He placed a large "X" on the downward slope. "Here's where you are," he said, trying yet again to get my attention. "You need to back down on commitments that require high-level cognitive and judgment."

"Time is running out," he said. "Things are going to get worse. Do I have to come over to your house and declare you incompetent? If that's what it takes, I will."

The words were difficult to swallow. I love Barry like a brother, but screw him, I raged in anger. Sure, he had my best interest at heart, but, you know, just screw him. Who does he think he is, a doctor or something?

"*Worse*, Barry?" I thought to myself, aping again a line from *Christmas Vacation*. "Take a look around you, Barry. We're at the threshold of Hell!"

That afternoon I tried to cut through my angst by mowing the lawn, about an acre and a half of it. Driving my sitdown, I was still stewing over what Conant had told me earlier.

"Time is running out?" I repeated to myself. "Really? Yeah, well, Barry, we'll see."

Trimming the slope behind the house, I noticed that my favorite watch, a gift from my wife, was loose on my left wrist. Within seconds, as I cut between the reedy locusts and a thick pine, the watch, to my horror, slowly slipped off my left wrist and fell to the ground. I witnessed the cutting blade suck the watch under the mower and spit out the remains; a small section of the watch band and a silver, oval watch frame were all that was left.

"Time is running out!" The words echoed through my brain. I've kept the oval watch frame and stretch of band in the top draw of my dresser as a reminder of vulnerability.

I was feeling particularly vulnerable at my buddy Paul Durgin's sixtieth birthday party in Milton outside Boston in late spring. The town and surrounding area is filled with overachieving Irish types from Boston who have dropped their "R"s and have learned to walk upright—surnames like Mulligan, Norton, Corcoran, Cunningham, Mulvoy, Forry, Brett, and Flynn. I'm comfortable with this lot, fully in my wheelhouse, but today I'm listing portside in the wake of more confusion, swamped by memory loss and the failure at times to recognize old friends. I used to work a room like a seasoned politician; they called me "the senator from Cape Cod"—always with a friendly hand out, piercing eye contact, a quip for all. But in the moment,

I'm feeling detached and isolated, a full spin cycle from extravert to introvert—a dizzying turnabout in personality. I'm comfortable in my own skin; it's just that now I don't want anyone in there with me.

And so I made the rounds as best I could, trying to reminisce with guys I've known for more than a quarter century, following a script that I've used many times before. I've learned, as a strategy, to keep the chat short, get to the point, move on, and hope that I'm not asked to retrieve information lost. The strategy is tiring, and often "just inches from a clean getaway," as Jack Nicholson jibed in *Terms of Endearment*, I get sucked into a black hole of conversation, a gravity pull for me that is smothering. After a fretful working of the room that afternoon, I retired to a seat of comfort—outside the Durgin house, behind the wheel of my car parked on the street. I sat there for an hour and a half, just grabbing the steering wheel, trying to understand what had just happened, and hoping to drive off the face of the earth, yet I knew I was stuck in the present. How did I get to this place?

Reluctantly, I returned to the party, feeling like a time warrior. Paul and his wife, Leslie, knew the drill.

"You back from your planet yet?" asked Leslie. "Yeah," I replied, "It was a wobbly trip!"

The flight back from San Francisco several months later with my daughter, Colleen, was shaky; lots of forceful air currents rocked the US Airways flight to Boston. I was there on business, and Colleen, as she has been throughout my life, was at my side. Doctors have advised me not travel alone. In between meetings, San Francisco was a blissful father-daughter bonding just months before her marriage to Matt Everett, a fine Baltimore lad with misplaced sports loyalties, at least in my silly parochial mind. But that's what I love about Matt; he presses forward against all odds.

So does Colleen. On the direct flight home from San Francisco the airline booked me next to an emergency exit in the front of the cabin; Colleen was in the seat next to me. The flight attendant asked if I was up to the task. *Hell, yes,* I thought. Colleen obliged. But it was not a good place for me. Somewhere over Chicago, I was disoriented from being on a plane for hours, and I had to take a leak. It happens. My mind told me that the door to the bathroom was directly to the right, the emergency exit; all I had to do was to pull up the lever. So I grabbed for it. Just seemed the right thing to do.

"*Daaaaaad!*" Colleen screamed in a cry that could be heard in back of the plane. "What the hell are you doing?"

With my right hand on the emergency exit lever, I realized from my daughter's chilling tone that this was not a good idea. And surely it wasn't. In a flash, I envisioned being sucked out of the plane with my daughter, along with rows two through thirty. Helluva way to end a good trip.

I envisioned authorities telling my wife: "Your nut of a husband decided to take a shortcut home, and things didn't work out well for the rest of the passengers. That really sucks, ma'am!"

Relax. I won't sit near the emergency exit anymore. Promise!

Dr. Conant's bell curve was beginning to resonate. The bell would toll again on a business trip to Martha's Vineyard while meeting clients at the Chowder House Tavern, elegantly appointed in oak, near the edge of pristine Oak Bluffs harbor. With its gingerbread and camp-style architecture, Oak Bluffs is a fantasy unto itself with its network of curving narrow streets. "Carpenter's Gothic," it is called here. In the mid-1800s, the town was the site in summer of huge revivalist-Methodist camp meetings in Wesleyan Grove, named after John Wesley, the open-air preacher and founder of the Methodist movement. I was in need of a big Amen that night.

Looking for my clients as I entered the Chowder House—where I've eaten many times—I saw a snug anteroom to the right that I had never noticed before. It was decorated much the same as the restaurant, with people sitting around the bar seeming to have fun. They were waving at me. I looked closer and saw my clients at a table in the corner. I waved back, trying to determine how to enter the room. I couldn't find the door. I knocked on the window, beckoning the clients to come get me. They started laughing. I knocked again. They waved back, almost taunting me. I kept searching for the door, and in frustration, worked my way to the men's room, thinking there might be access there. No luck. When I returned to the window, the clients were still waving and laughing. I knocked again, then my attention was drawn over my right shoulder. I was stunned at what I saw. My clients were sitting right behind me. I had been looking into a mirror, in the moment peering into infinity, the gateway to a parallel universe, in the vicinity of the Kuiper Belt.

The memory is still vivid. If you squint, you can see Pluto and beyond from the Vineyard.

"Memory is everything. Without it we are nothing," observed neuroscientist Eric Kandel, winner of the 2000 Nobel Prize for his groundbreaking research on the physiology of the brain's capacity for memory. Memory is the glue, Kandel said, that binds the mind and provides continuity. "If you want to understand the brain," his late mentor, eminent neurologist Harry Grundfest, counseled him, "you're going to have to take a reductionist approach, one cell at a time."

Cell by cell, Kandel took the brain apart. Had he dug a bit deeper, he might have found that memory isn't all that it's cracked up to be. While memory offers delineating context and perspective, it doesn't define us. Definition is found in the spirit, in the soul, but one must dig for it. "An unexamined life," Socrates once said, "is not one worth living."

I was in a circumspect mood on the way with Mary Catherine to snug Camden, Maine, to celebrate her sixty-first birthday in late

August 2013, stopping off for the night in Portland, a maritime city set on a hill downwind from the Atlantic. Early the next morning, outside the red brick Portland Regency Hotel, the seagulls were dive bombing the downtown in a mock scene from Alfred Hitchcock's masterpiece *The Birds*. The sun was bright at 6 a.m., lighting up the cobblestone streets; the air was crisp with a hint of fall on this pure, idyllic morning. Even the *Portland Press Herald* breathed of innocence. Its lead headline on the local and state page reported, "Dunkin' Donuts Tries New Paper Cup." No shit. It's a story about new paper cups designed to mimic plastic foam by keeping the coffee warm in the cup, "cool on the outside." I was feeling cool on the inside this morning, as I looked about me and began to drift, caught again in a time travel. Soft music from the Regency lobby drifted outside to a nearby park bench where I sat with my back to the sea. Oldies were playing. I heard the Lennon/McCartney song "Yesterday," and was drawn to it.

Yesterday, I was flush with hope; today, I'm adrift in thoughts and images I can't seem to control. They rule me. Often, I just go with the flow. I've acquired a few techniques along the way. One of them is to learn from nature.

You can smell the sea on the road outside Camden. West Penobscot Bay with the secluded archipelago Fox Islands in the distance at the edge of the Gulf of Maine frames a swath of blue that runs endlessly in a way to make one think the world is flat. The archipelago, with its jewels Vinal Haven and Hurricane Island, was first inhabited in 3300 BC by Native Americans called "The Red People." The rocky coast of Camden and neighboring Rockport, an artistic, cerebral town of about 3,000, if you count the living and the dead, is a place of mind-numbing perspective. Nature overwhelms here, bringing one to the realization of being surrounded by something much larger than one's essence. There is great security in knowing this, even more for those with Alzheimer's.

Sitting by myself on a porch in Rockport with white columns and 180-degree views of the bay, I come to understand that I'm not alone. This classic Maine cottage, owned by my brother-in-law,

Charlie Henderson, a retired Chicago money manager, stretches the definition of cottage with its 6,000 square feet of Down East elegance. It seems to me more of a biblical ark—300 cubits long, 50 wide, and 30 high—than a home. As I look out over a remnant of the world's animals, I spot the graceful flight of two ospreys. The majestic sea hawks, weighing about four pounds, with wing spans up to six feet, have a human element to them in instinct and in species. Ospreys are the single-living species in the animal kingdom that exist worldwide. A bird of prey, they mate for life, are nesting homebodies, tediously care for their young, and have voracious appetites: a diet of freshly caught fish. I watch the pair of ospreys practice diving runs over the bay. They fly in circles in tighter orbits, almost like the cone of a tornado, then they strike with wings tucked in an explosion at the surface of the bay. They snatch their prey with fighter-pilot visions from behind, and with sharp talons that act as fishhooks, lifting the prey to the heavens in aerodynamic flight with the fish headfirst. Then it's back to the nest for supper. The nest, the size of a Volkswagen bug, sits atop a spike on a fifty-foot pine with a commanding view of West Penobscot Bay. My brother-in-law tells me that the nest was destroyed four years ago in a pounding nor'easter. The mating ospreys rebuilt the nest the following spring, twig by twig. The mother, he says, sat in what was left of the nest, while the father flew in building materials. She was cawing at him as if to complain, "Wrong size!"

But, like humans, the eyes and instinct for survival of ospreys are often bigger than their stomachs. The Irish poet William Butler Yeats used the wandering osprey as a symbol of sorrow in his 1889 work, *The Wanderings of Oisin and Other Poems*. At times, its prey is so heavy that the osprey can't lift it. Their fishhook talons can't release, and they are pulled to the sea and drown.

Nature has taught me legions today. Even in death, survival is ever pursued.

Back on the Cape, days later at the end of a frenetic summer, I sit in my office with my collection of memories, and the sounds of silence are everywhere. Lessons of the journey invite the stillness. I've come now to understand that Alzheimer's is not about the past— the successes, the accolades, the accomplishments. They offer only context and are worthless on places like Pluto. Alzheimer's is about the present and the struggle, the scrappy brawl, the fight to live with a disease. It's being in the present, the relationships, the experiences, which is the core of life, the courage to live in the soul. It doesn't matter much to me anymore that I don't remember names or faces, that memory is a lost art, and that I must employ improvisations daily, the tricks of spontaneous intervention. I am always intervening on my own behalf, just to steady the boat—trimming the sails, looking for the *terra firma* of life, simply to discern where I am. Only to find that a higher power is at the tiller.

All too often, those with the disease have become voiceless, locked in their own insecurities and symptoms, and misunderstood by those who just don't want to go there. Like every man and woman, these time travelers in disease need guidance, acceptance, trust, and love. So, go there with them at times to Pluto, try to fathom their journey. It's not such a bad place. We can all get to Pluto; it's just that some of us are not coming back.

In a stretch, Alzheimer's is a form of cognitive dissonance. In a state of dissonance, individuals often feel "disequilibrium," frustration, dread, guilt, anger, embarrassment, anxiety. And so it is with Alzheimer's. All at once. Perhaps one might understand the denial, the deflection of Alzheimer's, like the ceramic elephant from Santa Fe in my office.

Within weeks of my return, the herd was thundering again in a series of chilling manifestations.

One day the elephant emerged again with sad words that a close college buddy from the University of Arizona, Pat Calihan, had died of dementia. A Phoenix native, Pat excelled in sports, friendship, and in life. He was an Irish storyteller, a mentor to many, a man with a tenacious work ethic and steadfast integrity. We shared many good times over the years on the playing fields, on the ski slopes of the Mogollon Rim, and in the pubs—talking about life, death, and all that happens in between. Pat was an everyman, with an innate ability to connect with people. A handsome dude, who in his youth had sunny blond hair and eyes the color of soldier blue, Pat had game. In college, we gave him the enduring nickname of "Whetto," and for reasons of political correctness, I won't disclose why. But the tag stuck, as his zest for life ever deepened.

Years ago, Pat intuitively knew something was wrong and tried to deflect it. Others close to him observed it, as well. The neurons weren't firing right, but still Pat fought on. In time, the diagnosis came like a death notice: an accelerated form of dementia. Pat, still "Whetto" in spirit, began to fade. He never gave up the will to live, until life itself snatched the will from him. As his obituary noted: "Pat was stricken in the prime of life with an ailment that eventually took away his cognitive abilities but never his thirst for life. But not his soul, not his being; never complaining, never compromising."

The end came after years in a nursing home. There were no ribbons, no television commentaries, no callouts. I heard about Pat's passing from my wife over Sunday coffee on the back deck. She had just received an email. Word of Pat's death took time to work through my neurons, trying to grasp what just had happened. I had lost a close friend that day, a brother in early life. His unwavering, loving wife, Becky, his children, his loyal brothers, and family at large, have lost a great champion.

How many more, I wondered? Too many, it turns out.

A month later, I lost another friend to Alzheimer's, a man named Hilly. I had visited him periodically to buck him up. His caregiver, a childhood friend, told me that Hilly, in his final days, couldn't discern the difference between breathing and eating. So, he gave up on both.

The news—the stark image of it—still stuns today. I didn't sleep all night.

When will the escalating deaths from Alzheimer's be enough to turn the tide for more research and a public outcry to make this monster stop? The time is now.

I haven't shaken the news, but instead have seized the blessing that Pat and Hilly, like my mother, are free now. The realization has been comforting, though disorienting in a series of aftershocks, like ghosts of past, present, and future in Charles Dickens's *A Christmas Carol*.

The night after Hilly's death, I had a dream, still imbedded in my mind. In the dream, I had moved to a new house. My wife took me there, and at first I thought I was back in Arizona. I wondered how she had ever convinced me to leave the East Coast, then I realized that I wasn't in Arizona. The landscape was green, pastoral with rolling verdant hills like the fields of Vermont, Maine, or Ireland—special places to me—tall oak trees, some hedges, blue skies. I worried how we ever got a mortgage for this mansion-like old stone home, given I have no bank credit. I asked Mary Catherine about it, and she told me that a caring friend had worked it all out. Not to worry. The house was rambling, and I talked to her about its great potential. Surprisingly, I was content here; it felt like home.

I then looked to the front yard—a wide swath of green grass, dotted with marble and granite tablets. I realized then to my surprise, I'm living in a cemetery, but I was fine with it. No fears, just peace. I then took a walk by myself, down a path on the right side of the house, surrounded by the most dense forest I had ever seen. I realized in the moment that I wasn't in a temporal place. It had the of feel of Lewis Carroll's *Through the Looking Glass*; the birds, the animals, and insects all talked, similar, at times, to hallucinations I've experienced in Alzheimer's. I engaged them. These were not demonic figures, and I enjoyed the conversation, fully relishing it.

I returned to the house, entering through the side yard. I was amazed at the number of tombstones I saw along the way and in front of me. Rows and rows of them, perfectly arranged. As I walked toward the front door of the stone house, I touched one of the tombstones in full confidence, patting it on the side and on top, saying to myself: *I'm good with this.*

When I returned to the house, my wife was gone. I was by myself. Then I woke up.

Days later, I told my friend Dr. Conant about the dream. We talked about it over coffee on his back deck overlooking Cape Cod Bay early on a Sunday morning in late summer, as a gentle southeast wind slapped the surf against the shoreline. The color of the bay was as blue as the autumnal equinox sky. After small talk of baseball and football, Barry and I moved to more pressing matters.

Barry now is fighting pancreatic cancer, and we spend much time together in deep discussion of life and death. He has a five-percent survival rate, although I keep reminding him that, ultimately, we all have a zero survival rate. I have manly love for Barry. While our perspectives are diverse in places, we meet at the tangent of friendship and caring, as all friends should, talking about the joy of being free of a disease, yet accepting what lies beyond. I've learned, over the years, that truth is a matter of perspective. We'll all find out one day who's right.

I tell Barry the story of my crusty country editor and mentor Malcolm Hobbs, who many years ago had wrestled with death. Toward the end, Malcolm told me that he wished he had a faith, that he was afraid of dying. As a rube twenty-seven-year-old, I told him that it was never too late to embrace a faith. Malcolm, a Renaissance man and an accomplished sailor, was the embodiment of an intellect that I sought dutifully. On his deathbed overlooking Arey's Pond in South Orleans, he told me of a dream of being swamped in a boat and reaching out for a secure hand. I told him to keep reaching out. The following morning, he said he had reached for the Universe and found a power far more commanding than he. Call it what you want, but Malcolm was at peace. The next day, as he was looking out over the pond on a frigid March day with a thin coat of ice on the roiling waters, a single white dory sailed from east to west. Malcolm, his wife, Gwen, and daughter, Janie, saw it in awe.

Malcolm immediately sat up in his bed.

"Dad," Janie said, "There's your dory. You sail it out of the river, into Pleasant Bay and out into the Atlantic; you sail that dory home."

When she turned back to her father, he was gone. Malcolm had sailed to the horizon and home.

As Barry and I look up from his deck, a single white dory is sailing gracefully across the bay. We are astounded. Barry then tells me a story about his late father, a minister, and how he relates now to his father in death as a magnificent blue heron. Within minutes, the white dory crosses the bay in front of his deck, and a resplendent blue heron sweeps across the shoreline.

Silently, we sit in awe, as we look out across the bay.

A week later, there is a knock at my office door. Standing in the threshold is a man in his early forties, dressed in an old-school flowing black cassock with a Roman collar, as white as the ridge board on my house. There is a peace, almost an angelic glow, to him. He looks like Father Chuck O'Malley in *Going My Way*, played by a young Bing Crosby. I'm thinking the Lord has called me home. *Extremaunción* to go! But the man has no oils or candles.

I look closer. He looks elusively familiar, but I still can't get my bearings. He calls out my name and introduces himself. It is James Smith, a former reporter I trained twenty years ago at *The Cape Codder* and *The Register*, one of the oldest continually published weeklies in America. James is now studying to be a Catholic priest in Nebraska. Two decades ago, we were part of a Bible study after work in the newsroom; some shunned us for it. James tells me that he has read a newspaper story about my illness and felt compelled to visit; he also tells me that his father is dying of Alzheimer's. He has come for a purpose; clearly he has something to say. We talk about the notion of detachment, an end-life divesting of material, and intellectual possessions. Disentanglement, he counsels, results in purity of spirit. This seminarian is a student of scholar Albertus Magnus, St. Albert the Great, as he is known in parochial circles. Magnus was born in the thirteenth century; the German friar is considered among the world's greatest intellects. He was the mentor of the brilliant Thomas Aquinas and taught Aquinas that memory is the coin of temporal life. Dante, in his *Divine Comedy*, places Magnus and his pupil Aquinas in the class of the greatest lovers of wisdom.

Albertus, James tells me, practiced poverty of the mind when he learned late in life that he would lose his memory. There were no tests for Alzheimer's then. James reads to me from his iPad. It is an excerpt from Albertus's teachings, compiled by the late theologian Réginald Marie Garrigou-Lagrange, considered the twentieth century's greatest student of Albertus and Aquinas. The excerpt is a bit dense for me, but meant to take hold. "The goods of the intellect are our knowledge, our talents. . . . We must learn to ignore curiosity, vain glory, useless natural eagerness ... placing ourselves at the service of God, detaching ourselves from our own lights."

James reads on from Garrigou-Lagrange: "Our memory inclines to see things horizontally on the line of time that flees, of which the present alone is real, between the past that is gone, and the future that is not yet. . . . But the chief defect of our memory is what scripture calls the proneness to forget God. Our memory, which is made to recall to us what is most important, often forgets the one thing necessary, which is above time and does not pass."

I come to realize that it's fitting to forget myself, while embracing the light from wisdom, putting on what St. Paul calls "the mind of Christ" when he writes to the first Christians in Corinth (1 Cor. 2:16).

God's mind doesn't atrophy, though mine will someday, but only in body.

James leaves, and I sit alone again in silence, surrounded by memories of photos, news clips, and memorabilia from the last seven decades. But memory isn't everything, just the glue of one's life.

My Elmer's bottle is empty, and so in Alzheimer's, I reach daily for the paper clips of the mind, a reserve of mental fasteners to hold the dots of a thought together as the brain functions like a laptop frozen in a software pinch, displaying a disturbing rainbow-colored icon that spins at high speeds, declaring the computer is not engaged. Everything is shut down.

My brain, on this day, is not responding. The rainbow icon is spinning again. Back in my office, the imagery of my memory, I look for reinforcement in a picture of my mother on the wall; the picture of my grandfather is behind me. I think about what's to come. Dismissively, I start writing the "B-roll" of my obit in a staccato style, mimicking apocryphal obits that newspaper buddies and I used to draft over a few beers after a deadline, a style that William Randolph Hearst would relish: "Dead. That's what Greg O'Brien is today."

But today is not the day. I am caught again in the mirror of infinity—seeing the past, confused in the present, and preparing to head to Pluto, Sedna, and beyond for the final staging, at peace with revelations of the present, the security of not having to hold onto the past.

The wind has shifted again. The rusted iron cod on the weathervane at the gable end of my barn is pointing to the southwest, yet another warning of foul weather fast approaching from the nor'east. I sit alone in a high-back Elizabethan chair, the same seat occupied at my parents' dinner table on Sunday nights in Eastham. I am deep into solitary, probing thought. Inside the mind of Alzheimer's isn't such a bad place to be on this cloudy fall day. There's a clarity to it, as I await the sunrise of a new morning, secure that the sun will set at dusk, hoping to see it rise yet again, knowing one day it will not, as I drift further out into the Milky Way looking for my mother.

PART TWO

BEYOND
a Diagnosis

16

New Horizons

New horizons come at a cost—physically, spiritually, and principally out in space. In deep space, as in Alzheimer's, the question becomes: What next?

To probe deeper into the Milky Way, one must finesse the Kuiper Belt on the galaxy's outer edge, dodging more than a hundred million ancient icy masses and particles, the Placentia of our universe, and maybe even ducking nomadic rogue planets untethered to a star, or rogue stars untethered to the galaxy. The National Academy of Sciences ranks probing the Kuiper Belt the highest priority of solar system exploration.

NASA's intrepid spacecraft *New Horizons* has explored beyond imaginable reach with a historic flyby in July 2015 of the dwarf planet Pluto, coming within 7,700 miles of the icy sphere after traveling 4.6 billion miles, and now heading deeper into the Kuiper Belt, then out into interstellar space, drifting in an endless sea of the cosmos in the hopes, perhaps, of landing in the palm of God's hands. All this assumes that *New Horizons*, the size of a baby grand piano and carrying the ashes of the American astronomer Clyde Tombaugh, who discovered Pluto, can also avoid a spate of isolated black holes, celestial bodies with gravitational pulls so intense that light cannot escape. Roosevelt would be some impressed.

Pluto, equally spellbinding with a surface temperature of minus 400 degrees Fahrenheit, is a word picture of new horizons: with its nitrogen ice glaciers; Big Bang-induced nitrogen rivers; water ice mountains and the likelihood of ice volcanos; a hazy atmosphere that paints a blue halo around the planet; and now the possibility of an underground icy sea beneath the planet's "heart" region, about 62 miles deep and containing as much water as all the earth's seas and a salt content similar to California's Dead Sea, according to planetary scientists studying *New Horizons'* findings. Yes, Pluto has a heart, formed primarily by huge glaciers of nitrogen ice the shape of a heart, spattered across almost half the planet's surface. To observing scientists, the celestial body clearly speaks today from its heart, as those in the depths of Alzheimer's.

The parallel lingers.

While liquid water is a vital ingredient, Pluto is not a prime candidate for life, though Massachusetts Institute of Technology planetary scientist Richard Binzel told the *Huffington Post*, "One is careful to never say the word impossible."

What's possible now is that Pluto might have its planet status restored. A group of NASA scientists have proposed a new definition of what determines a planet, which the International Astronomical Union (IAU) is reviewing. The IAU makes such determinations; earlier it stripped Pluto of its planetary standing because "it has not cleared its neighboring region of other objects," the only one of three planet criteria that Pluto does not meet.

The question of Pluto's very existence has been debated from the start. What we cannot discern, we often fear, then deny.

New Horizons has discovered astonishing revelations of Pluto, once viewed as just a speck of light—yet another striking example, as it is with Alzheimer's, of the need to explore beneath the surface. The findings of *New Horizons* have reinforced within me a metaphorical analogy between the dense isolation of Pluto and Alzheimer's. With greater education, perhaps Pluto does, in fact, reclaim its planet status, the little engine that could. If there was ever a more perfect Alzheimer's metaphor, it's the dwarf planet Pluto and the Kuiper Belt. If you want to understand the isolation of Alzheimer's and other dementias, just look at the stark photos and illustrations online, black holes and all, an alternate definition of which is "a place where people and things disappear without a trace."

It is the mission of Dr. Rudy Tanzi to do the impossible—to fight like hell so those with Alzheimer's don't disappear without a trace. Dr. Tanzi, a renowned neuroscientist, a professor of Neurology at Harvard, holder of the Joseph P. and Rose F. Kennedy Endowed Chair in Neurology, serves at Massachusetts General Hospital in Boston as the vice-chair of Neurology and director of the Genetics and Aging Research Unit. He is also chairman of the groundbreaking Cure Alzheimer's Fund Research Consortium, one of the world's finest Alzheimer's research initiatives.

Dr. Tanzi has become a close friend. His expert advice and supplemental recommendations, beyond prescribed medications, have helped to keep my head above water. Regarding supplements, he recommends plant-based omega 3s, DHA and EPA, which support a healthy functioning of the brain and cardiovascular system, and Niagen, which supports cellular health in the brain. Worth a Google.

Rudy knows the starkness of Pluto. He has co-discovered three of the first known Alzheimer's disease genes, and has identified several others in the Alzheimer's Genome Project, which he directs. He has published nearly 500 research papers, and has received the highest awards in his field, including the Metropolitan Life Foundation Award and Potamkin Prize. In addition, he received the 2015 Smithsonian American Ingenuity Award, and was named to the 2015 list of *Time* magazine's "100 Most Influential People in the World." Tanzi also has co-authored several books; among them: *Decoding Darkness*, *New York Times* bestseller *Super Brain*, and *Super Genes*. And has been named by *GQ* magazine as a Rock Star of Science; in his "spare" time he takes off his lab coat and plays keyboard with the iconic band Aerosmith, with Aerosmith guitarist Joe Perry as part of the Joe Perry Project, and with singer Chris Mann. He has recorded with Johnny Depp and performed with Iggy Pop and Zak Starkley. Tanzi's close friend Perry is a founding father of the Rock Stars of Science program, whose mission encompasses fundraising and outreach for research for life-threatening diseases. At Aerosmith sessions, Tanzi has been directed to play like "a drunken church lady."

Isn't that special…

Tanzi, whose research is energized by his keyboard play, observes, "If I don't play music…my creativity is just not at peak."

If anyone can unravel the plaques and tangles of Alzheimer's with peak performance, it will be Tanzi. Not long ago with colleague Doo Yeon Kim, Tanzi created what has been termed "Alzheimer's in a dish"—human brain cells in a petri dish that cultivate the markers of Alzheimer's, making it possible for scientists to discern the Pluto-like features of Alzheimer's and better comprehend countless state-of-the-art drugs that might curb this mind-blowing disease.

Who better on earth to place one's trust in? I will roll dice with Rudy any day! Alzheimer's is deeply personal to him; it stole his grandmother. Ever sanguine, Tanzi, when asked if there would ever be a cure for Alzheimer's, told the *Boston Globe*, "Cure is an interesting word."

My thesaurus says that "interesting" is a synonym for "thought-provoking."

Looking below the surface in thought-provoking ways, one has to dig, literally scrape, for a cure. Rudy has the dynamite in hand. Yet while a cure, or partial cure, is on a new horizon, it is not within grasp at the moment. There are numerous, impressive clinical trials in the works, and major pharmaceuticals, like Biogen, Eli Lilly, Otsuka, and others, are working overtime with a degree and mix of success.

George Vradenburg, co-founder and chairman of the distinguished Washington, D.C.-based national and international advocacy organization UsAgainstAlzheimer's (usagainstalzheimers.org) and also a good friend, has said that the first person cured of Alzheimer's will come from a clinical trial. Tanzi agrees. And they are correct. But it's hard to put a smiley face on this.

Tanzi and Vradenburg are a tag team on research and political fronts. I think of them in some ways as the World Wrestling Association champions of the late '80s, the "Brain Busters." Vradenburg also is co-founder of the Global Alzheimer's Platform (GAP) Foundation (globalalzplatform.org) and a conveyor of the Global CEO Initiative on Alzheimer's Disease (ceoalzheimersinitiative.org). He has testified before Congress about the global Alzheimer's pandemic, and was named by Obama Administration U.S. Health and Human Services Secretary Kathleen Sebelius to serve on the Advisory Council on Research, Care, and Services established by the National Alzheimer's Project Act. He also is a member of the World Dementia Council.

There's not a minute to waste, as the soul-searching NOVA/PBS documentary *Alzheimer's: Every Minute Counts* details. Produced and directed by Emmy Award-winning Elizabeth Arledge and Emmy Award-winning executive producer Gerry Richmond, the film is a wake-up call about the national threat, medical and fiscal, that Alzheimer's poses—one of the most critical health crises facing the nation and the world. The documentary explores the dire social and economic consequences unless a medical breakthrough is discovered. The film comes on the heels of another ground-breaking NOVA/PBS documentary, *Can Alzheimer's Be Stopped?* Produced and directed by Emmy Award-winning filmmaker Sarah Holt, the documentary explores the work of key medical researchers as they gather clues to reconstruct the molecular chain of events that ultimately leads to dementia, and follows top researchers, like Tanzi and others, into the field as they develop leading theories of this cryptic disease.

In the documentary *Every Minute Counts,* Tanzi states, "Alzheimer's is the biggest epidemic we have in this country. I'm shocked that people are not panicked about what this disease is going to do to the country or to their families…. It's only going to get worse, because right now we have no drugs that can stop the progress of this disease…. Over the last five years there has been much more awareness of the huge problem that Alzheimer's represents in our society, and we're starting to see the benefits of that. It's still a drop in the bucket. Given how big this problem is, given how much we know, what we can do, and how little we're doing with the knowledge we have, we need 10 times more (resources). We need billions of dollars per year thrown at this disease."

Notes Vradenburg in the documentary, "Alzheimer's is an epic disease. It will take us down. This disease will take us down. I think it's no question that in fact Alzheimer's will be the financial sinkhole of the 21st century."

Still, Vradenburg and Tanzi remain hopeful about the future, assuming that federal appropriations increase dramatically, along with participation in clinical trials.

Far more volunteers are needed for a range of clinical trials, available in medical, research, and pharmaceutical centers around the world, and through organizations like the Alzheimer's Association, UsAgainstAlzheimer's, and the Cure Alzheimer's Fund, and others.

"This is a battle, I believe, we're going to win because we're going to lose so many along the way," says Vradenburg in an interview. "Research will give us some insights, but to develop state-of-the-art medicines to delay the symptoms of Alzheimer's and ultimately stop the disease, we will need legions of individuals in clinical trials. This is just the beginning of the beginning of the fight; we have now engaged with the enemy, which has had its run of the field. We've hardly picked up our weapons, but we have begun to engage."

The path to a cure is mind-bending and fraught with disappointments and setbacks. So what does "victory" look like ultimately? Depends on one's perspective. In spite of the best intentions of some of the brightest minds in the world, no one at this point clearly knows. All the more reason that every minute counts. Success, it's been said, has many fathers. Perhaps victory ultimately is defined with medications to slow the progression of the disease, either before or after the onset of symptoms. While that's encouraging, many of those imprisoned in the throes of the disease with terrifying symptoms are not looking for an extension, a "weekend pass," an even slower death. We'd choose a ten-year sentence over a life term.

The focus rightly needs to be on intervention and prevention at the earliest stage, if possible.

Alzheimer's, Tanzi says, can begin with brain pathology when one is 40 years old or earlier, decades before the onset of symptoms that can run progressively another 15-25 years, taking one into their 80s or 90s. If you peel back the 5 million Americans "diagnosed" with Alzheimer's today, the number stricken is probably double or triple that, which might make Alzheimer's close to the top killer in the nation. Many with the disease in early stages are undiagnosed, under-reported, or doctors decline to tell patients of a diagnosis, given that there is no cure. Alzheimer's, recent studies suggest, has moved from the nation's sixth deadliest killer to the third. Alzheimer's is now the leading killer in England and Wales, both of which have better reporting systems.

"While our life span is increasing, our brains are not keeping up with it," says Tanzi.

From 1999 to 2014, deaths in the U.S. from Alzheimer's rose by more than 50 percent, and the death rate is expected to continue to climb as the nation's aging population and life expectancy increases.

In the meantime, to help contain the beast, what's good for the heart is good for the brain, Tanzi notes. In summary, a combination of exercise, sleep, a good diet, and social interaction may be the best medication available today to stem an onslaught of Alzheimer's.

"Regular exercise is the number one preventative; it helps stop brain inflammation, a big part of this disease," Tanzi said during a recent panel discussion in Boston in which we both participated.

"Exercise induces the birth of new stem cells in the short-term memory area of the brain."

The second most important shield, Tanzi adds, is sound sleep—seven or eight hours a night, "mental floss," as Tanzi calls it, noting lack of proper sleep has been linked to cognitive decline.

Many assume that when one sleeps, the brain slumbers as well. But that's not the case, says Tanzi, who notes that the brain is far more active in sleep than during daytime. Healthy sleep, he adds, is needed to hit the "save" key on memories, processing a bolus of information and stimuli encountered in daily activities. "Deep sleep is a time in the sleep cycle when the brain cleans itself out and recycles brain toxins," he says. "Deep sleep is the only time the brain does not produce amyloids that create plaque and disrupts brain functions. I used to pride myself on just four or five hours of sleep a night. Now I religiously get seven or eight. If not, I might as well be smoking, or sitting on a couch at night eating two bags of potato chips."

Tanzi says a healthy diet also is critical in fighting Alzheimer's, most notably the Mediterranean diet that has been shown to be most effective in reducing Alzheimer's risk—more fiber, more olive oil, less butter, more fruits, nuts, less red meat, more fish, vegetables, and other sources of protein. So watch the chips!

Tanzi also urges to keep socially and mentally active.

"Constantly learn new things, not just playing brain games," he counsels in scientific terms. "Every time you learn something new, you're making connections between the nerve cells, increasing synapse and building up a synaptic reserve. Loss of synapse correlates most with a degree of dementia. For a healthy retirement, a synaptic reserve is as essential as a financial reserve. An active lifestyle will also help in managing and reducing stress, which causes inflammation of the brain—the production of toxic brain chemicals. Studies now show that stress management and forms of meditation help fight the biomarkers of Alzheimer's."

The race to fight the biomarkers is an all-out sprint, but could someday, many predict, end at a perilous intersection of medicine and science—"artificial intelligence," and that's not necessarily a good thing. All the more reason world governments need to dig deeper to appropriate critical research funding. Playing God and Frankenstein are at polar opposites for a cure in the natural.

While artificial intelligence—technology that mimics or one day exceeds human reasoning—is programmed to achieve directed goals, some critics are concerned about harmful ways of achieving those goals. Computers have no soul, just a mission, not to mention the autonomous weapons armed with artificial intelligence and calibrated to annihilate. As humans, it's been said, we preside day-to-day over the planet not because we're the toughest, fittest, or swiftest, the animal kingdom dominates that, but because we're the most intelligent. Move over, *I, Robot* is on its way, coming to a neighborhood near you someday. Theoretical physicist and cosmologist Stephen Hawkings warns that the rise of robots, hence artificial intelligence, could be disastrous for mankind. We all await the verdict. I'm not convinced that robots are the remedy, nor are others.

I have faith in the natural, and am inspired by individuals like Stephen Wiltshire, a nationally renowned British artist with autism, who was mute as a young boy. Wiltshire can draw from memory landscapes in exact detail after viewing them once. Experts believe that unique wiring between right and left hemispheres in the brain allows Wiltshire and others like him to tap into creative reserves. I am also intrigued with what experts call "neuroplasticity" or brain plasticity, a natural process of building new pathways in the brain when neurons go silent—in short, the potential for neural networks to alter connections, recruiting the brain.

And then there's what's called "endless memory." Take the remarkable case of savant-like Marilu Henner, award-winning actress, producer, author and radio host, best known for her role as gutsy, spicy Elaine O'Connor Nardo on the sitcom *Taxi* from 1978 to

1983, winner of 18 Emmy Awards. Henner has the ability to recall the slightest detail of nearly every day, endless memory. There are only a few cases worldwide of this extraordinary capability called Highly Superior Auto-Bibliographical Memory, H-Sam as it's sometimes called. I've had the pleasure of meeting Henner, author of *Total Memory Makeover*, which attempts to help others unlock memories. Henner, inspiring in a natural way beyond belief, is a thinking machine.

"Recalling memories is kind of like karaoke," she once told CNN. "You know the first one is hard, then you can't get the microphone away from people. You start opening up those memories, and it's just a floodgate…"

Greek myths are replete with stories about "thinking machines" and artificial beings, like Pygmalion's Galatea, the bronze robot of Hephaestus, and the Talos of Crete—an ancient urge to become more godlike that persists today. While artificial intelligence began as a discipline to create computers and software capable of intelligent behavior, the science has now expanded to the implantation of memory chips and chasing metaphors of the mind. Juggling the balance between cutting-edge science and ethics is a perilous high-wire act without a net. Faced with a choice of natural intelligence or artificial, many of us with Alzheimer's would chose to go quietly into the night, as science expands to new horizons of the artificial, wrought with the unpredictable. Imagine the possibility of a memory chip in the brain, surfing the internet, downloading novels, and thinking faster than a speeding bullet, more powerful than a locomotive. Look…up in the brain, it's a bird, it's a plane; no, it's a robot, super intelligence. Think of the domination, the extension of it.

There are some whacky stories today of robots getting married, and closer to home some news agencies are turning, at times, to "robo-journalists." Reports CNN, "They don't call journalists 'hacks' for nothing. At large news agencies where speed is crucial, template-style stories have long been used for company results, allowing journalists to simply key in the relevant facts and numbers, and fire off the dispatch. Often disparagingly referred to as 'churnalism,' some of the larger media organizations . . . have now turned to robots to take the grind out of formulaic dispatches."

Surely, this will drive the "fake news" vigilantes batty.

Then there's "human gene editing" on the world's horizon, "a once unthinkable proposition: the modification of human embryos to create genetic traits that can be passed down to future generations," the *New York Times* reports. The "ethical mind field" could lead the boutique design of babies—much smarter, healthier, more attractive, and far more successful individuals than nature can produce. The technology, pursued aggressively in countries like China and Sweden, might one day result in a "master race," perhaps a modern-day version of *Flowers for Algernon.*

Consider also the futuristic hypothetical process of Whole Brain Emulation (WBE) or "brain uploading" to a digital platform, a perceived process of scanning one's long-term and short-term memory into a computer that could run a simulation model of the brain, considered virtual reality, a "life extension," by the researchers.

Shoot me in the head, please...

Where are we heading in the name of science? Are such implantations and manifestations substitutes for natural cures? I wish I was smart enough to know; the questions need to be deeply probed.

Cure is an interesting word.

In the 1966 Daniel Keyes novel, *Flowers for Algernon*, later adapted to the Academy Award-winning film, *Charly*, starring Cliff Robertson, a laboratory mouse named Algernon undergoes surgery to increase intelligence by artificial means. Robertson's character, Charly Gordon, is a severely intellectually disabled adult who endures the same procedure, which triples his IQ, becoming a genius, stunning everyone, including his teacher Alice Kinnian, played by Claire Bloom. The two ultimately fall in love, a romance of frenetic turns. In the end, Algernon's high intelligence begins to diminish, and the mouse dies. Charly then comprehends that his brilliance, too, is fleeting, and he withdraws. In the final scene, Alice watches Charly playing with children in a community playground, relapsed to his former self.

There's a bit of Charly in all of us in Alzheimer's and other forms of dementia; the natural overwhelming the artificial on new horizons. Like the Pluto spacecraft itself, we're all on a journey to unknown places. There is purpose, often at times when we don't think so. My life now has become a series of anecdotes, revelations in this journey, as I learn from others, taking copious notes in the place of the soul, as angels visit and the demons chase—teaching moments, as with all my brothers and sisters in this disease. We mirror one another. Life instructs in its narratives, if one listens.

New horizons come at a cost.

17

The Demons Were Chasing

The demons were chasing, faster and faster. I could hear the screeching howls, the pounding pursuit through a canopy of thick oak and red maple trees that enshroud Lower Road beside a dense, choking groundcover of honeysuckle and myrtle. Like the sea fog that rolls in at intervals over the mud flats, the demons were disorienting.

I had to sprint, a full-out panic dash, to avoid capture at sundown. The heart was pounding; the sweat pouring. The monsters were gaining on me, ready for the pounce. As a hazy spring afternoon gave way to dusk in pastoral Brewster on Outer Cape Cod, a numbing fog crept in like a headless horseman—first in misty sprays that tingle, then in thick blankets that penetrate the mind, disorientate the senses, rising slowly from the base of the neck to the forehead. Alone, I was enveloped in fear and full paranoia; it had a smell of wind chill from a raging North Atlantic storm, the kind of nor'easter that takes the breath away. In the moment, there was no escape. The mind plays tricks.

At full gait, I hurried past Brewster's fecund community garden with its impenetrable stalks of corn that stood in sturdy platoons, dashed by a forest of moss-covered locust trees bent in grim serpentine forms, then sprinted, feet barely touching the ground, past the ancient cemetery of sea captains where Rhoda Mayo was buried in 1783; Dean Gray in 1796; and Rev. Otis Bacon in 1848, who "fell asleep in Jesus," as his gravestone declares.

Where was Jesus now? The demons were advancing as a blazing red sun dipped into Cape Cod Bay to be doused like a candle. Faster and faster, they chased. Today, I beat them with every ounce of will in me. But they will be back with a vengeance. Alzheimer's plays tricks on the mind.

My life, once a distance run, is now a race for survival.

There was a time before my diagnosis that I ran six miles a day along bucolic back roads of the Outer Cape, at least one at a six-minute mile pace. Not bad for a guy then in his late 50s. I ran for the simple love of it; the solitude was soothing, listening to the caw of herring gulls, the chirp of peepers, the cry of black-bellied whistling ducks. Now all I hear is the chilling hoots of a barred owl. My mind is dead to the song of shorebirds as I run to jumpstart my brain at the end of the day, a process akin to crank starting a chainsaw after it has sat overnight on a New England deck in February. You gotta rip at it to get it. So I rip; I run until my legs give out along these country roads that have given way to a frightening labyrinth of confusion that echoes muscle memory to the haunted forest of Oz. Just follow the yellow brick road, I tell myself. We're off to see the Wizard! Yet the Wizard has no cure. Still, I look for the signposts.

My progression of Alzheimer's advances as the lights go faint in the brain.

So I run from the demons of illusions, confusion, rage, and ongoing depression. My daily running routine has become symbolic of the chase, a race ultimately I will lose. Running for me flicks the light back on; it calms the rage, like letting steam out of a boiling teakettle. Running helps to reboot my mind so I can do what I love most— write, think, and focus; it restores physical and mental stamina. If I'm not running, I'm moving backwards in Alzheimer's, into the hands of a pack of forbidding demons.

The demons now have chased me inside. I no longer run on back roads where I get wholly lost in fears and confusion. On a recent Christmas, I was given a family gift of glow-in-the-dark running attire, resembling a Department of Public Works (DPW) vest and pants; the gift that keeps on giving, I was told. The family, concerned that I'd get lost, wander off, or get hit by a bread truck, was pleased with the giving. I was pissed! The gift came with phosphorescent sneaker laces that made me look like an alien from *Men in Black*. Again, more loss of control.

Then there's the "Where's Waldo" app, an iPhone GPS application that my wife and kids obtained to determine my location at all times, "for my own good," of course. For me, it was yet more loss of control and freedom, but reassurance for family that I wouldn't fall off the edge of Cape Cod, as Columbus and crew feared centuries ago on a broader scale.

I wish the world were flat; no dizziness then. My family makes me dizzy enough. In my hometown of Rye, New York, near the train station to Manhattan, is a restful tavern called the Rye Grill. At an extended family gathering there a few years ago, my wife told my siblings and some close family friends about the "Where's Waldo" app. Instantly, they all wanted a copy. Again, it angered me; more loss of control. Some of my brothers, sisters, and friends were giddy about tracking me, all wanting the app to determine my course to the bar, bathroom, buffet table, and beyond. They were all yucking it up.

So I did what any respecting Irishmen would do after a close childhood friend at the function told me he had to drive north a few miles to Connecticut to pick something up. I asked him to take my iPhone with the "Where's Waldo" app as a diversion.

"That ought to fix 'em!" The Irish never get mad.

In an instant, my buddy was gone, up Route 95.

"Oh my God!" roared family and friends monitoring my trajectory. "Greg is on Route 95 heading north."

I waited by the door of the Rye Grill as those monitoring my GPS progress came sprinting out.

"I'm not dead yet," I told them. "So don't screw with me…"

I've retreated now inside to the treadmill at the gym in Orleans where I must hold onto the railings so I don't lose my balance. The monsters have followed me here. They taunt me with loss of self, greater rage, and thoughts of suicide.

Early on a damp fall evening about two years ago, the rage inside was crushing. I was determined to outrun these fiends, hot on the chase. Survival was then, as today, defined as an extreme sprint, a personal record. So I asked a young, angelic-looking woman at the counter to clock my run.

"No one will believe this," I told her.

She obliged.

I held the railings tight, looked straight ahead, and imagined the run of my life. I was going to beat these demons today, kick their ass. At the half-mile mark, my timer—the slight, honey-blonde woman— informed me my time was three minutes, five seconds. Not fast enough, I thought. Not fast enough. My pursuers were gaining. "Not today," I kept telling myself. "Not today!"

A minute later, the young woman, concerned at the pace, asked me, "Mr. O'Brien, should you be doing this?"

"My dear," I replied, panting hard, running crazy fast. "You're asking me the wrong question. The questions is: could you be doing this when you're 60?"

She cheered me on. "You run like Superman," she said. At the stroke of a mile, my time was a personal record of five minutes, twenty seconds. I beat the monsters that day, and impressed a young woman. "Faster than a speeding bullet…more powerful than a locomotive."

I'm unable now to run as I once did, as the day I set my personal record at the gym. Alzheimer's breaks the mind, then the body down. But running has become my best friend, and doctors have told me to ramp it up.

Researchers believe that running may enhance mood, and for those with mild to moderate Alzheimer's, it may also improve some brain functions that affect daily living, according to an article in the December 15, 2015 issue of *Runner's World*. In "Exercise May Be the Best Weapon Against Alzheimer's," Alison Wade reported: "And for those at high risk of developing the disease, physical activity may do even more: A growing body of research indicates regular cardiovascular exercise can protect the brain and delay the onset of Alzheimer's symptoms, improving both cognition and quality of life."

At a recent Alzheimer's Association International Conference, Laura D. Baker, PhD, an associate professor of gerontology and geriatric medicine at the Wake Forest School of Medicine, presented study results that suggest exercise might be able to do what drugs so far cannot in those at high risk for developing Alzheimer's: slow the progression of the disease. Wade reported: "[Baker's] study revealed that after six months, participants who built up to exercising at an elevated heart rate for 30 minutes, four times a week, improved their cognition and had decreased levels of phosphorylated tau protein compared to those in a stretching-only control group. Scientists use tau protein levels as a measure of how Alzheimer's disease is progressing. The protein naturally increases with age in everyone, but in people with Alzheimer's, it increases considerably more. In Baker's study, the exercise group saw a slight *decrease* in their levels after six months."

No drug currently approved has had the same effect.

So I run. I will run until I drop.

The demons were back again months later with a vengeance.

I was driving in the early evening along Stony Brook Road, about a half mile from my house, a primal place, as it meanders through the scrub oak, pitch pine, and kettle hole remnants from the last great ice age. Interrupting the solitude like the crack of a shotgun, a deer darted across the road—or at least what my mind told me was a deer. I am not sure, nor are my doctors. Flashback 25 years ago when a buck destroyed the front end of my Toyota station wagon, I instinctively turned my reliable yellow Jeep to the right to avoid an oncoming crash.

The Jeep hit an embankment, crashed through a granite stone wall, went airborne about 15 feet into the parking lot of Our Lady of the Cape Church, crashed meteoric impact, rolled twice, ripping off the top of the roof—my head hitting the windshield with such a force that it splintered the glass, strewing boxes of the first edition of *On Pluto*, like cards dealt at the Bellagio in Vegas, into the rain-soaked parking lot of the church.

My head was numb and bleeding; Pluto was never closer. Within minutes, the local police and an ambulance were on the scene. I was quickly strapped to a gurney, raced to the hospital, and told that I should not have not walked away from the crash, the third time I had escaped a certain death.

My son, Conor, at the time was at home in the family room, and noticed a police officer walking down our steps to the door. Conor thought the worst. "I couldn't breathe," he told me later. "I opened the door and burst into tears, without the officer even saying a word. God bless him, the officer instinctively knew the fear and said: 'Your Dad is ok.' It was so terrifying seeing you in Cape Cod Hospital that night…"

The crash occurred in the parking lot of the church where we had my mother's funeral after she had succumbed to Alzheimer's.

Do you believe in angels?

My brother Tim does.

Weeks later, I got a text from him. "You'll never believe what just happened…"

I called him immediately. Driving in the middle lane north of New Haven on I-95 in Connecticut on an icy highway, the car in the right lane skidded into Tim's yellow Jeep, pushing it into the passing lane where it collided with another car. It was a sandwich of a crash, one that Tim should not have walked away from; his yellow Jeep was totaled and the front axle snapped in half. Tim was told the angels had favor upon him.

Mom, in death, was making a point, protecting her boys in the consequence of frightful accidents. Two yellow Jeeps, the color of angels, bought to captivate a mother in her final days, were both gone. She no longer needed the protection; we did. She was speaking from Heaven.

There are consequences in life for everything, as there should be, and my personal physician and a surrogate brother, Dr. Barry Conant, in consult with Brewster Police Chief Dick Koch, revoked my right to drive at night after the accident, just to be sure, given ongoing progressions of the disease. It was a stunning loss of freedom for me, a loss that others in this disease suffer eventually.

Barry and I meet often over coffee to talk about life and the pitch count. Barry also is a role model for me and others shipwrecked in this fight and other bouts on the shoals of medical trials.

Shipwrecks ever stir the soul. The intense isolation of being lost at sea is deeply penetrating. As I stare up over morning coffee at a watercolor of the British schooner *Walter Miller*, which was stranded and wrecked in a dense fog on Nauset Bar off Outer Cape Cod in the late 1800s, I can't help but think of the hopelessness of the moment.

Cape Cod is a graveyard for shipwrecks. Since the early 1600s, more than 3,000 ships have run aground in the treacherous shoals of the Cape's Great Outer Beach, from Provincetown to Chatham. Yet, turning despair into hope 121 years ago, the villagers queued up in a fierce nor'easter to shoot a rope line from the beach to the *Walter Miller* to attach a breeches buoy—a crude rope rescue device with an ancient leather harness—to rescue the crew, pulling them to shore, heave-ho by heave-ho.

I am having breakfast today with Barry, one of the modern-day Outer Cape villagers. In the roiling waters of Baby Boomers bracing for end times, Barry and I are both shipwrecked, feeling the isolation of grounding on the shoals of inveterate disease. There is no breeches buoy for the two of us, no heave-ho from the shore; the rescue rope goes out only so far.

And so we talk casually over scrambled eggs about the shifting sands of life and forgotten promises of a generation. However, the elephant in the room is the collective poignancy of the moment. "My goal, as I exit, is to be in harmony with the divine," says Barry.

I nod in quiet agreement.

Our regular Saturday breakfasts are akin to an encounter in *Tuesdays with Morrie*, only with both of us in the role of Morrie. Two guys trying to beat the curve, dead men still walking. Barry, at 60, has pancreatic cancer with a 12-percent chance of survival within the next three years; he also has a defibrillator in his chest, an inherited heart condition.

And so, the two of us press on. Today is a roundtable of future promise, not failures of the past, for which there are many. We are card-carrying members of the once-invincible Baby Boomer generation.

The doctor and the patient, we are cut from different cloths, yet we recognize the parallels between us. Look between two facing mirrors, and one can see a seemingly endless line of images fading into the distance. In principle, it's called "looking into infinity." Each mirror reflects the image into the other mirror, bouncing these reflections back and forth into infinity—gateways, some speculate, to parallel universes.

Barry and I today stand at the gateway. Together, we embrace the moment in a reflection of the past, with anticipation of what is to come. "Every day now, I feel that I'm put in a different classroom to learn a particular thing," Barry says, as we share a third pot of coffee. "That's what keeps me going—probing the heart beyond rote rules and regulations." The son of a strict Baptist minister from Long Island, New York, Barry calls himself a "recovering, fundamentalist Baptist, who has become Unitarian in his understanding of the divine." The father of two, he is an avid fisherman on Cape Cod Bay, where at low tide the water flows out for almost a mile with the pull of the moon, exposing soft ripples of mud flats, just below the surface, flush with steamers, quahog, and razor clams. Years ago, he sought to catch as many fish as possible. The bigger the trophy the better.

He is different now. The cancer has changed him, softened the drive of this Hemingway prototype of *The Old Man and the Sea*. He now throws as many fish back as he lugs to his backyard grill overlooking the bay. Live and let live. Barry has the eye of an eagle and the soul of a pastor. He watches intently for the laughing gulls, black gulls, and terns that dive for baitfish, sand eels, and baby herring, known in these parts as bay anchovies. He knows that the bluefish and stripers will chase the bait. Barry says you can fish on the flats for two hours—an hour before and after low tide—without having to worry. The tide, as it is with aging, creeps in deceptively.

Looking out at the horizon, Barry says one cannot discern the tidal flow, and if caught unaware, the swim back is a long haul in waters where Great Whites have been spotted. "Not a place," counsels the doctor, "for a guy like you with Alzheimer's."

"But if you're careful and going out in the early evening, the sunsets are indescribably beautiful," he says. "The sun dips into a watery horizon, and as the candle is extinguished, the light fades up."

So it is with life, he notes.

Barry and me, the doctor and the patient, we learn from one another, as the roles keep reversing in this conversation.

"I accept that my life today is not a long-term plan," says Barry. "I think we are all eternal souls that, for the moment, are given mortal and physical bodies to learn and to understand the universe, to be more at peace with what we have been given this day.

"We are part of a greater, eternal whole, but the vast majority does not recognize this, allowing themselves to be distracted by self-imposed, day-to-day stresses, and exploiting unhealthy behaviors to muffle the voice of the god inside them—to stifle the search for a place beyond memory." I can relate, for I am gripped with memory, the loss of it, as I strive to speak and write from the heart, not the head, as I once did. I chase now a freeing spirit, much like a gifted athlete "in the zone," or a master artist with a brush and a kaleidoscope of colors within reach. Perseverance separates the artist from the dabbler. As you lose self, one finds self—the dichotomy of two opposites happening at once. The bright guys might call this quantum physics. I call it the journey from the embryo to the soul.

Barry is searching himself, a path perhaps more discernible for those with cancer, Alzheimer's, AIDS, ALS, Parkinson's, Huntington's disease, or any number of vile diseases that attack the soul as well as the body. "I hope to be at peace if the cancer takes me out, remembering that my soul will remain eternal in a different plane of existence, still learning and resonating even more with the divine," he observes.

Barry says he tries to ignore fear, rising above it.

I tell him that I am motivated by fear. But today we find each other along this journey, seeking the essence of truth, trying to separate the real from the imagined. A favorite Old Testament scripture, I note, is Isaiah 6:8: "Then I heard the voice of the Lord saying, 'Whom shall I send? And who will go for us?' And I said, 'Here am I. Send me!'"

Ultimately, whatever direction we are sent, our timelines are in place, the tumblers are clicking. We are grateful for the tick.

And so, I ask Barry, what he would do if he knew today was to be his last?

Barry says he hopes all his regrets would be gone, all his apposite goodbyes delivered to family and friends. "I'd like to be able to say a loving, yet temporary goodbye to my wife and kids, then wade out into the flats of Cape Cod Bay, remembering who and what I am."

I tell him that I'd walk the beach, a place that has always given me solace. Maybe I'll see him casting a line.

Barry and I have coffee together frequently; it's the equivalent for me of a doctor's visit. I hate the sterile feel of a doctor's office, and Barry knows it. One recent summer day, he invited me to the Snowy Owl, a funky coffee shop just down the street from my house that he frequents. It was the first time I had been there. Named after a yellow-eyed, black-beaked bird with thick plumage and heavily feathered talons, the Snowy Owl has the look of a rustic barn inside, with 200-year-old reclaimed wooden planks that line the walls and ceiling. The place is always packed with locals, and the noise at times can be thunderous. Barry noticed my confusion, incapacity to connect the dots, and suggested we sit outside on a long stone wall. Halfway through the conversation that began with a discussion about family, sports, fishing, then corresponding health issues, I spotted a fleet of wild roosters prancing toward me along the top of the wall, the comb of their necks distended like bristles. Barry didn't flinch; didn't notice a thing. I was distressed, and started thinking again of hallucinations that have haunted me. The roosters kept coming. Barry kept talking. I kept sweating. I looked at Barry, gazed back at the mirage of roosters, then said abruptly: "What the shit, Barry? Do you see the roosters?"

"What roosters?" he replied.

"These creepy birds coming for me," I said.

Barry shook his head, looked down at the ground...then started laughing like a little kid.

The roosters were real, part of the barn vibe, and my buddy Barry was just having fun with me. I've always encouraged him to reinforce a sense of normalcy. His laugh made me laugh, the howl of a guy desperately fighting cancer, made me laugh at my own disease. It was a guy moment.

But not everything in life is funny. Not long ago, there was another shipwreck in Barry's life. Cancer returned after four years at bay; this time two nodules were found in his chest, a biopsy had revealed. I had emailed him at Christmas to tell him what an incredible role model he is for me. I didn't hear back. Then weeks later he told me of the discovery and efforts to remove the cancer.

In an email, he wrote, "I did not want to worry you, especially during holidays...so I chose not to share this saga with you. I just didn't see the point in dumping unwelcome news on your life. You certainly have plenty to keep your limited resources tapped out.... If next week's scan shows bad news, I will probably plan to stop working soon. Unlike you, I don't want to work til I drop. I want to have some time and energy for some other things before I get too sick to enjoy them, but I still fervently hope in a year's time that you and I will look back at this few months as having been only a temporary setback and I'll be cancer-free again. I hope and pray you manage to continue to cling to your sweet spot...and I hope and pray I continue to beat the odds with my disease. I want to be around to correct any spelling errors you make quoting me...Love you, Barry."

Good news as of this writing. Barry's cancer has not returned. I keep praying.

Shipwrecks stir the soul.

I gather strength in the journey from many, as do my brothers and sisters in this disease. Another cornerstone of support for me is an old friend, Bob Mumford.

Irish playwright George Bernard Shaw once said about our existence, "Life is no brief candle…. It is a sort of splendid torch, which I've got hold of for the moment, and I want to make it burn as brightly as possible before handing it to future generations."

Bob burns bright today, a remarkable torch to family and friends, as the winds of life seek to douse his spark. I met Bob more than 30 years ago when we were young bucks on Cape Cod; I was a cub reporter, and Bob was a brilliant transportation expert on this fragile spit of land whose population in summer swells to the size of Boston. There's only one way on and one way off this peninsula—a dead end, the shape of a blacksmith's fist and forearm. It is a "wild and rank place," wrote Henry David Thoreau after walking our beaches in the 1850s: "A man may stand there and put all of America behind him." The land here narrows to a seagull swoop; so one has to know their way around to expound on traffic.

Bob still knows his stuff. Age has blessed him with great sagacity; he's now putting all of America—life as he once knew it—behind him.

Months ago, walking on the lip of spring into the eclectic Chocolate Sparrow café on the Outer Cape in Orleans on a tempest of a March day, Bob at a distance looks the picture of health. A handsome man in the fifth decade, his smile is engaging, his handshake strong, his body language poised.

Yet there is something different about him. He is wearing a tight blue ski cap, covering what appears to be tiny white suction cups attached to the head; he's carrying a canvas satchel, the size of a small toaster, with a battery pack and chords that snake beneath the ski cap.

"Every day's a blessing," Bob declares, knowing I'm unaware of his denouement.

"How are you doing?" he asks openly regarding my diagnosis of early-onset Alzheimer's, a disease that he knew robbed my family tree.

"Every day's a blessing," I respond in kind.

I am stunned as Bob takes off his cap.

I fumble for a response, and can only find the words to say, "My God!"

Bob's head is shaved; it's covered with electrodes that on cue, he explains, zaps what is left of a rare, terminal brain tumor. The process is called Novocure; it produces an electric field that disrupts and destroys the cancer cells as they are dividing.

A section of Bob's tumor, as much as possible, was removed last summer at Dana Farber Cancer Center in Boston, along with about 75 percent of his cranium, the part of the skull that encloses the brain. Called the "braincase," the cranium, research tells me later, protects the brain and supports facial structures such as the eyes and ears, holding them in place to collect sensory information most efficiently.

It is hard to imagine losing a "braincase," like an egg rolling off a table.

After the operation when Bob was handed his battery pack lifeline, he asked doctors how long he had to cart it around.

"From six months to forever," he was told.

"How long is forever?" Bob asked.

It's a question many of us ponder today.

Yet Bob, a champion of a man, is sanguine about his state of mind and dreadful memory loss, a mindset we both share. It is dispiriting to lose a thought in a second, 86,400 seconds in a day, not knowing when the next lapse will occur; to stand exposed, and yet stand one's ground, to begin to grasp in fundamental, naked terms, who one really is—the good, the bad, and the ugly. The ugly is haunting; the many things one would like to take back over the years, but cannot—feelings of failure and transgression.

As Baby Boomers, Bob and I are coming of age. Over coffee at a corner table, we reflect on the past. We always thought, until now, that better days lay ahead. Now Bob and I must work to redefine ourselves, as the shadows of life creep in like a fog rolling toward the shoreline. Death by a thousand cuts? We don't see it that way.

"Unfortunately, life is a fatal disease," Bob opines.

I nod my head. "It is what it is," I say.

Aren't we all a bit crazy, swimming against the odds?

The father of two incredible children, Bob was diagnosed a while back after his beautiful, caring wife, Sarah, and friends noticed something was deeply wrong. Bob was off his game, not remembering, losing at times his sense of self.

"You have a problem," doctors told him after tests confirmed that he had a rare glioblastoma multiforme (GBM) brain tumor with only 8,000 known diagnoses, a survival rate of one percent, and the house betting against surviving an operation.

"I dodged a bullet," Bob tells me in full gait, gratified to have survived the procedure and be able to "eat, think, and talk," the basics of life.

"I told my doctor, 'Make sure I come out of this.'"

Bob speaks from the heart, a journey one takes from the cradle to the grave, accelerated by mind-numbing disease.

A lesser man might have sought an easier way out. Not Bob. He defines "fight." Look the word up in Webster's and you might find a synonym that says, "See also Bob Mumford."

Bob indeed is a role model. Years ago, having witnessed firsthand the painful, terrifying slow demise of my grandfather, my mother, and my uncle from Alzheimer's, a death in slow motion, I sought an exit strategy and failed at it—learning, as Bob exemplifies today, that the real measure of an individual is not the stock portfolio, the business card, the material possessions, or good looks, but the fight in one to get up off the mat after getting knocked on your ass. Lying down is a position of defeat. Bob has reinforced this in me. He stands tall, swimming against the odds.

Such challenges are motivation to dig deeper into a cognitive reserve. The process of fighting off symptoms—whether cancer, Alzheimer's, ALS, AIDS, autism, heart disease or any number of vile illnesses—is exhausting, and yet exhilarating, when one succeeds in a forceful fight for clarity.

The conversation between us now moves to nature, as it often does in these parts, to herring and the olfactory phenomena displayed in Atlantic herring, as they make their annual migration at the strike of spring. The fish repeatedly are flushed back by cascading water, hitting their heads on rocks, yet instinctively climbing the ladder again and again. Bob and I relate to that. We are moving by reflex, rather than conscious thought, with an accelerant of humor.

Laughter is a powerful antidote to pain. A good laugh, doctors say, reduces tension and can leave muscles relaxed for up to forty-five minutes. Laughter boosts the immune system, decreases stress hormones, and triggers the release of endorphins—the natural drug of choice.

Bob's grin obscures the blue ski cap. It's another victory for us. And so we live to fight another day.

But that was then. Weeks later, Bob died after a valiant fight. His candle burns brightly in spirit, leading others to light.

18

"Ya Gotta Believe!"

Perhaps more than any individual, Ralph Branca, the legendary Brooklyn Dodger pitcher, taught me about perseverance, unconditional love, and the will never to give in—a lesson for all to follow. Branca pursued endurance as a worldview, even when his memories were fading.

There was a time many years ago when Brooklyn was the world.

Flatbush, Prospect Park, Greenpoint, Gowanus, Bay Ridge, Bensonhurst, Cyprus Hills, Bedford-Stuyvesant, and other sections of the iconic borough that defined America at a time when the Hudson River was the dividing line between east and west. In his enlightened history, *When Brooklyn Was the World, 1920-1957*, author Elliot Willensky captured in freeze frame a time when the street was an amphitheater—stoop ball was king; the Fuller Brush Man had the confidence and swag of a dignitary; jacks and jump rope ruled; neighbors actually spoke to each other; and "stores on wheels" sold fresh-baked goods and fruit washed down with a swig of seltzer.

Norman Rockwell, eat your heart out…

In 1920, the BMT subway reached Brooklyn's outer edge, linking Manhattan to the heartland then of this nation, home to hallowed Ebbets Field in Flatbush at 55 Sullivan Place, which opened in 1913 and sadly closed in 1957 after the Hudson became just a river. A sweet spot in its day, the 35,000-seat Ebbets was home to the venerable Brooklyn Dodgers, who captured, for a time, the sports imagination and the resolve of a country.

Enter Ralph Branca, June 12, 1944, a strapping, giant of a man, a gifted pitcher from the mound to his Italian soul. In so many vital ways, Ralph, who wore number 13, personified Brooklyn, and embodied the national pastime—the will to press on—when a single pitch of his in 1951 to New York Giant Bobby Thomson, the "Staten Island Scott," ignited "the shot heard around the world," an epic slip in sports history, a home run that lifted the Giants in a pennant-winning game.

History can be cruel.

There was another shot heard recently round the baseball world and beyond at the stroke of midnight just before Thanksgiving 2016 in Rye: Ralph Theodore Joseph Banca was called up to pitch on God's team. The saints are cheering wildly; 13 is a lucky number in Heaven! A career once defined by a high inside fastball has come to eternal life.

"One of the greatest guys to ever throw a pitch or sing a song is [no] longer with us," Branca's son-in-law Bobby Valentine, former Mets and Red Sox manager and a man himself of baseball accomplishment, tweeted at Ralph's passing. "In his 91st year on Earth he left us with the same dignity and grace that defined his every day on Earth."

Amazing grace, how sweet the sound…

Born in Mt. Vernon, the 15th of 17 children, Ralph Branca was far more than a gifted ballplayer. But for those who read the backs of baseball cards, Ralph was a 20-game winner, a 3-time All-Star, with an 88-68 win/loss record during 12 seasons—829 strikeouts in 1,484 innings, and a career .379 earned run average (ERA). Branca never saw color in baseball, just heart. On opening day in 1947, Jackie Robinson's major league debut, Branca lined up on the field beside Robinson while other players refused to because of Robinson's color. They became close friends on the field and off. "Jackie was all alone," Branca observed, as quoted in Ian O'Connor's perceptive ESPN reflection on Branca. "I was only doing what I was taught to do." That year, Branca had a 21-12 record and a 2.67 earned run average (ERA) in 280 innings pitched. He earned his first All-Star appearance.

The box score of someone's life, as we all know, just tells part of the story.

After the crushing pitch to Thomson in 1951, Ralph was comforted by Father Pat Rowley, a Fordham University priest, a cousin to Branca's then fiancée, soon to be wife, Ann.

"Why me?" Ralph asked. "Why me?"

"God chose you because he knew your faith was strong enough to bear this cross," Fr. Rowley responded.

Many years later in an ESPN interview, Branca said, "That really was a very big relief for me. I realized they sent in the best man they had, and Thomson beat me that day."

God has brought his best man home—the Lord's hand-picked emissary to those who ever took a third strike in life or gave up a home-run ball, teaching them by example that it's always dark before the sun rises.

Wrote Marty Noble of MLB.com with the announcement of Branca's passing, "The game—no, American society—is diminished by the loss of a man of such integrity, heart and strength."

Branca had great heart, off the field, as much as on it. His daughters Patti and Mary are testimony to that. We all grew up together.

Ralph was a father figure to me, and to many others growing up in Westchester County, just outside the glow of baseball, celebrity, and the New York media. We were his "boys," and all the better for it—hanging out at the Branca house, listening to baseball stories, but more importantly being schooled by Branca about the need for love, forgiveness, self-deprecating humor, and for pressing on against all odds—lessons none of us will ever forget. We will carry them to the grave, as our coach did.

Yes, Branca was as much a coach in life as a famous baseball player. He used his renown to teach others. He filled a gap for me in surrogate ways at a time when my father was distracted with raising and financing 10 children. As the oldest boy, I kinda just went my way; Ralph was there at times to catch me in the net.

Catch is an operative word here. Over time, I became Branca's backyard catcher, or as daughter Patti calls it, "Ralph's personal catcher." I was a shy, reticent kid then, filled with uncertainty, a journeyman catcher, but Ralph listened to my baseball stories as if I were Yogi Berra: narratives about our Senior Babe Ruth All-Star team that won the New York State championships two years in a row, with trips to the divisional World Series tournament. Ralph never blinked, just listened.

In the late 1960s, well beyond his retirement, Branca was looking to get back in shape in the hopes of pitching batting practice for his buddy Gil Hodges's team, the 1969 Miracle Mets, which won the '69 World Series in the eighth year of the franchise against the Baltimore Orioles. "Amazin' Mets," coined Casey Stengel, who managed the team in its inaugural season through 1965. And so, we worked out regularly, pitcher/catcher, on the Rye High School field.

Ralph could still throw hard. Pop! The hollow of my left hand can still feel the zing through the catcher's mitt. Muscle memory. Ralph frequently took me to Yankee and Mets games—his catcher in tow. We talked about the strategies of winning ball games; little did I know at the time that Ralph was instructing me about life. I was a nobody, yet to Ralph, I was his battery mate, and Ralph wanted to teach. He was a coach.

Ralph knew I always wanted to play pro ball, my boyhood dream; only thing keeping me back was the talent. One day after a particularly grueling workout in the early fall of 1969, Ralph told me he was going to pitch batting practice the next day to the Mets at Shea Stadium.

"You're coming with me, and you're working out on the field," he announced, as a father would proclaim.

The next day as declared, Ralph pulled up in front of my house on Brookdale Place to take me to Shea. I was told to wear dress pants, a collared shirt, and to bring my baseball gear in an athletic bag. Neighbor Phil Clancy, an old Dodger fan, was peeking out the door as if the Second Coming were at hand. He kept poking his head in and out, thinking he would be turned into a pillar of salt. Ralph was bigger than life.

Days later at my mother's repeated urging, I scribbled copious notes of the Mets experience, then pounded out the notes on my Royal typewriter, still in my office today. The notes were put in a plastic box for safekeeping. When Patti emailed me shortly after her father had passed away, I opened the box. The memories were overwhelming.

"Hello, Mr. Branca," the security guard at the door to the Mets locker room said. A sign on the door forewarned: "Private. Keep Out." Fully intimidated. I read into it: "Greg, this means you…"

Stepping into the Mets locker room, as a young man, felt like I was walking into Lewis Carroll's *Through the Looking Glass*, where nothing would be what it is because everything would be what it isn't.

Once inside, there was no Mad Hatter, but there, head on, were the likes of Tom Seaver, Jerry Koosman, Ron Swoboda, and many other Mets stars. On the wall in the back of the room was a sign painted in big black letters by pitching ace Tug McGraw. It was inscribed with the team motto, "Ya gotta believe!"

I was believing….

Ralph excused himself for a minute, popping into an adjoining office for some small talk. "Hey Greg," he yelled minutes later, "come on in. I got someone I want you to meet."

I shuffled in.

"Greg, this is Gil Hodges," Ralph said, explaining to Hodges that I was his catcher, now playing baseball at Fairfield University. "It's just a small college, Mr. Hodges. I'm just honored to be here."

"Greg's pretty fair with a glove," Ralph replied. "Hey, ah…Gil," Ralph said (I realized later a set-up in advance), okay if Greg works out on the field with me today?"

"I have a small problem," Hodges said.

"Mr. Hodges," I replied. "I'm just thrilled to be here."

"No," said Hodges. "I have to get him a uniform; no one is allowed on the field working out without a uniform."

Wow!

Within minutes, the equipment manager brought in a neatly pressed Mets uniform, number 53, legendary Eddie Yost's uniform, then a third base coach at the end of an incredible career. Branca and

I dressed in locker room stalls. Seaver's locker was to my left.

"Okay, gentlemen, let's go," minutes later Hodges shouted, walking through the locker room, clapping his hands.

Ralph and I walked out with about 15 other players, down a dark, concrete tunnel toward the dugout. The sound of our iron spikes dragging along the floor was deafening. At the end of the tunnel stood an imposing but friendly figure. I couldn't see who it was. He was slapping players on the butt with his mitt as they stepped up into the dugout.

My eyes focused at I got closer. I was stunned. It was field coach Yogi Berra!

Berra looked me square in the eye; perhaps he thought I was brought up from Triple A for the pennant drive. "Let's show some hustle," Berra shouted, as he whacked me with his glove.

"You bet, coach!"

I was pinching myself. As I walked onto the field, I was gawking like someone looking up at the ceiling of Grand Central Station for the first time.

"Why don't you go out and shag a few flies during batting practice," Branca said, probably a bit discomfited that I was looking like a rube.

I was directed to the outfield, thinking a bunch of ball boys were roaming the perimeters. To my surprise, the Mets starting National League All-Star outfield Tommie Agee, Donn Clendenon, and Cleon Jones were running sprints on the warning track. Jones came up to me to introduce himself.

I quickly explained profusely that I was this little shit catcher, a nobody, and just here as a friend of Ralph's, my tryout in believing in dreams.

"Well, let's see if you learned anything," said Jones with a smile.

The first ball was hit right at me, about 12 feet to my right. "Go get it, rookie," Jones invoked. I jumped at the chance, feeling as though I had cinderblocks attached to both feet. Somehow, I managed to position myself beneath the ball and catch it. That felt good. Soon I was one-handing catches, and hitting imaginary cutoff men in the infield; I even one-hopped a ball to third.

Do you believe in miracles? Yes, when in the company of Ralph Branca!

Later, Branca summoned me to warm him up for batting practice, to the right of home plate, back near the box seats where young kids, as I once did, reached over the waist-high concrete wall to get an autograph. After Ralph walked out to pitch batting practice, a young kid called out to me with a baseball in hand.

"Sir, would you sign this?" he asked.

No one had ever asked for my autograph, but in a moment of triumph I obliged.

In those days, sadly gone, entire teams would sign a single baseball. So I flipped the ball over, looking for Seaver's and Koosman's signatures, then signed my name. Flipping the ball back over again to avoid incrimination, I handed it back.

My dream complete, Ralph had delivered like the messiah.

Fast forward to many years later. Other dreams turned into nightmares with my diagnosis of early-onset Alzheimer's.

"Why me?" I asked Ralph. "Why me?"

There was no hesitation. "God has plans for you. Get off your ass and keep fighting," he urged, as his own memory began to fade and functions were shutting down. Ralph was a private man; he didn't talk about the ninth inning of his life, but we both understood. "It's all about the fight, about encouraging others to fight."

A few weeks before Branca's death, I received a call from his daughter Patti, saying her father was failing and that I should call him. I did immediately. We had a good talk—the exit interview, the tough goodbye delivered from the heart. Ralph, as usual, was more interested in how I was doing than talking about himself. "Keep fighting," he urged me. "Don't you dare give up…"

Surrogate father to son, we came full circle; I've stored those words in my heart.

After learning of Ralph's death, I woke my son Conor in the morning to tell him. Ralph had reached out earlier several times to Conor as a mentor, as he had done with me.

"Dad," Conor told me, stunned at the news. "I just had a dream about Ralph: you, me, and Ralph were all playing baseball."

Ralph, on the way to Heaven, chose again to reach out to someone in need of encouragement, as he had decades ago with me. A perfect game…

19

Winter Solstice

The light is starting to fade.

Much has been written about the "Longest Day," the June solstice, heralding the summer solstice; it has become a metaphor for Alzheimer's. Yet for me, the Winter solstice, the shortest day of the year, is a far more powerful allegory for dementia. Others in the disease feel the same, deep into the darkness.

"Deep into that darkness peering, long I stood there, wondering, fearing, doubting...," wrote Edgar Allan Poe.

For all creatures of the earth, nothing is as fundamental as daylight, which blooms new memories and sheds light on life itself. The darkness can be numbing; isolation warps the mind.

On the rim of holiday celebrations and year-end resolutions, the tilt of the earth 23.5 degrees from the sun summons the Winter solstice when the sun is lowest in the sky, reflecting a scant nine hours and 32 minutes of daylight—the shortest day of the year, a time of inner reflection for all of us.

The sun's purposeful journey across the sky, from shortest day to longest, has been measured since early time, and manifested in such mystic monuments as Stonehenge in England and Machu Picchu in Peru.

For many, this solstice—derived from the Latin *sol* (sun and *sistere* to stand still)—can be a black hole of depression and intense loneliness, brought on by deprivation of sunlight. Seasonal Affective Disorder, SAD, they call it. The ancients struggled against the ravages of winter and sought ways to celebrate the solstice, seeking greater spiritual meaning and celebration in the abyss. Among them: Newgrange in northeastern Ireland dating back to around 3200 BC, a grassy burial mound rising from an emerald field with small openings to the sky and chambers beneath that flood with sunlight precisely at the Winter solstice. Or consider the ancient Mayan stone building in Tulum, Mexico, which contains a small breach at its peak, producing a starburst effect when the sun rises on this day.

As the sun hugs the horizon on the shortest day, there is no celebration for those of us with Alzheimer's or other dementias— SAD on steroids. We stand still in the darkness. While the longest day, the Summer solstice, has become a metaphor for the sunrise-to-sunset challenge of Alzheimer's, the shortest day is symptomatic of the denouement of the disease—ever present at dusk.

Medical experts call the Alzheimer's phenomenon of end-day confusion and restlessness "sundowning," a period of increased uncertainty, agitation, and drifting in a fog as light fades to black, a time of greater rage and mood swings in the shadows of the mind.

With the development of Alzheimer's and plaques and tangles in the brain, theorists suggest that there may be a disruption at sunset in what doctors call the "Suprachiasmatic Nucleus." This is the tiny region of the hypothalamus responsible for controlling bodily rhythms to keep the body on a 24-hour schedule.

In Alzheimer's, we tend to wander.

I was up again at 4 a.m. the other night, one of five nocturnal ramblings that early morning. The new me, paucity of sleep. Picking my way in the dark in the familiar territory of my home, I fumbled into the bathroom as I felt the numbness creep up the back of my neck like a penetrating fog, slowly inching to the front of my mind. In the moment, it was as if a light in my brain had been shut off. I was overcome by the darkness of not knowing where I was or who I was. So I reached for my cell phone that substitutes as a flashlight, and called the house. My wife, deep asleep in our bed just 20 feet away, rose like Lazarus from the grave to grab the phone in angst, fearing an early morning call of a car crash involving one of the kids, or the death of an extended family member.

It was me, just me. I was lost in the bathroom.

The stress of Alzheimer's, for those diagnosed, and for their caregivers, is deadening deep into the darkness, out to Pluto. One never knows who's going to show up in the early stages of this disease: the new me, or the old me? Will I be on or off today?

I'm off on days when I suffer at the hand of the "Black Dog."

Robert Bly captures such darkness in his poem, "Melancholia," in his book of poetry, *The Light around the Body*:

"A light seen suddenly in the storm, snow
Coming from all sides, like flakes
Of sleep, and myself
On the road to the dark barn,
Halfway there, a black dog near me."

The bite of the black dog can be worse than its bark. To some, the black dog is man's best friend, a faithful companion in the rear of a pickup truck, particularly on Cape Cod, Nantucket, or the Vineyard. To others, it is a metaphor for the shadows of depression. Depends, as always, on one's perspective. I was bitten early in life; the hurt never goes away. All I know is that I can't sleep at night, haunted by demons of depression that keep me captive in the early hours.

Robert Lewis Stevenson in *Treasure Island*, perhaps one of the finest works in English literature, cast the black dog as a pillaging pirate, a harbinger of violence, with two fingers missing on his left hand. Eighty-four years later, putting the best face on imagery, master sailor Robert Douglas on Martha's Vineyard befriended a black lab, boxer mix aboard his schooner the *Shenandoah*, calling his mate the "Black Dog" after Stevenson's swashbuckler. For 16 years, Douglas and his companion were inseparable, ultimately the inspiration of a celebrated tavern and accessory chain, anchored in Vineyard Haven, which bears the name The Black Dog.

Still, the black dog is haunting for me. In 16th-century English myth, it was associated with the devil or a hellhound, a nocturnal apparition whose appearance was regarded as a presage of death, a guardian of the underworld. There is no hyperbole in this for those who live with depression, the fear of melancholy. Actor Robin Williams, who courageously fought these monsters, knew it all too well. While Williams's suicide shocked the world with piercing questions of "How can this happen?" his death cut deep for the 19 million who suffer at the hands of the black dog. According to an autopsy report, Williams also had Lewy Body Dementia, which could have contributed to his decision to die by suicide.

The wholesale misunderstanding, in lay terms, of depression and dementia is greatly distressing. It is not a mood swing, a lack of coping skills, character flaws, or simply a sucky day, a month, or a year; it's a horrific, often deadly, disease. Many, like Williams, choose to deflect the relentless in-your-face assault of these demons, hoping to stare them down for as long as possible. It's a lonely, numbing gaze, a confrontation that sometimes one cannot win. Losing is not failure; it is evidence of the fight. Williams, just a year younger than I, fought valiantly against depression and dementia. He is a hero in his defiance of disease that roams boldly at will, often taking no prisoners.

In depression, accelerated in dementia, there is no off button. No Hollywood scenes the likes of *Moonstruck*, a Norman Jewison classic where Loretta Castorini, played by Cher, slaps Ronny Cammareri, a beguiled Nicholas Cage, then slaps him hard again, commanding, "Snap out of it!"

You can't snap out of depression. Even Winston Churchill used the ever-present "black dog" as his daily symbol of despair. Reflecting on his depression, he wrote: "I don't like standing near the edge of a platform when an express train is passing through. I like to stand back and, if possible, get a pillar between me and the train. I don't like to stand by the side of a ship and look down into the water. A second's action would end everything. A few drops of desperation."

Like Robin Williams, Churchill used his affliction for good; in his case, as a battering ram against Hitler in World War II. In the book *Churchill's Black Dog, Kafka's Mice, and Other Phenomena of the Human Mind,* psychiatrist Anthony Storr observed how Churchill marshaled his depression to enlighten political judgments: "Only a man who knew what it was to discern a gleam of hope in a hopeless situation, whose courage was beyond reason and whose aggressive spirit burned at its fiercest when he was hemmed in and surrounded by enemies, could have given emotional reality to the words of defiance, which rallied and sustained us in the menacing summer of 1940."

Churchill's depression, observers have suggested, allowed him to assess fully the Nazi menace and recognize in the process that conciliatory gestures—the policy of England at the time—would only embolden Hitler. Thus, as prime minister, he altered the course of history, attacking Hitler head-on, using his black dog to his advantage. Sic him!

From the start of recorded history, many leaders and creative types, artists and writers, given to mood and anxiety disorders, have used the black dog as a lens to the soul. Eugene O'Neill, Tennessee Williams, and Charles Dickens all appeared to have suffered from clinical depression, as did Ernest Hemingway, Leo Tolstoy, and Virginia Woolf, to note a few.

Comprehending depression is as confounding as the question comedian George Carlin posed many years ago: "If God is so powerful, can He make a rock so big that He can't pick it up?"

Depression is heavy; it is complicated, the cause of a range of factors.

"It is often said depression results from a chemical imbalance, but that figure of speech doesn't capture how complex the disease is," according to a health report from Harvard Medical School titled *Understanding Depression.*

Research suggests that depression doesn't spring from simply having too much or too little of certain brain chemicals. Rather, depression has many possible causes, including faulty mood regulations by the brain, genetic vulnerability, stressful life events, medications, and medical problems. It is believed that several of these factors interact to bring on depression.

My depression was brought on as a young man. Looking back, I felt at times lonely, worthless, desperate, and confused. I was an "A" student, a jock, a good-looking kid, the funny man at family gatherings and parties. Still, I felt useless. I spoke to my parents about it and they told me that I'd get over it. Years later, I found out my father was on depression medication and my mother had succumbed to it as well. Earlier, her brother had taken his life in a depressive state. Finally, I saw a doctor and was diagnosed with clinical depression—again not code for a bad day, but a frightful state of mind.

The black dog can be provoked by other diseases, doctors advise. It stews in the defective tangles and amyloids of Alzheimer's disease.

The black dog roams within me as I look for its leash to try and rein in the beast and, in a way, make good from evil, a far better guidepost.

✴

The reining-in process for depression amid the steady onslaught of Alzheimer's is volatile at times. Moments of rage and the dropping of F-bombs are not personal choices for those in Alzheimer's. It's an uncontrollable disease, like Tourette's in some ways, a loss of synapse in the hippocampus part of the brain—a forgetting, a dismissing, of the difference between private and public. The hippocampus functions as a "memory gateway through which new memories must pass before entering permanent storage in the brain," the Memory Disorders Project at Rutgers University notes.

Damage to the hippocampus from Alzheimer's, and from head injuries, Rutgers states, can result in a memory deficit in the brain, a loss of ability to form new memories, although older, long-term memories may be safe. "Thus, someone who sustains an injury to the hippocampus may have good memory of his childhood and the years before the injury" but diminishing short-term memory since. This can also trigger a loss of taste and smell, and the inability to process sound. A healthy brain filters noise. Experts call it "the cocktail party effect," the ability to distinguish relevant sounds and conversations from background noise. With damage to the hippocampus from Alzheimer's, other forms of dementia, and head injuries, staying on task is a crap shoot: relevant sounds and conversations are often obfuscated by background noise, causing an incredible disconnect to the point of wrath, then withdrawal.

Researcher Laura Colgin draws the analogy of a radio. Think of your brain like a radio, she suggests: turning the knob to find your favorite station, but the knob jams, and you're stuck listening to something that's in-between stations. "Just like radio stations play songs and news on different frequencies, the brain uses different frequencies of waves to send different kinds of information," adds Colgin, researcher at the Kavli Institute for Systems Neuroscience and Centre for the Biology of Memory at the Norwegian University of Science and Technology (NTNU).

Says Vitaly Klyachko, a neurobiologist at the Salk Institute in Southern California, synapses by their nature, protecting against an overload, do not transfer every type of information they receive. In fact, he notes, only 10 to 25% of the signals that a neuron receives will be transmitted across the synapse; the rest are "dropped" much like a cell phone call.

So when the brain goes haywire, this vexation can cause inordinate rage and angst out of gut frustration, as was the case for me recently at the proper Harvard Club in Boston on well-heeled Commonwealth Avenue, during a Cure Alzheimer's Fund symposium. My friend Dr. Tanzi was the keynote speaker and was brilliant and spellbinding, as usual. All the Ivy notables were gathered at a reception afterwards on the second floor of the Club, with its high ceilings and mahogany walls, an over-abundance of brain power in the room.

The noise in the reception hall was deafening to me, a melding of voices, common in Alzheimer's. It got louder and louder, as I stood with some friends, trying to take it all in. My attention was directed at one individual just a few feet away. Dressed in the deep blue of a Boston banker, I'm sure he was not speaking any louder than anyone else in the room, but my brain focused on him, telling me that he was shouting in shrill rants, like the piercing stabs from the movie *Psycho*.

Finally, I couldn't take it. I walked up to the man, a stranger to me, tapped him on the shoulder, interrupting his conversation, and declared, "Would you shut the *fuck* up!"

There was silence.

"*Uh-oh,*" a friend next to me said, separating me from the group, as another companion attempted to explain to the startled gentleman what had just happened. Best face I can put on this is that it was an unscheduled classroom exercise, a demonstration, if you will, in real time, after my friend Tanzi's speech.

I was escorted downstairs to a couch in the lobby to calm down. Lisa Genova, a good friend and the author of the *New York Times* best-selling *Still Alice*, who holds a PhD in neuroscience from Harvard, sat with me. When I suggested minutes later that I go back upstairs, Lisa, far smarter, calmly cautioned, "Why don't you just sit here a bit…"

Vociferous receptions, stressful, time-sensitive situations, and large gatherings can be the bane of those with Alzheimer's. One has to try to find the humor in it as a coping strategy. Another case in point is a Nantucket Airport drop-off.

I spend much time on Cape Cod, Martha's Vineyard, and Nantucket these days, given that doctors don't want me to drive. I walk a lot now on the Outer Cape and Islands, getting picked up by friends and caring souls. Perhaps they think I'm the "village idiot."

I often travel to Nantucket by plane or fast ferry, an hour boat ride from Hyannis, often with attorney John Twohig, a former partner at Goulston & Storrs in Boston and now executive vice president of New England Development. John is in a fleet of guardian angels, a mentor to me, and a damn nice guy. His mother-in-law, who lived with John and his family for six years, died from Alzheimer's and John gets it. He also gets the fight in me, and has kept me focused with communication and strategy projects, as has his wife, Susan Nicastro, another attorney. We make a good team, and I am thankful for that.

Racing to meet a plane back to Hyannis one day not long ago, with John at the wheel of a rental car, me riding shotgun, and two elite architects from Cannon Design in Boston in the back seat, I suggested what my brain told me was a way to save time. We were late, in jeopardy of missing the plane. As John pulled in front of the airport to drop us off, unload all of our presentation materials, and then park the rental car, I said, "Why don't I just take the keys and you drop off the car."

So I reached for the keys in the ignition as we were rounding the entrance at full-speed. Pretty smart, I thought. Don't ya think?

"I may have a problem driving and parking the car if you take the keys," John replied, knowing neurons had just misfired. "I'll have to push the car..."

"Ok," I said wholly embarrassed, "then maybe it's not such a good idea."

The two architects in the back seat turned white. John glanced in the rearview mirror and saw them exchange looks like "Who are these guys?" Their body language clearly suggested they were looking for an ejection seat.

John and I laughed like little kids; we've been down this road before. The architects realized that something in the moment had gone sideways with me, but that all was good. Later, they learned about my diagnosis and one of them even read my first book. It brought us closer. We laughed some more about it to the point later where, over coffee, one of the architects forgot what he was about to say and his colleague asked him, "Have you been drinking from Greg's cup?"

Close friends say I've been drinking from Larry David's cup. David is a paradigm for loss of filter. Yet the Emmy-winning comedian, actor, playwright, producer, and the genius behind *Seinfeld* and HBO's *Curb Your Enthusiasm* is refreshing and invigorating in his brusqueness. He says what we all want to say, but often can't, until the prefrontal cortex goes awry. The prefrontal cortex, doctors say, is the section of the brain that filters, mostly keeping at bay inappropriate thoughts, comments, or actions. Researchers at the University of Pennsylvania have proven that inhibiting this filter can boost unfiltered, creative thinking. While the creative genius in David can turn the switch on and off, many of us in Alzheimer's play the role daily without premeditation or a script, a common manifestation—often blunt, rude, and crude in our language and advances, discarding social norms. Words, images, and actions that otherwise would be caught in the prefrontal cortex flow freely in the sewer of this disease. Many think of Alzheimer's as just a loss of cognitive abilities, poor judgment, short-term memory loss, depression, disorientation, rage, and delusions at times. All of these symptoms and the timing range in individuals. The "filter thing," as we call in it our family, the personality shift, caused by changes in the brain, has now climbed into the front seat, grabbing for the wheel.

Larry David is among a cadre of heroes for me as I try, after the fact, to laugh at loss of filter. Conceded David, "I'm a walking, talking enigma. We're a dying breed...I don't like to be out of my comfort zone, which is about a half an inch wide."

So we go with the flow. It can be a bumpy ride.

Like the time in a *Curb Your Enthusiasm* episode on a plane when David gets up from first-class seats, parts the blue curtain separating the wealthy from the holy unwashed, and heads to coach bathroom because the first-class bathrooms are occupied. He is immediately confronted by a woman in her seat, who had been told earlier that she could not use the bathroom in first class.

"We have our different areas," the woman tells David, halting him in his tracks.

David apologies. "I'm so sorry they did that. That's terrible!"

"Thank you for understanding," the woman replies.

"While I understand, and I empathize with you…I'm still going to use the bathroom," David insists.

There is pushback from the woman. "Oh, so you're in first class, and you can do whatever you want to do…you get on first, you get free drinks, you get a hot towel."

"I'm not a first-class person, I'm coachy," David replies, telling the woman she has it all wrong.

"But you're not acting coachy; you're acting first classy," the woman says, escalating the exchange to the point that they both begin mimicking caricatures of first-class and coach passengers.

Finally, David storms off to the second-class bathroom and urinates.

Not long ago, neurons in my head misfired again in public; this time at Boston's Logan Airport on a trip to Los Angeles with my wife—blanks due mostly to the shrill noise and seizing confusion of flying. I wasn't acting "first classy," and was suffering from the isolation of feeling somewhat useless (as I often do now). There was a time when airlines actually offered customer service: you go to the counter, flash a license, drop off a bag, then head to the gate, maybe with some extra time for coffee and a bagel.

No longer.

The ticket counters now are flush with kiosks that look like the George Lucas robot R2-D2. Out of body overwhelmed, I felt like I needed access to the nuclear code just to get a boarding pass. I used to be the guy—you know, the guy, the husband, the father, the guy who fixed things. I wanted to be *the guy*! Now I was reduced to an agitated state of disarray, no longer the star quarterback of the family. That position now fell to my wife, Mary Catherine.

"It's broken," I yelled at her, as she fidgeted with R2-D2 to get the boarding pass and bag tags. That's all I could think to say to reassert that I was still in charge. But that train, to mix a metaphor, had left the station.

"See, it's broken," I yelled again, as the brain cells short-circuited.

At airports now, one is supposed to have their quiet voice. I was raising my voice like a wave about to crash on the shoreline.

"No, it's not," Mary Catherine shot back, clearly stressed that I was in a launch countdown, as she tried frantically to engage R2-D2.

"The damn thing is broken!" I replied in a voice that was attracting attention of other travelers and nearby TSA.

Within seconds, a stern, stout woman approached me.

"What's wrong," she quipped, attempting to back me down.

Don't go there, I thought!

"It's broken. The damn thing is just broken."

"No, it's not!"

"Yes, it is…"

Stretching the definition of polite, the woman bumped my wife over to the right and worked the robot, her fingers hitting keystrokes like a master pianist.

Instantly, R2-D2 spit out boarding passes and bag tags.

With an air of smugness, she handed the bag tags to me.

In full gate confusion, I replied in a booming voice, "What the hell am I supposed to do with this?"

"You *PUT* them on your bags," the woman said in a voice that drew out that second word with the greatest of sarcasm.

Challenged and not to be outdone, I stepped toward the woman, looked her directly in her eyes, violating the private zone space, and said with annunciation:

"Well, am I supposed to fly the *FUCKING* plane, too?"

Holy shit. Alarms were going off. Passengers were glued to the confrontation. Other associates assembled like the posse. *No Fly List*, I was thinking. *No Fly List…*

My wife stepped in. She was the guy now—you know, the guy. Horrified at what had just happened and wondering how much longer she could absorb such invectives, as common with me now as daylight, she explained to the woman that I have medical issues that provoke the carpet bombing of F-bombs—in the moment, the only way I can articulate the pain and fear of a light going off in my head.

While all was not likely forgiven, we were allowed to proceed to the gate.

"You need to watch your husband closely," the woman told Mary Catherine. "He should be on a pitch count."

The flight home from L.A. was equally eventful. And I looked to find the humor in it.

In addition to other progressing symptoms, I have lost continence, to the point where I never wear light pants out of embarrassment. The brain is not sending signals that it is time to go to the bathroom, explosions of a different significance.

Several hours in the air on the flight back to Boston, somewhere over Chicago, my wife turned to me and in the tone of a disciplining mother at the end of her tether, commanded: "GO TO THE BATHROOM."

Childlike, I replied in a four-year-old tone, "NO!"

"Gooooo to the bathroom!" she said.

"No," I said abruptly, attracting the glances of passengers around us.

"Go to the bathroom or you'll pee in your pants," she replied.

More eyeballs.

"I can't," I said. "The flight attendant's cart is blocking the back of the plane."

"Then go to the bathroom up in first class." Mary Catherine was now on verge of an explosion herself.

"No way," I said. "Going through the curtain that separates us from first class is like going through the veil in the ancient Jewish temple into the Holy of Holies. I'll get struck by lightning."

Passengers in the four rows ahead and behind me put down their laptops, yanked off ear phones to channel into this conversation.

"Go to the bathroom," she insisted.

I finally obliged and with great care stepped through the curtain that separates the privileged from the holy unwashed.

"I have to use the bathroom," I said sheepishly, as confusion swayed. "I know I'm not supposed to be here, but it's an emergency. Can I take a pee?"

The flight attendant sighed, rolled her head like she was in a Pilates class, then said, "Just make it quick."

"Where's the bathroom?" I asked, now in full gait turmoil.

"Right behind you," the woman said, as if I was a dunce. Little did she know...

In a full gait of confusion, piercing shrieks were playing again in my head.

There was a door on the left and a door in the middle. I didn't know which one to grab. I contemplated both. In my muddle, I visualized the old Monte Hall TV game show *Let's Make a Deal.*

"Do I take the door on the left or the door in the middle, the door on the left, or the door in the middle?" I mused.

I chose the door in the middle, and placed my hand on the knob. Bad choice. The CAPTAIN'S DOOR!

Holy shit! More trouble.

Reading the horror in my face, and realizing brain cells weren't firing, the flight attendant, like a master drill sergeant, directed me to the door on the left, then marched me back to my seat.

"Please sit," the woman said sternly, walking away. "And don't get up again! Never again!"

Mary Catherine looked up in a Pilates head roll herself.

"Okay, what the hell did you do?" she asked.

Passengers tuned in again. Must see TV!

"You almost got me thrown off the plane," I whined.

"WHAT DID YOU DO?" she said, raising her voice.

"I put my hand on the captain's door," I finally admitted.

"You what?"

"I put my hand on the captain's door!"

There was a collective gasp from rows 8-12.

"Okay, that's it!" Mary Catherine replied. "From now on, pee in your pants..."

Good news was that I was back in my seat, no flight marshal had cuffed me, and the plane sped to Boston lickety-split.

Such unraveling is occurring more and more now. At times, it's hard to find the humor in it. Sleeping on the couch the other night, having been anaesthetized by the push and pull of CNN and Fox News coverage of a world gone nutty, I awoke to a hallucination on the edge of an oak coffee table next to the couch. There I saw a small demonic, green creature taunting me. Fully awake, my instinct was to swipe at the demon and it would go away, as hallucinations have in the past. The demon remained, and the taunts got louder. I swiped again, then again. The apparition lingered. At first, I was terrorized, then angered, so enraged that I lifted my right leg off the couch and crashed it down on the demon with such force that it splintered a quarter-inch glass covering on the table. The force of the loud crash cut through a pair of thick jeans and broke the skin just above my ankle. There was no demon, only my hallucination, and a humiliating explanation to my wife the following morning on why the glass was shattered. Bad news any way you slice it. That Sunday morning, I picked up the pieces of the broken glass, took them to the town dump, and tossed them into the recycling bin.

The thought crossed my mind of jumping in myself.

There was always good news with our striking Labrador Retriever "Sox," named after the Boston Red Sox. Sox has been a good guidepost for me in my journey. Animals, particularly dogs, can sense illness in people. Dogs have a farfetched sense of smell. Unlike humans who have approximately 5 million scent receptors, dogs have anywhere from 125 to 300 million scent receptors, depending on the breed, according to animal experts. Dogs, having such an acute and accurate sense of smell and a high level of awareness of the types of energy surrounding them can, at times, detect illnesses, including epileptic seizures, cancer, and dementia. Experts suggest that the canine's ancestral grey wolf's pack survival depended upon the instinct to know which member of the pack was sick.

Sox knew I was sick; a faithful caregiver, she stayed at my side at the house at all times, a sentry on watch, often licking my face like a mother trying to heal. I frightened her with my rage at times and spitting expletives; she would cower, but always return as if to say in dog talk, "I understand." Will Rogers had it right when he wrote, "If there are no dogs in Heaven, then when I die, I want to go where they went."

Life for all of us is filled with the unexpected, and on a Super Bowl Sunday, I had to call a family audible, amidst the Ooh-Rah of the game, a wrenching down-and-out, an end life pattern I will never forget, a twisted ending that shook my soul.

Changing a play at the family scrimmage line is an intense ordeal. At 14, Sox was at the end of her rope. I had to break the news to the family that our stunning yellow Lab, who had defined us with unremitting faith, hope, and love, was going to die that night. Failing kidneys, internal bleeding, and neurological complications were overcoming her, and I was to be the executioner.

There are no playbooks for such talk. I had to scramble. For most of my adult life, I've made a living with words; now they escaped me— blanks, just blanks, as I fought off my own incapacity to connect the dots. In recent years, the family has witnessed my own progression in Alzheimer's; now Sox, who had been a family caregiver of sorts, was failing. The metaphor was unavoidable.

"It is time," my wife Mary Catherine and I told our adult children, Brendan, Colleen, and Conor, who in many ways were raised by Sox. I could hardly get the words out.

Later that evening, instinctively, I fumbled for ways to keep Sox alive for another day at the emergency animal hospital on Cape Cod where she had been taken. The caring veterinary physicians were willing to oblige, but stressed that Sox was in great pain and would likely die alone otherwise.

That's all I needed to hear. Sox would pass peacefully on my lap.

"Sox's functions are shutting down," the attending physician explained, "and she has neurological issues of confusion and disorientation."

"What do you mean?" I asked.

"It's as if Sox has dementia, Alzheimer's," the doctor explained, unaware of my diagnosis. "That's the best way to explain it."

"She has WHAT?"

My wife and I were stunned. Sox and I had come full circle.

Our loss is no more heartbreaking than that of other individuals and families in our place. So I write in the midst of our own grief to give collective voice to a bonding, brand loyalty, that lasts a lifetime and beyond.

Sox, a purebred female with boundless verve and devotion, was a "Sweet 16" birthday present for my daughter Colleen, who had been lobbying for a dog for years, and now is a teacher in inner-city Baltimore, soon to be a first-time mother, and me a rookie grandfather.

"Daddy, please!" she would ask with a gaze that melted my heart.

An old salt of an investigative reporter, I probed breeders throughout New England and found one outside Boston with a newborn yellow Lab, the color of my daughter's hair. The Lab had been spoken for, but, on reflection, the prospective owner, a cancer victim, wanted the pup to have a secure and loving home, and passed Sox on to us. When presented with her birthday present, our daughter beamed with the energy of pounding surf on the Cape, as she held this wiggly ball of fur in her hand.

It wasn't long before Sox became the alpha female in the family, the gender opposite of the barreling Labrador retriever in the celebrated movie *Marley & Me*, an adaptation of John Grogan's fine book. Sox darted through screen doors, peed on the wide pine wood floor in the family room, shed hair faster than Donald Trump, and ate just about everything in sight. When we had to correct her, she bowed her head in shame, sheepishly peering up with soft brown eyes to see if the lecture was over. Early on, Sox had the oomph of a racecar, running in circles around our house until she collapsed in exhaustion. We used to call these laps the "Sox 500."

Like Marley, Sox also flunked her obedience class in Chatham. The trainer was not impressed.

But we always were, as over the years she stole our hearts and taught us about life and how to love unconditionally, and to growl when needed, not to bite. Endearingly simple and a contradiction of sorts, Sox had the gut instincts of a savant and the curiosity of a kindergartener, She always waited for us by the door, wagging her tail in delight as if we had been gone for a year; she could catch a tennis ball in mid-air, and fielded grounders like an All-Star shortstop; she picked up sticks in the backyard like a master landscaper; and Sox, I believe, sensed that I had medical issues and was always by my side at home, licking my face for reinforcement or lying with me on the couch; she was faster than a speeding bullet, and able to leap tall buildings in a single bound...

Sox had religion, too. When she occasionally slipped away from the house I often found her down the street in the church parking lot at Our Lady of the Cape; maybe she thought she could light candles for us. Do dogs go to Heaven? Many years ago, Pope Paul VI consoled a tearful child with the hope that it might be possible—the reference more recently was incorrectly attributed to Pope Francis. Perhaps Sox hedged her bets.

Sox also loved the salt water and the beach. In summer, she would sit on guard at the bow of my boat on Pleasant Bay, her face pointed at the sea like Leonardo DiCaprio in *Titanic*. On ocean excursions to the outer beach, Sox always would devour the sand, then run up to the shoreline and drink as much salt water as she could. We scolded her every time, but she didn't care. Sox knew best. That is, until one day when she coughed up what seemed like a gallon of the Atlantic, and pooped sand on someone's blanket.

There were the tender moments. Sox was on Crosby Beach with Colleen and her husband-to-be Matt Everett when he proposed. A moment frozen in time.

The end was no surprise; we saw it coming for many years—loss of weight, loss of hearing, loss of energy, and great difficulty walking. Still, she was in the moment. When the kids were young, Sox would leap up the stairs to their bedrooms at night, making the rounds like a duty nurse. When she could no longer climb, Sox would patiently wait at the bottom of the stairs until they awoke.

As her health deteriorated, our roles changed. I became the caregiver for Sox. She didn't sleep much at night, awakening about every two hours to urinate in the backyard. The water was going right through her failing kidneys. So for months I slept nearby on the family room couch, just so Sox knew she was not alone. At regular intervals, I walked her to the backyard and we peed together, and afterwards I fed her as much as she could eat. She poo-pooed the dog food, so I gave her boneless Perdue chicken and meatballs. Still, you could see her ribs, yet she wouldn't give up while she had a prayer. We bonded in new ways.

It wasn't until later in this full-circle walk with Sox that I learned about dog dementia, formally called "Canine Cognitive Dysfunction/Dementia," or CCD. Sox was a poster child for the disease with progressing symptoms. I had been in denial, as many do in Alzheimer's: her pacing in circles, incontinence, getting lost in familiar places, unable to retrace her steps back into the house, staring off at times into deep space, not responding to directions she once knew, and sleeplessness at night. I promise, she didn't drink out of my bowl. Sox, the caregiver, had met me in my place.

When I saw our champion that Super Bowl Sunday night at the emergency animal hospital, I knew in my heart it was time to let go, though I struggled with it. Sox just lay motionless on the floor, staring at my wife and me. She knew the end was near. The kids, sucked into a black hole of emotion, all wanted to say goodbye, so we FaceTimed with Brendan, Colleen, and Conor. We all felt as though the wind had been knocked out of us.

Colleen was first to console Sox, a time when love speaks louder than words. She could hardly talk.

"Is she in a lot of pain?" Colleen asked quietly. You could hear her reach for breath. Sox was reaching, too.

"She's going to sleep, honey, where there is no pain," I told her.

"Can I see her one more time, Daddy, please?"

I cradled my iPhone above Sox, and she made eye contact immediately, those piercing brown eyes that said to us: I'm not leaving; I'm just going away.

"Daddy, please kiss her for me..."

Conor, the youngest in the family, was overcome in numbness.

"Can you just scratch her head for me?" he asked. "Can you give her a hug?"

The moment gave new definition to FaceTime.

Brendan, the oldest, closed the loop.

"Love you so much," Brendan said, with my phone on speaker next to Sox's ear. "Hey, it's me, buddy, Brendan..."

It's hard for one to catch a breath, releasing raw emotion.

"I love you so much, Sox! You're the core of this family. You made me smile; you made me so happy. Dad, I'm so sad...I'm so freakin' sad."

The words trailed off.

"My head is throbbing," Mary Catherine told me as she said her farewell to Sox in this sterile, yet imitate, six-foot-by-six-foot room.

"Goodbye, sweetheart," she told Sox. "I love you!"

In seconds, I was alone with Sox—one-on-one, just as the day I brought her home. I lay next to her on the floor, rubbing her head.

Dammit, this hurt! Sox knew it, that inner sense.

"I love you," I told Sox repeatedly in a soft voice as I held her close. "It's ok, just let go, let go, Daddy loves you..."

Moments later without notice, Sox suddenly stood up for one last time, in defiance of death. She licked my face, then turned in three tight circles, licked my face again to say goodbye, then lay down, never to get up again.

The attending doctor entered the room with two syringes, one to relax Sox, taking all pain away; the other to let her go. With Sox in my lap, her head resting on my right knee, the first injection was administered. Slowly, Sox leaned her head back toward me and appeared to smile, as if to say her pain was gone. With the second injection, the doctor told me to keep talking to Sox.

"Hearing is the last thing to go," the doctor said.

I told my angel Sox how much we loved her, how much she was a part of our family, that we would never forget her. I hugged her tightly. She was at peace.

The doctor then put a stethoscope to Sox's heart, and softly uttered two words I will never forget.

"She's gone..."

Angels abounded again not long ago in Phoenix in the form of an Uber driver named Kenny on a night F-bombs would rain in the desert. My son Conor and I flew out from Boston to the Valley of the Sun for an extended family wedding and for a week of writing. Mary Catherine joined us later.

It was a long, confusing trip that stretched Conor's patience beyond the snap of a rubber band. As I've explained, I don't fly well these days. Mary Catherine had emailed my doctors earlier to get some tranquilizing drugs, insisting I take the "stun gun pills," as I called them, to level me out, the sort of stuff they give dogs before flying in crates.

"Thank you for all you do for Greg. Your support and friendship means so much to us," she emailed one of my doctors. "One of the many things Greg suffers from more and more is rage and outbursts while in frustrating settings. It is worse when traveling; all offering too much confusion for him. I'm surprised his outbursts haven't gotten him on the no-fly list yet!

"Doctors earlier prescribed 50 milligrams of Trazadone to calm the rage, but Greg says it makes him 'loopy,' and won't take it. Do you have any suggestions of any other medication that Greg could take while traveling? We have two trips coming up—one to Phoenix and one for our 40th anniversary. I just want to be sure I am thankful for the 40 years before I get on that plane with him!"

With pills in hand and in typical Mick form, I assured Mary Catherine that I would take the pills, then didn't, just upped my dosage of Aricept, Namenda, and Celexa. Hey, I took a biology course in high school.

Conor and I flew Southwest, one of my favorite carriers, but had to transfer through Atlanta. A long day. By the time we got to Phoenix, I was on edge. Couldn't wait to get the hell out of the airport. Phoenix is a fine airport, but in baggage claim they keep changing the carousels where bags are deposited. An announcement for Baggage Claim Area One becomes Baggage Claim Two, then Three, then Four. Not a good drill for someone with Alzheimer's.

I always wait at the bottom of the chute where the bags first pop out so that no one steals my bags. They have large, purple "Greg O'Brien, On Pluto" identification tags, made for me by close friend Leslie Durgin to ease the torment of cascading luggage on wheels that race like Pamplona's Running of the Bulls.

Conor usually waits on the other side of the claim area because my bag anxiety greatly frustrates him. But, no problem: bingo, this time my bags were out first! I grabbed them, looking carefully, almost anally to make sure they were mine. They were. Conor got his bags and we raced for a cab for the 15-minute ride to the Hilton Squaw Peak Pointe, a place we've stayed on visits for almost 20 years. I'm quite comfortable there, nothing changes: the incredible Lazy River tube ride, the water-view miniature golf, the Western ambiance of the Hole in the Wall and Aunt Chilada's restaurants, the relaxed room layout, and inspiring views of Squaw Peak. Nothing changes here, an incredible place, and I don't like change.

When we arrived at the Pointe lobby, the front desk, as usual, was accommodating, placing us in the best room possible with a pool view. My cell phone was vibrating like a cheap sex toy. It was my wife back on Cape Cod. Mary Catherine had been awoken by a call from Southwest Airlines: I had taken someone else's bag. My brain at the time told me the bag was mine, but upon later inspection there was no comparison.

I took the Lord's name loudly in vain at the front desk, alarming patrons in line behind me who might have feared the hotel was executing late-night arrivals. Conor cringed.

I called my wife, and she gave me the bad news.

The call had awakened Mary Catherine, and she was a bit groggy.

"How do I exchange the bags?" I asked.

"You'll just have to figure it out," my sleepy wife said.

Click! I hit the off button on the iPhone...

An expletive rang out!

Conor apologized to the front desk, then I explained I had a bit of a rage and anxiety problem, given my diagnosis. The kind gentleman said he would help us. Like General Patton, he summoned an elite Uber driver named Kenny, a native of Jordan and one of the most accommodating and calming individuals I've ever met. Realizing that Conor and I were close to the dividing line, the gentleman at the front desk told Conor to take the bags that were ours up to the room and relax, and said that Kenny would take me back to Sky Harbor Airport for the exchange of errant bags, and wouldn't let me out of his sight. Promise! Along the way, I apologized to Kenny for my rants. We talked about Alzheimer's; Kenny seemed to understand. He had lots of questions. Perhaps the disease was in his family. He was trying to calm me. I told him that a sense of humor, perseverance, and faith were keys to living with Alzheimer's, although I couldn't find the humor of the night. I told him about my favorite nephew, another Kenny, Kenny McGeorge, who fights autism like a champion.

The phone rang. It was Southwest Airlines.

"We have your bag, Mr. O'Brien, and we need the one you took right away! The passenger is here with us, and his bag has medication that he urgently needs."

"So does mine," I said.

Does it get any worse? The anxiety was exploding.

"Just head to Terminal Four, the South Side and we'll meet you there," the woman explained, in a tone suggesting that finding a strange terminal at night in a big city was as easy as grabbing a Sprite Zero out of the fridge when you wake up thirsty at night. "Just hurry!" she insisted. "Hurry!"

"Holy shit," I said, jumping back into rage, "where the (expletive) is Terminal Four and the South Side. I'm from the East, not the South! Do you think I have a compass in my freakin' pocket?"

Instantly, a gentle and reassuring hand reached back from the driver's seat. It was Kenny.

"Greg," he said with his soft Jordanian accent, "I'll take it from here."

Kenny, with the aplomb of a character in a Larry David sitcom, grabbed the phone, and patiently made arrangements for the handoff on the South Side curb of Terminal Four. But by the time we arrived, cars were backed up on the South Side for about a quarter mile. Not to be deterred, guardian Kenny swung into a parking garage above the terminal, and swiftly walked me to the curb, with the aberrant bag in hand. The Southwest representatives, two of them, were waiting for me like soldiers. In my heightened imagination, the moment had all the rasp of a prisoner exchange at the "Bridge of Spies," Glienicke Bridge in Berlin, a small steel structure crossing the Havel River that links Berlin with Potsdam, the front line of the Cold War for several years. In 1960, CIA U-2 spy pilot Francis Gary Powers, who was shot down while flying a reconnaissance mission over Soviet airspace, was exchanged there for a Soviet spy. Glienicke Bridge, notes History.com, was the setting for some of the most notable high-value prisoner exchanges between the Soviets and the West.

Not many words were exchanged on the curb, one handoff for another. The Southwest representatives were relieved, but I'm sure a bit exasperated with me. I asked to speak with the passenger who had waited with such patience. I apologized to him, a kind black man who seemed more concerned about me than about his bag. We exchanged gentlemen hugs.

Seconds later, walking away with my bag in hand, Kenny reached out again.

"Greg, I'll take it from here," he said, grabbing for my bag.

Later the following night, as I told friends in Phoenix about the exchange, in the middle of the conversation, I got a text from my nephew Kenny, as I often do at night, asking how I was doing. Nephew Kenny, in his late 20s, will often text me as much as 15 times a day. He's learned like me to write and speak from the heart.

Minutes later, I got another text from Kenny; it looked like he had changed cell phones.

"Hi, Mr. Greg, how are you? It's Kenny."

"When do you work at Safeway, bagging groceries?" I asked.

"I work *all* day tomorrow," he responded.

"Conor is with me, and we'd like to come by the store to see you," I texted.

"Sure, what time?" he replied.

There is a pause in transmission.

"U know who's this?" Kenny asked. "It's Kenny the driver from last night!"

Both Kennys have incredible senses of humor. Kenny the driver was just having fun in the moment, just messing with me, knowing it was another case of mistaken identity. We all laughed about it.

I adopted Uber Kenny for several days, needing a driver in Phoenix to maneuver the "bumper car" mindset of the city. The perfect choice. When he took my wife and me back to the airport later in the week for the return flight, we talked about the various incidents, laughed, and exchanged gentlemen hugs. Leaving the car, my attention was drawn to Kenny's rearview mirror. A silver chain with a cross was hanging from it.

My mother was no more perfect than anyone's mother. In my mind, though, she brimmed in gifts and with love. She was a superhero. Yet, at times, she seemed troubled.

When I was a teenager, I noticed her often standing at the kitchen window overlooking a corn patch with Rye Brook in the distance, meandering out to Long Island Sound. She was engaged in conversation. I wasn't sure with whom. At first, I thought it was a way of deflecting the stress of raising a brood of kids with a collective attention span of a young, yellow Lab. The disengaging increased: misplacing objects, loss of memory, poor judgment, seeing things that weren't there, and yes, the rage, warning signs years later that I began noticing in myself.

Mom today is still with me in spirit, that realm between the present and the past, between life and death. She had my back again a few months ago in an encounter on stage in Beverly Hills where the Golden

Globe Awards are presented. I had been asked to speak before 1,000 Hollywood celebrities at an Alzheimer's fundraiser and Hollywood revue, called "A Night at Sardi's." It was the final performance of this annual event. The stars were out that night in clusters.

The evening was hosted by David Hyde Pierce from the award-winning TV show *Frazier*, and featured performances by the cast of *The Big Bang Theory*, Joey McIntyre, Jason Alexander, and Grace Potter. Seth Rogen and other A-listers presented as well.

Backstage before my speech, I was incredibly nervous. Few get to stand in this place. I told myself to calm down, that I'm doing this for my mom, for all she had taught me.

I then heard a soft, confident voice that said, "You rock! Greg, you just rock this!"

And so I did. I rocked it, reading from a prepared speech.

At the podium, I noticed a woman standing behind me to the right. I felt that she was there for encouragement and support. I had a good, calming feeling about it. Several times I wanted to turn around to see who it was, but felt inside: "Just stay focused, stay focused!"

After my speech, I turned around, and the woman was gone.

Later, I asked my wife, "Who was the woman standing next to me?"

My wife paused. "Greg," she said. "There was no woman. No one was on the stage with you."

I insisted, "The woman behind me to the right, who was she? There was a woman standing behind me...She told me to rock it!"

"Greg," my wife replied, "there was no woman..."

I asked again.

"There was no woman," my wife replied, absorbing what had just happened.

The spirit of my mother, I believe, was on the stage with me, and perhaps the souls of others consumed by this demon called Alzheimer's. They must have had a kick-ass after-party. Wish I could have been there.

My mom was always one for emphasis; she never thought I got it. Immediately after the speech, a good friend in the audience, Elizabeth

Gelfand Sterns, producer of the movie *Still Alice* and a close associate of Maria Shriver, sent a text to another good friend, Lisa Genova, author of the best-selling *Still Alice*. Elizabeth wrote in a text, copied to me: "Greg is a rock star!"

Two days later, at Los Angeles International Airport, in a restaurant while awaiting a flight back to Boston, my wife gasped as she looked up at a television commercial on the screen above us. The caption on the TV commercial read, "For those who rock..."

Then the following Sunday, I was asked to speak at an Alzheimer's walk along Cape Cod Canal before hundreds of participants. I followed my mother's script to urge others to walk in faith, hope, courage, and humor. As my wife and I passed the starting line of the walk, there was a woman to the right holding a sign and waving it at me. I didn't recognize her, but took a photo on my iPhone. The sign read, "You Rock!"

The tears welled up.

Do you believe in angels?

20

Seeking Redemption

"We all long for Eden, and we are constantly glimpsing it: our whole nature at its best and least corrupted, its gentlest and most human, is still soaked with the sense of exile."
—J.R.R. TOLKIEN, *THE LETTERS OF J.R.R. TOLKIEN*

I am soaked today in exile, as are others in this disease, as Alzheimer's ensues—one foot on the terra firma we call reality, the other south of Eden, a realm beyond the physical. But what is reality? I always thought I knew.

When the brain—our perceived essence—begins to shut down, the spirit pursues, I'm finding. The physical now seems a veneer to me, a façade, a made-for-TV movie. On the cusp of this new reality, I seek to rid myself of this body, slowly moldering like my mind, yet I'm still conflicted with leaving family and friends behind. So I straddle in my search for Eden.

It's the journey from the cradle to the grave.

"You've connected with something," a good friend said the other day. "I wish I could go with you."

"Not sure where I'm headed," I responded, noting that the world beyond seems at times far more unfeigned than the world before me.

In his best-selling book, *Proof of Heaven*, Dr. Eben Alexander, a renowned Duke University and Harvard-trained academic neurosurgeon, made the connection on a brink of death, spending seven days deep in coma from a devastating brain infection and finding the "hyper-reality of the spiritual realm," the place of the soul. "Our spirit is not dependent on the brain or body," he told *The New York Times* in an interview. "It is eternal, and no one has one sentence worth of hard evidence that it isn't."

Strong words from a doctor who earlier could not reconcile his knowledge of neuroscience with any belief in Heaven, God, or the soul. Dr. Alexander, in *Proof of Heaven*, writes of his journey beyond this world, encountering "an angelic being who guided him into the deepest realms of super-physical existence. There he met, and spoke with, the Divine source of the universe itself." Today Dr. Alexander believes "true health can be achieved only when we realize that God and the soul are real, and that death is not the end of personal existence but only a transition."

Not long ago, as noted earlier, I experienced a similar near-death experience at Cape Cod Hospital's Emergency Room, having lost close to eight pints of blood and embracing a tunnel in the search for a light at the end. Hey, I'm no Einstein, but the man once said that we "should look for what is," and not for what we think should be.

And so I try to make sense of losing one's mind. I am encouraged about the prospects of plumbing the depths of the soul, which, I suspect, has no color, political preference, or ideology, just mere enlightenment. It is the search for that enlightenment that keeps me and others whole when cerebral and body functions fail. Decades ago, as a young, brash journalist, I thought I had all the answers, and that my job was to impart such wisdom of my terms, my narrative. I know now in Alzheimer's that I clearly don't have the answers—greater motivation now to sift the real from the imagined, a vetting for me confounded by fighting off the misperceptions and the progressions of this disease. I don't trust my brain anymore, so I follow my heart.

I know, like all of us, I will die without the answers, but I will run the race of knowledge. In the process, I seek redemption from my enemies, family, friends, and from God, or however one defines the universe or omnipresent. I'm hoping redemption is in my quiver, as I've come to realize on the backside of my 60s, that I'm a bigger transgressor than most, having committed every sin imaginable, other than murder and adultery, and having been tested in both. I'm no Puritan, no altar boy, just a guy striving beyond my grasp for what is real. Alzheimer's has brought me to this place—pursuit of truth, wherever that takes me. And I've come to understand that if you want redemption, you have to give it.

In the journey, I'm inspired by many, among them retired award-winning *Philadelphia Inquirer* sports writer Bill Lyons, who was diagnosed with Alzheimer's several years ago. His wife, Ethel, a "warrior woman," has battled cancer and emphysema. In the first of several columns about his battle with Alzheimer's, Lyons in a piece headlined: "My Alzheimer's Fight: Never, Ever Quit," wrote:

> In the winter of 2013, with the February cold bone deep, I sat in one of those cramped and sterile little examining cubicles in the Penn Memory Center and listened to the man in the white lab coat ask if I knew what Alzheimer's was.
>
> "Death by inches," I said.
>
> "And you have it," he said.
>
> I'm pretty sure the world stopped at that moment, and then there was a roaring sound, like a freight train barreling through my brain pan. I sat there, frozen, and I remember thinking what a crummy job this poor guy's got.

Lyons has personalized Alzheimer's, calling his intruder, "Al." I've taken to the name myself.

At first glance, "Al" is somewhat of a submissive, disarming, forgetful sort, who over time takes on the persona of a Hannibal in *Silence of the Lambs* in a grisly swath of mass murders. "Al" unwittingly may be here to teach our generation something, as collectively we wrestle with losing car keys, forgetting where the car is parked, walking into rooms with no clue of why they are there, and other, far more wrenching disconnects to come. Some call it age, "Al" calls it taking no prisoners. But as Baby Boomers in their 50s, 60s, and 70s take their final laps in life, there is a sense of urgency among many to do more good on the way out, create new memories. Good often comes out of striving through imperfection.

"Al is an insidious and relentless little bastard," writes Lyons, "a gutless coward who won't come out and fight. Instead, he lies in ambush in my brain, and the only way I can put a face on him is to look in the mirror...I should very much like to kick Al's ass."

So would I, and thus have given "Al" another moniker: "Mr. Fucker."

Lyons in his eloquent columns writes that he's not alone in this struggle; neither are others with this taboo of a disease, thanks to faith, selfless family, friends, caregivers, doctors, researchers, and a spate of national, regional, and local support groups. But when the light in the brain goes out, as Lyons knows, often without notice, and synapse is firing wildly like a sniper, we often withdraw to the bunker, lashing out in gut anger, retreating to our inner selves, keeping our heads down below the tracer bullets.

My anger at Mr. Fucker is rising within, yet often misplaced, spraying uncontrollable ire in all directions, usually at loved ones— my wife, children, friends, and at God. I'm angry at God.

Feeling a bit like a modern-day Job, I had a WTF talk with the Almighty the other day. I was enraged!

"Do you know who I am?" I shouted at God from the heart. "Do you have a clue? You gave me clinical depression as a kid, then you gave me cancer, then Alzheimer's; you also gave me walking pneumonia, spinal stenosis, scoliosis, and degeneration of my spine. I have no feeling now in my feet up to my shins, and my immune system is in the toilet. WTF!"

There was silence, as I pondered my outburst, knowing in my heart that I want a God of discipline, almost like legendary New England Coach Bill Belichick: "Just do your job!"

I shouted out again in primal anger to the Lord, "Do you have a freakin' clue who I am?"

Those who live by the sword, die by the sword when calling God's bluff. I instantly heard a brusque response in my heart from the heavens, with a salutation I use daily:

"Yes, *dumbass*, I know who you are. I made you! And I have you right where I want you…"

"Good then," I said, stunned at the response, thankful I wasn't turned into a pillar of salt. "I guess then we can move on together."

I am flushed with the shame of my language, hurling profane epithets at God in anger that would likely raise hairs on the back of Beelzebub's neck. I've been told that the Lord has big shoulders, and embraces straight talk from the heart. But still, I feel the force of Irish guilt. Alzheimer's, I've come to understand, must be fought on both medical and spiritual grounds; I am humbled by such grace.

Not to take myself off the hook, profane language can be common in Alzheimer's and other forms of dementia—an expression of gut rage and loss of filter, along with hitting, grabbing, kicking, pushing, throwing things, scratching, screaming, biting, and making strange noises, all part of the loss of control in this disease. I don't fear at this point that I would hurt anyone. I just worry that I will hurt myself in these moments of overpowering anger, like punching though a glass window, as I've been tempted to do in the past. There is a medical term for uncontrollable cursing. It's called Coprolalia, the involuntary and repetitive use of obscene language, as a symptom of mental illness or organic brain disease. I've sought medical assistance in this regard, and recently had a come-to-Jesus talk about anger with my pastor, about the sheer loss of control and the subsequent guilt. The cursing, the utter blasphemy, for me is like pounding a large nail into a piece of wood; you can remove the nail, but it still leaves a hole.

Pastor Doug Scalise strikes me more as a jock than a minister. Perhaps that's why I drift toward him. At 52, he's in good shape—thin, compact, and can move laterally with ease. A former Colby College centerfielder, a captain of his team in Waterville, Maine, he now plays in a Cape Cod wood bat league for those over 40. He can still hit the curve and the slider, instincts he brings to the pulpit. Pastors must deal with all sorts of rotations and spins. At Brewster Baptist Church on bucolic Main Street, he oversees what he calls a "big tent" church that serves the full range of political, cultural, and social perspectives—all joined together in the cohesion of faith. No one is judged here; we just worship. An ecumenical sort myself, I attend services here as well as the Catholic church down the road. But don't tell my relatives in Dublin, for I'll be stoned. I've also attended services at a synagogue and spoke once at the Unitarian Universalist Church. So I guess I've hit for the cycle.

Pastor Scalise's office speaks to his love of parochial sports. He's a home boy. To the right of his desk is an autographed Boston Celtics Larry Bird jersey; to the left of his desk is an autographed photo of Ted Williams, "the splendid splinter." With Scalise at his desk, it's a trinity of sorts. You can tell a lot about a person from an office. Also framed on the walls are diplomas attesting to Scalise's spiritual side—a Master of Divinity from Boston University and Doctor of Ministry from Northern Baptist Theological Seminary in Lombard, Illinois.

Like all of us, Scalise knows his time on earth is fleeting. Recently, he had a brush with death, an often-fatal heart condition called the "Widow Maker," 98 percent blockage of the anterior interventricular branch of the left coronary artery. He felt severe chest pains after a workout, and emergency surgery at Cape Cod Hospital saved his life. "We all have a shelf life," he tells me, as I reach out for guidance. "We're designed with built-in obsolescence."

Scalise indeed knows what it's like to walk through the Valley of Death. In fact, he has a copy of the 23rd Psalm in his office: "Though I walk through the valley of the shadow of death, I will fear no evil…"

The verse speaks to all of us.

"You can't helicopter over the valley," says Scalise. "You gotta walk through it. Mountain hikers know this. The valley is dark and often you can't see around the next corner; you just have to keep walking."

"Alone?" I ask.

Scalise, a man of with considerable wisdom, points to a photo of a flock of high-flying geese. With the juxtaposition of the photo, it appears the geese are flying past the moon. While we're all told in life to soar like eagles, he says, geese fly even higher in flock "V" formation.

"It's a study of teamwork," he adds. "Geese in formation take turns in the lead, breaking the wind; others in the flock draft off the lead, with each bird honking encouragement and benefiting from the bird in front. They all take turns at the front, the hardest role. It's an exercise in leadership. No one is left alone. And so it should be in life."

The pastor knows why I'm here, the evangelical equivalent to a dark confession box. I'm more comfortable in the light.

I tell him about my WTF talk with God and my intense anger at the Almighty; he reminds me of Mary Stevenson's poem, "Footprints in the Sand," and fury when one perceives that the Lord is not watching: "The times when you have seen only one set of footprints, is when I carried you."

Scalise likes to talk in parables. He tells me about a woman in his church who just died of Alzheimer's, and that when she lost the ability to speak, she and her husband could communicate through expression in the eyes through her soul. "The heart is too deep for words," he says.

He then tells the story of another parishioner on his deathbed, surrounded by family, praying for him. The man couldn't speak either; eyes closed, he was unresponsive. "All of a sudden he sat up in bed, lifted up his arms as to embrace or take a hand, then fell back into his bed. He was gone, he was home."

"Never stop speaking from the heart," Scalise tell me. "When the body weakens with disease, the heart—the soul—grows stronger. It survives for eternity."

I'm assuming now that Pastor Scalise is trying to distract from my anger, assuage me, or buck me up from my deep-seated guilt of fracturing the Third Commandment. But he's not going there yet. He tells another story; this one about the classic Jimmy Stewart movie *It's a Wonderful Life*. "In the movie," he says, "there's a little framed piece on the wall in George Bailey's office in the Bailey Brother's Building and Loan. Most people never see it. Director and producer Frank Capra cut to the framed piece twice, just for a few seconds. It read: 'All that you can take with you is that which you have given away.'"

I press the issue with him, questions anyone in the early stages of Alzheimer's would ask. I tell him about terrifying ongoing dreams where I'm in combat or fighting off an evil presence. "I had a tough one last night," I tell my pastor, noting the dream is reoccurring. "Someone, or some evil entity, was trying to break in the front door of the house, and cracked the door open; I kept pushing back, yet the satanic apparition was able to float through the door. Scary confrontation. I kept swinging at the apparition, which laughed at me, and looked straight into my soul. I didn't back down, but it deeply scared me. My two boys were in the room. The apparition disappeared.

"What's happening to me, why am I so angry, and what do I give away? I got nothing now." I ask.

"You have a right to be angry," he tells me. "It's okay to be angry at God. The book of Psalms is filled with such raw emotion, asking the Lord to 'rouse thyself.' We all think God is sleeping at times. Wake up, we say, get on the job! The anger is understandable, yet misdirected in places. God, I believe, doesn't impart disease, but the Lord will use illness to bless. In illness, we have to look for the blessing, the lesson of giving thanks and gratitude for what remains."

He then stares at me like a pitcher backing down a baserunner, "God has work for you; it's not your time. That will come. But not now. You have work to do!"

"So keep the faith," says Scalise, no pampering, no feeling sorry. He pauses, then refers to Shakespeare's *Hamlet* with the ease of a college English professor. He describes a scene where Hamlet and Horatio are walking in the courtyard to see if the ghost of Hamlet's father will appear on the castle ramparts, as soldiers have been reporting. Horatio is skeptical. Hamlet is hopeful, and presses the issue: "There are more things in Heaven and earth, Horatio, than are dreamt of in your philosophy."

Weeks later in a sermon, Scalise reinforces the point, which has application for all who listen. He quotes from Apostle Paul's Letter to the Romans:

"...We boast in our hope of sharing the glory of God. And not only that, but we also boast in our sufferings, knowing that suffering produces endurance, and endurance produces character, and character produces hope, and hope does not disappoint us, because God's love has been poured into our hearts through the Holy Spirit that has been given to us."

Scalise tells the congregation it has a choice when walking through the "Darkest Valley" times of tribulations that can make or break us. "Don't squander the opportunity," he counsels, urging the flock to walk in endurance, hope, and love. "Grow through what you go through," he says, offering a parable of a carrot, egg, and coffee beans in boiling water.

"A young woman," he says, "went to her mother and told her about her life and how things were so hard for her. She didn't know how she was going to make it, and wanted to give up. She was tired of fighting and struggling. It seemed as one problem was solved a new one arose. Her mother took her to the kitchen. She filled three pots with water. In the first, she placed carrots, in the second she placed eggs, and the last she placed ground coffee beans.

"She let them sit and boil without saying a word. After a while she turned off the burners. She fished the carrots out and placed them in a bowl. She pulled the eggs out and placed them in a bowl. Then she ladled some coffee into a mug. She asked her daughter, 'What do you see?'

"'Carrots, eggs, and coffee,' the daughter replied. Her mother brought her closer, and asked her to feel the carrots. The daughter did, and noted that they were soft. The mother asked her to take an egg and break it. After pulling off the shell, she observed the hard-boiled egg. Finally, the mother asked her to sip the coffee. The daughter smiled, as she tasted its rich aroma.

"Then the daughter asked, 'What's the point?'

"Her mother explained that each of the objects had faced the same adversity, boiling water, but each reacted differently. The carrot went in strong, hard, and unrelenting. However, after being subjected to the boiling water, it softened and became weak. The egg had been fragile. Its thin outer shell had protected its liquid interior. But, after being through boiling water, its inside became hardened. The ground coffee beans were unique, however. After they were in the boiling water they had changed the water.

"'Which are you?' the mother asked her daughter. 'When adversity knocks on your door, how do you respond? Are you a carrot, an egg, or a coffee bean?'"

Pastor Scalise looks up.

"Which one are you?" he asks the congregation.

I'm ducking in the pew, thinking he's speaking straight at me.

Pastor Scalise is dialed into me. A follow up sermon is about trials in life and standing firm in one's faith. "Trials come to all of us," Scalise this morning from the pulpit, "the question is what will you do when facing a trial—what will your response, attitude and approach be?" Paraphrasing from the New Testament Letter of James, he adds, "Faith matures by what it endures."

Scalise goes on to tell a parable about a farmer talking to a passerby about his soybean and corn crops. Rain at the time was abundant, and the fields were fertile, Scalise notes, adding that the farmer's comments to the man were surprising.

"My crops are especially vulnerable," he told the man. "Even a short drought could be devastating."

"Why?" the man asked.

"While frequent rain is a benefit," the farmer said, "during such times of rain plants are not required to push roots deeper in search of water. The roots remain near the surface. And a drought would find the plants unprepared, and quickly kill them."

Message received. My roots need pushing, I'm coming to realize.

Scalise concludes his sermon with a quote from the distinguished African-American scientist and inventor Booker T. Washington, who wrote: "No man should be pitied because every day of life he faces a hard, stubborn problem...It is the man who has no problems to solve, no hardship to face, who is to be pitied...He has nothing in his life which will strengthen and form his character, nothing to call out his latent powers and deepen and widen his hold on life."

Faith learned the hard way, I'm finding, is the way out of exile and the path to Eden.

Next stop: Switzerland.

21

Switzerland or Bust...

The Swiss Alps rise from Lake Geneva like chariots of fire—a vertical rise analogous to the prophet Elijah's ascent to Heaven. The hallowed Alps were formed 34-to-23 million years ago as the African tectonic plate nudged into the European plate, pushing the plates onto each other, akin, the experts say, to pushing up a pile of rocks, or thrusting two mounds of sand toward each other on the beach.

Perfection in the natural way.

Lake Geneva—far below the majestic peaks of Liskamm, Weisshorn, and the Matterhorn—glistens in the sun. The shape of a croissant, with a surface area of 223 square miles and a depth of more than a thousand feet at the deepest level, this glacial lake, the largest natural lake in Western Europe, gives new definition to inspiration and the conception of new memories. While Switzerland is known for neutrality—a historic appeasement of the French, Germans, and Italians to preserve a peace within—there is nothing neutral about this view.

I was invited to Switzerland in the fall of 2016 with Mary Catherine and Conor to speak in Lausanne on Lake Geneva before a world health conference on Alzheimer's, *Lausanne III: The Road to 2025: Delivering Next Generation Alzheimer's Treatments.* Each year, the Lausanne Dialogues convene international medical doyens to promote innovative strategies in Alzheimer's research, regulation, and access. It was first held in 2014 as a response to the challenge articulated at the UK G8 Dementia Summit to stop Alzheimer's by 2025. This goal was reinforced at the First World Health Organization Ministerial Conference on Global Action Against Dementia in 2015. Stopping Alzheimer's by 2025, a bold initiative, requires innovation, collaboration, and creativity, the willingness to learn critical lessons from other diseases, and listening to those living with Alzheimer's—one of the reasons I was asked to speak at the request of George Vradenburg, a driving force behind the Lausanne Dialogues.

The Lausanne Dialogues are organized under the auspices of The Organization for Economic Cooperation and Development (oecd. org), one of the world's largest, most reliable sources of comparable statistical, economic, and social data, monitoring international trends, collecting data, analyzing and forecasting economic development, and investigating evolving patterns in a broad range of public policy area. The Lausanne workshop is supported by the State Secretariat for Education, Research and Innovation SERI, Switzerland, The Global CEO Initiative on Alzheimer's Disease (CEOi), and Alzheimer's Disease International (ADI).

Clearly, I was out of my league, on stage with medical experts and brainiacs from around the world from Nigeria to Japan, Australia to England, Germany to Switzerland, and beyond. All I could think of, as I was called to the stage to speak, were lyrics from "If I Only Had a Brain:"

> *I could wile away the hours*
> *Conferrin' with the flowers*
> *Consultin' with the rain*
> *And my head I'd be scratchin'*
> *While my thoughts were busy hatchin'*
> *If I only had a brain*

With apologies to the late Ray Bolger, the sinuous, peripatetic Scarecrow in L. Frank Baum's *The Wizard of Oz*, for those of us with Alzheimer's—the early, middle, and late stages—the disease is a ride over the rainbow. Our heads are full of stuffin'.

Thank God for prompts and notes, yet another real-time example of perception not always resembling reality. I told the distinguished assemblage with great trepidation that I couldn't talk about complicated medical issues, for all I did in high school was cut up a frog. But I spoke to them in laymen's terms about living with Alzheimer's in faith, hope, and humor, and the various strategies required to ply the currents of this disease.

"My hope," I concluded, "is to connect some of the dots of Alzheimer's." I then read a stanza from William Earnest Henley's classic poem, "Invictus:"

> *In the fell clutch of circumstance*
> *I have not winced nor cried aloud.*
> *Under the bludgeonings of chance*
> *My head is bloody, but unbowed.*

"There are great parallels," I said, "between Henley's Victorian poem and those living with Alzheimer's today. Henley concludes his seminal work about the throes of unthinkable struggle, 'I am the master of my fate; I am the captain of my soul.'"

We all seek to be captains of our soul.

There was a disconnect on the way to Lausanne. "Al" was bearing down, and I was demoted to the rank of private.

The Delta jumbo jet from Logan Airport in Boston landed in Amsterdam on its way to Geneva for the first leg of the trip. Amsterdam Airport Schiphol—the main international airport of the Netherlands, in a country where anything goes, certainly not the kind of place for someone grasping for the thread between perception and reality—is a cornucopia of humanity. It has all the ambiance of the Cantina bar scene in the original *Star Wars* in the pirate city of Mos Eisley on the planet Tatooine. As trivia aficionados observe online, the Cantina "is the haunt of freight pilots and other dangerous characters of various alien races...and sometimes a band of musicians named Fibrin Dan and the Modal Nodes."

Dot-dot, dot-dot...da-da-dot; dot-dot, dot-dot...da-do-la-dot...

Amsterdam Airport, at first glance to an individual easily confused, is horrifically distressing: busy, buzzing, loud, lots of alien languages, and striking native dress, an etiological ordeal. Then there's the incessant, mind-bending announcements of flights, delays, transfers, and cancellations in tongues that make ancient Babel sound like an entry Spanish 101 quiz. *"Come, let us go down and there confuse their language, that they may not understand one another's speech,"* it says in Genesis 11:6.

The core of the Kingdom of the Netherlands, Amsterdam and its airport are impressive by all rights, yet a clear disconnect for me. The voices, the noises, the diverse languages reverberated in my mind once again like the stabbing violin of a horror film.

I had to leave.

"I'm the hell outta here," I told my wife, heading to any place perceived as sanctuary outside the terminal. "I'm done, just freakin' done."

"You just sit; you just SIT!" she shouted.

"Then I'll pee again in my pants."

"Fine," she said, then after quick reflection instructed Conor: "You go with your father to the bathroom. Do *NOT* let him out of your sight!"

I was under house arrest, no escape, indisputably in line for a "Pet Passport" that allows animals to travel easily between member countries without undergoing quarantine. Mary Catherine was probing for the paperwork. Thoughts of flying in a cage were illuminating. Stand down...So I did.

Finally, we boarded the flight to Geneva, then an hour and a half train ride to the resort town of Montreux on the northeast side of Lake

Geneva in the canton of Vaud at the foot of the Swiss Alps, the self-styled "Swiss Riveria." It was to be a staging area for the cerebral climb to Lausanne. I sat by myself in quiet reflection on the upper level of the train as it thundered past remarkable countryside approaching the Alps in *The Sound of Music.*

Montreux rises gently above Lake Geneva in tiers to vernal heights covered with woods and vineyards that shelter from north and east winds. Below along the lake, you can find fig, bay, almond, and mulberry trees, even cypresses, magnolias, and in places palm trees thriving in Mediterranean warmth. The town, liberated in 1798 by Napoleon, has distinct architectural styles—the most notable, the "Belle Époque" buildings of the grand hotels built at the turn of the 19th and 20th centuries, accommodating predominately to well-heeled English tourists; Queen Victoria was an admirer of Montreux and visited many times. Over the years, Montreux has given shelter to the likes of: English playwright, composer, actor, and singer Noel Coward; author F. Scott Fitzgerald's wife, Zelda; Russian composer Igor Stravinsky; and Empress Elisabeth of Austria and Queen of Hungary.

A prime example of Belle Époque architecture is Le Montreux Palace with its yellow awnings and lush gardens that run down to the lake with views of the French Alps in the distance. The sprawling, imperial Montreux Palace is fully elegant, yet calmly welcoming in assiduous service of the Swiss style. So why not stay a few days among the European elite, I pondered. Hey, as a constituent of the great unwashed, I got plenty of money, it's just tied up in debt.

And besides, the Montreux Palace is a good place to get lost.

Our room was as expected—gracefully, elegantly appointed, museum quality, with a balcony overlooking the snow-capped Alps. The beat below of Avenue Claude-Nobs was enticing. I wanted to explore.

"Not so fast," I was told by my wife, the commandant. "You stay put in the room; look out from the balcony, write, read a book, or just stare at yourself...Conor and I will take a look around and come back for you. *Stay here!"*

And with that, the two exited the room. The door shutting behind them had the resonating cling of an iron cell in a prisoner of war camp.

"Green light," I thought! "Green light...I got the green light."

Alzheimer's has a way of rendering one cerebrally color blind; a red light, a stop sign, becomes a green light. Go for it, often just because someone told you that you can't. *The Great Escape* for me. Steve McQueen, a.k.a. Capt. Virgil Hilts, the "Cooler King" at Stalag Luft III, would be proud. Alzheimer's in its apparitions has a way of bringing one back to the illusion of movies—some fanciful, some thrillers, some psychological nightmares. The trip to Switzerland and accompanying disconnects had moved the dial further for me than ever before.

In a blink, I was out the door, with iPhone in hand to respond to a room check from the commandant. I dashed to the right, away from the main elevator, to avoid detection and a trip back to the "cooler." At the end of a long, isolated hall with oil paintings on the walls dripping in rich history, I spotted a remote stairwell. This was not to be a staircase to Heaven. I descended to what I thought was the lobby with the speed of a downhill skier, skipping four steps at a time. I was free in the moment.

The stairwell seemed to have no ending, an abyss of a downward spiral. At the bottom, there was no lobby, just white sheets draped over furniture, empty room after empty room. The place had the smell of mildew, as if someone had tried to extinguish the flames of hell. My mind was racing. I was lost; delusions were in full gait. I ran up to the next floor. Same frightful panorama. My cell phone couldn't connect, no signal. Dammit, no signal! Can you hear me now, I cried within? In a flash, Le Montreux Palace had become the Overlook Hotel in Stanley Kubrick's *The Shining*, and I was writer Jack Torrance seeking haunting solitude to create. "All work and no play make Greggie a dull boy..."

My racing imagination took me to new depths—to the end of the hallway, to what I imagined were rivers of blood and two freaky twins dressed like dolls, ghosts of the murdered Grady Twins. "Come and play with us…"

"Hell no!" I shouted, racing back up and down the stairwell, rifling for reality.

Reality was found on my third trip back to the basement. I heard more voices. In the words of Jack Torrance, "Things could be better…Things could be a whole lot better." Ultimately, they were. I came upon two tall, thin guys dressed as bellmen. I was afraid to ask what hotel they worked at, or to see if they had robot legs. The two led me down a maze of dank hallways, then to a door. "Step *away* from that handle." I felt like screaming. Too late for that. The door opened, and the grace of God came streaming in. Lights in my brain that had been flickering in this early stage were now at full power. I was back in the exquisite Montreux Palace lobby, having been furtively lost in an isolated section of the hotel, apparently closed for the off-season.

My cell phone was now vibrating in my pocket. It was the commandant.

"Where the hell have you been?!" she yelled.

"I was in hell," I replied.

What was tantamount to imaginary ankle bracelets awaited my return to the room; a benevolent front desk clerk led the way. "*Stay put*" had escalated from a command to a death threat.

Two nights later, two days before the Lausanne Dialogues, lights in the brain went out again. At about 2 a.m., I raced out of the room, speech in hand. "I'm late," I shrieked. "I have to give my speech."

"Go back to bed," both Mary Catherine and Conor shouted. I was wholly awake now.

"Bullshit," I responded, running out into the hallway fully dressed, taking a left, not a right to the netherworld. I lost my way again. Giving up the ghost minutes later, I sat on the floor of the hallway, speech in hand, my head bracing the far wall, eyes to the ceiling. Thank God the Grady Twins were sleeping.

Conor, warden in training, finally caught up with me. "Holy shit, Dad! Back to the room..."

Forty-eight hours later, the half-hour train ride from Montreux to Lausanne, along the shores of Lake Geneva, was uneventful other than celestial splendor at the hands of the Almighty. Still, I was shaking off the symptoms of synapse disconnects. Disembarking the train and hailing a cab to the Starling Hotel near the SwissTech Convention Center in Lausanne—not far from École Polytechnique Fédérale de Lausanne (Swiss Federal Institute of Technology)—would prove challenging. Conor was all over it with his iPhone apps and extras. Mulish Mick that I am, two suitcases in hand and carting a backpack, I was intent on finding my own way.

"Stay with us," Mary Catherine yelled.

"Not gonna happen," I said in the muddle.

Green light, green light. I headed up a separate staircase to the street. We were divided yet again by hundreds of people and a wide, congested thoroughfare that seemed to provoke piercing horn-blowing and road rage. In an instant, my mind took me back to in the pirate city of Mos Eisley on the planet Tatooine.

"Stay put," Conor instructed Mary Catherine. "I'll find him." The two whipped out the "Where's Waldo" app on their phones; there I was, a blip on the screen. Conor then crossed the thoroughfare like Moses parting the Red Sea. His piercing glare almost burned my corneas; I thought he was going to fit me with a child harness and leash. Who are the parents now?

Strike three! And I hadn't even given my speech yet. We drove in the cab to the hotel in silence. I would be redeemed that night at a special speakers' dinner held in downtown Lausanne at the posh Lausanne Palace on Rue du Grand-Chêne in the chandelier-adorned Ustinov Room, surrounded by some of the brightest minds on the planet. I could only digest every other word, and that's just off the menu. But Mary Catherine and Conor were suitably impressed, and chatted up a storm with the intellectual elite. I thought I was home free. Later, the "good night" part back in the Starling Hotel room didn't go so well. I mouthed off again to my wife, as the confusion, rage, and darkness of the last few days crested. Caregivers bear the brunt of this disease when those of us afflicted are out on Pluto.

We all got up early the next day as if nothing had happened. In Alzheimer's, every day is filled with new sets of trials. After dressing in a stylish blue suit, I started wandering the room. "Put your shoes on," my wife instructed. "I can't," I said to myself, "someone is standing in them." It's happened before. I walked toward the apparition, and in a puff it was gone.

My speech before the Lausanne Dialogues went well. I followed my prepared script about living with Alzheimer's, the fight to stay on the planet. "My life slowly is changing," I said in conclusion, "yet it remains the same, a slow demise of who I once was. On bad days, I feel a shadow of myself. Like Lewis Carroll's *Alice in Wonderland* where 'nothing would be what it is, because everything would be what it isn't.'

"Alzheimer's," I also remarked, "is a cunning, calculating killer. Perhaps Ernest Hemingway said it best, 'The world breaks everyone, and afterwards, some are strong in the broken places.'

"Be strong in the broken places…"

I done good. But little did anyone know at the Lausanne Dialogues the ugliness of what had transpired days earlier. Even the brightest are capable of a drive-by, unable to penetrate the unfathomable darkness of this disease. And that's as terrifying as the disease itself.

We left Lausanne late in the afternoon after the speech and panel discussion, taking a train to Geneva for the flight back to Boston early the following morning, and staying the night at the Starling Hotel branch at Geneva International Airport, a short walk from the train. We all desired to tour downtown Geneva, a city that hosts the largest number of international organizations in the world, some of the best museums, and world-class architecture.

"How do we get there?" Mary Catherine asked the receptionist at the front desk.

"Bus number five," the man said hurriedly.

That didn't sit well with me. "How do we find bus number five?" I inquired.

"It's just around the corner," replied the man, distracted with check-ins. Without looking up, he pointed left to a hotel exit. "Not far from here."

"So is Paris," I said in a loss of filter.

I got the glower from my wife.

We headed stage left, out the side door, to a quiet country lane, more suitable to golf carts than a city bus line.

"So this is 'around the corner,'" I interjected, race-walking in search of a bus stop that I was convinced didn't exist, part of the paranoia of this disease. The disconnect deepened as numbness, as it does often, crept up the back of my neck and enveloped the mind. I was fogged in again. My pace quickened as I tried to pinpoint "around the corner." Soon I was running; not sure why, but I was running, faster and faster away from Conor and Mary Catherine. "This is bullshit," I kept saying in symptomatic rage that now comes on without notice. "This is bullshit."

My mind was racing; I felt we were lost, and I wanted out of this nightmare.

I took the first left-hand turn, heading out to what seemed like a busy road. I came upon two middle-aged women along the way and asked where the bus stop was located. They looked at me like I was from Pluto.

"Bus-ssss Stop-pppp," I said drawing out the words.

No response. They didn't comprehend. They thought I was just another crazy American, which I am.

So I kept running, with Conor and Mary Catherine farther and farther in the rearview mirror.

Then it began raining buses. I saw several of them whizzing in the distance ahead. Amen! I ran faster. Conor and Mary Catherine now chased after me with a pace that suggested they feared the world was flat and that I might fall off, perhaps to their delight. One of the buses came to a screeching halt at the side of the road on its way to busy, bewildering downtown Geneva. I sprinted toward the side door and jumped in, grabbing the first empty seat—safe at last, safe at last. The only fly in the ointment was that Conor and Mary Catherine hadn't caught up yet with the bus. Seconds later the side door closed. I looked up, and I saw them huffing and puffing, faces planted against the window of the door, looking in with horror at me.

I noticed Conor turning to Mary Catherine and staring at his mother in deep thought. Later he confided that he was thinking: "Hey, what's the worst that can happen? Dad will get lost again, but he's a survivor. Someone will figure it out for him, and Mom and me will get a needed break...."

*Nah...*flushed with Irish guilt and in primal response mode, Conor literally forced the bus doors open to get his mother and then himself on board. We were a family again. "All good?" I asked. Neither wanted to talk to me, until after a first round at a tavern downtown.

Cheers!

I had pushed them to the limit. On my next international trip, if there ever was one, I was told, we'd be accompanied by a squadron of kickass handlers. "Do you get that?" I sheepishly shook my head like one of those cheap toy Chihuahuas that look out the rear windows of old Chevys.

"Ah, it's all part of the experience," as Clark Griswold would say.

Early the next morning, we all flew back to Logan Airport, collectively with a greater understanding of the progression of Alzheimer's and a full appreciation, on all fronts, for what we had just experienced—the remarkable beauty of Switzerland, the grace and intellect of the Lausanne Dialogues, the unremitting struggle to stay in the moment, and how that touches those one loves, and those on the way.

Boston or bust…

22

Sweet Adeline

Sweet Adeline,
My Adeline,
At night, dear heart,
For you I pine.
In all my dreams,
Your fair face beams.
You're the flower of my heart,
Sweet Adeline.
—RICHARD H. GERARD

Abiding "Sweet Adeline," a ballad written in the late 1800s under the title, "You're the Flower of My Heart," became a hit when performed in 1904 by the Quaker City Four. The song became so popular that John F. Fitzgerald, "Honey Fitz," the father of Rose Kennedy and maternal grandfather of John F. Kennedy, made it his political theme song during his tenure in Congress and two terms as mayor of Boston. Honey Fitz sang the ballad at scores of political and social happenings as well as on the radio, venerating the name Adeline in barbershop quartet fashion.

Teutonic in origin, the Latin translation of Adeline is "noble, or of nobility." It was a common name in the Middle Ages, then faded from usage until the Gothic Revival of the mid-1700s. The song's popularity amplified over the years, becoming a favorite of the Irish at last call. Mickey Mouse even serenaded Minnie Mouse with "Sweet Adeline" in a 1929 Disney cartoon.

Hold that thought.

My daughter, Colleen, noble in all ways, had the principled heart years ago to leave the refuge of her Washington, D.C. job as a security analyst for a consultant to Homeland Security to teach needy children in the inner-city of Baltimore. She took a sizeable pay cut, taught her students to walk in love and hope, married a fine Baltimore guy, Matt Everett, whose family has lived in the city for generations, and then got pregnant, our first grandchild on the way. All in due time.

I always thought I was too young to be a grandfather; now I'm wondering why I waited so long. In this journey, I've worried privately that I'd never get to hold a grandchild, a common fear in early-onset Alzheimer's. I was losing ground in my desire to remain here. After word of her pregnancy in the spring of 2016, I reflected quietly on the day I gave my precious daughter away. She was an extraordinary bride in all ways. The wedding reception at the Ocean Edge Resort and Golf Club overlooking a panorama of Cape Cod Bay was spectacular in its venue and guests that numbered more than 200. Lots of confusion, disconnects for me, too many voices, so surreptitiously I took breaks outside the ballroom and stared blankly at the bay, looking out at Pluto and pondering how other fathers diagnosed with this disease fought off symptoms on their daughter's big day. Friends and relatives came looking for me. On cue for my invocation, I tried to capture the mood of all fathers in the room, in a speech I wrote days earlier on a ferry ride across Vineyard Sound to Nantucket, with tears streaming down my face:

Words have sounds.

We hear words. Not just read them.

Run.

Breathe.

Reach.

Live.

Celebrate.

Faith.

Forgive.

They all have meaning in sounds. In the composition of the mind. Scholars call it onomatopoeia—formation of a word from a sound associated with it.

The word today swirling around my head is: Change. As a verb, Webster's defines change as "to make or become different." As a noun, change is defined as "the act or instance of becoming different."

We are here today on the precipice of change, the making and the instance of it. Becoming different.

While my mind agrees with Webster's definition, my heart says otherwise.

I've never done change well.

The sounds I hear when I think of change: the first cry of a beautiful little girl entering the world in the delivery room of Boston's Brigham and Women's Hospital; Colleen's laughter at walking Brewster flats as hermit crabs tickled her toes; her anticipation as she climbed for the first time those steep steps of the yellow school bus on her way to kindergarten; the cheers on the softball field as she turned a double play; the stench of the old Boston Garden as we watched Disney on Ice together; the swing of "Sweet Caroline" at Fenway; sitting in Tom Brady's personal suite for a Pats game at Gillette Stadium; the rip of my heart as she left for Elon University, and I felt in change there was something terribly wrong; the first time she brought Matt Everett home with her, and I felt something was terribly right.

Winds of change are swirling today. My mind is an old school carousel of Kodachrome slides of Colleen's life, all arranged in chronological order. I can hear the click as one slide advances the other.

I can't stop these flashes and sounds of color. Nor do I want to.

Marriage, to me, is reaffirmation of God's plan. We, as parents, are caregivers, caretakers in the nest for our children. They belong to God, our father. Our job is to nurture, to love, to direct, to refine, to support—all in imperfect ways—then to let go, and let God. When love comes from the heart, not the head, it is perfect.

The letting go part, however, is difficult for all of us. But the spreading of wings results in beautiful, soaring flight.

So Colleen and Matt soar today, as you leave the nest, soar as high as you can. Fly side by side. Help, encourage, and love each other endlessly in flight. A picture worthy of a gold frame.

You begin your family album today. The first click was the "I do."

Now it's "we do," the first person plural. You have become one. That is a change. A good change: becoming different, but in remarkable ways. The winds of change have cleared the canvas. You paint your own picture now, a stunning picture in words, in romance, in children, in challenges, in flight, and in words from the heart.

Words have sounds. We hear them.

I love you, Colleen, with all my heart...

Flash forward to Colleen's delivery, November 11, 2016. She sent a text at midnight saying her water broke. Mary Catherine was in bed, heading to Baltimore at first light; I let her sleep. I had been told earlier by several family members, close and extended, not to come to Baltimore for the delivery, that I would be a persona non grata, yet another distraction. "Remain home and don't forget to go to the bathroom," I was instructed. So I stayed on the Cape with Conor, under house arrest.

"Keep the faith, breathe easy," I texted back to Colleen, not clearly remembering what "water broke" meant. Like a slip and slide, I thought the baby was heading down the shoot. Not by a longshot.

With Mary Catherine in Baltimore later that morning and Colleen and husband Matt at Greater Baltimore Medical Center, I got another text at noon. "No new word yet," my wife wrote.

No word? Really? The baby was in the chute.

At 2 p.m., there was another terse text. "Colleen pushing at 2 p.m."

Great, I thought. "Matt, oil up the catcher's mitt!"

No word. Radio silence.

Finally, I texted my wife at 4 p.m. "What's up?"

"No new word, that's all I know," she replied.

"That's bullshit," I texted back in a fit of loss of filter. "I need a new word."

I was justifying my house arrest.

Alzheimer's, in so many ways, is an altered state where paranoia reigns. The Alzheimer's Association, alz.org, will tell you: "Individuals with dementia may become paranoid as a result of false beliefs, or delusions, symptoms of the disease…. Although not grounded in reality, the situation is very real to the person with dementia. Keep in mind that a person with dementia is trying to make sense of his or her world with declining cognitive function. Examples of paranoia are accusations that someone is poisoning their food or stealing their money, or statements such as, 'My spouse is an imposter.'"

I was thinking Mary Catherine was an imposter.

I texted her again at 5 p.m.

"Any new word?" I was desperate, channeling myself.

There was no response. Dead silence.

In my paranoia, I began thinking something was critically wrong. Colleen's water broke at midnight; this was 18 hours later. Holy shit! Really? "They are hiding something from me," I feared. "They just don't want to deal with me in an emergency." I was pissed, moving toward yet another rage. Little did I remember that Mary Catherine was in labor with our first son, Brendan, for about 22 hours at Boston's Brigham & Women's Hospital.

At 6 p.m., I called my wife. "What's up, I need to know now!"

"I have nothing to tell you," she said curtly, clearly annoyed at my persistence.

"I need to know if something has gone wrong with Colleen or the baby," I insisted.

"There is nothing more I can tell you," she said.

"Fine," I replied. "Then I'm heading down now to talk to the doctors!"

"Oh, no *you're* not!" she said.

"Yes, I am!"

Click. The phone went dead.

Within minutes, Mary Catherine, unbeknownst me, convened an emergency session of the College of Cardinals, available siblings, to talk me off the third rail. Seconds later, I received a call from my older sister Maureen, a tough Irish lady and a baby nurse at Northern Westchester Hospital in Mt. Kisco, New York.

"You stay home," she ordered sternly, like a field marshal. "You just stay home! Look, we all know that you know a lot about writing, politics, and Alzheimer's, but you know squat about delivering babies. You stay home. Got that?!"

Reassured by my sister, I responded, "Do you still love me?"

"Yes, but you stay the fuck home!"

I needed to reload, so I asked Conor to take me to the gym to work off the rage. We ran on treadmills, side-by-side. About a half hour into the run, Conor reached over to hand me his iPhone. I thought it was a sports score. I didn't have my glasses.

"What's this about?" I asked.

"Congratulations, you're a grandfather," he said, showing me a text just sent with a photo of my granddaughter.

I started crying. A beautiful baby, eight pounds, eight ounces, Adeline Mae Everett, entered the world in noble fashion. The name Adeline, I wanted to believe, because she came from nobility, half a member of the Brian Boru clan, an Irish king who concluded the high kingship of Ireland. Mae, as family history would have it, is the proper name of my maternal grandmother's sister, Mae Clancy, a first-generation Irish American, who married, then was whisked off to a Carmelite convent in Peekskill, New York, after something horribly went wrong with the marriage. At the 1876 Abby of St. Mary, now abandoned, the nuns took a vow of silence. Enough said. We were never told about Mae's past, though on visits as young kids, Mae and her Carmelite sisters, who all made Eucharistic hosts at the abbey, would be allowed to speak for the day. To my knowledge, no one ever spilled the family beans.

And to my knowledge, Adeline Mae Everett, with a healthy set of lungs, has never taken, nor will ever take, a vow of silence.

$$\underset{\diagup}{\cancel{}}$$

The trip to Baltimore the following month on Christmas Eve 2016 to see my Adeline for the first time was both electrifying and unnerving. As you now know about me, airports can be my undoing. Too much noise, confusion, and people in uniforms yelling stuff. Loading laptops, backpacks, belts, winter coats, shoes, paper clips, cell phone, and small change onto a conveyor belt can be disconcerting with petulant travelers queued up and sighing behind you. I usually yell out something stupid, like "this sucks..." Not the kind of exchange TSA likes to hear. "Excuse me?" I often hear.

"Oh, my husband is just having a bad day; he has a medical issue," my patient wife usually explains, then turns to me and stares a penetrating stream of lasers into my corneas.

On this particular morning, the conveyor belt was herky-jerky, stopping and going because the dumbasses ahead of me (*there I go again*) had bottles of water, mouthwash, shampoo, and other verboten liquids in their carry-on. Given my head shaking and muttering through the metal detector, I was patted down. I don't like strangers touching me. I was out of sorts. Once released, I waited on the other side of the conveyor belt for the bolus of what I had shipped. Without notice, a single shoe shot out. It was my wife's, a tan Sperry topsider. Out of body, lights in the brain dimming, I was thinking body parts now were on the way. I turned to my right to look for a cop, then saw my wife limping with one shoe. Remember when you were scared about losing a child, a family member, thinking they were lost, abducted, whatever, then shouting at them in relief when they're found? So I threw the shoe toward my wife...

Conor immediately sent Colleen a text: "Can't wait to see you and the baby! Bells are ringing! The wonderful Christmas spirit is upon us! Oh, Dad threw a shoe at mom going through security. Merry Christmas! When does Santa stuff his fat ass down the chimney tonight?"

My bad. Caregivers offer grace.

Finally, we arrived safely in Baltimore, staying downtown on the harbor, not far from Colleen and Matt's home in the handsome Roland Park section of the city and near ancient cobblestones of historic Fells Point—ballast for schooners and "Baltimore Clippers" that plied the blustery oceans of the world. Established in the mid 1700s, Fells Point was a classic shipyard that built and supported dozens of privateers in the War of 1812 that preyed on British shipping vessels. The British retaliated, calling Fells Point a "nest of pirates," an enflaming moniker that eventually led the British to attack Baltimore Harbor and mercilessly bomb Fort McHenry, an assault that inspired Francis Scott Key to write the poem, "Defence of Fort M'Henry," later to become known as "The Star Spangled Banner." During the battering, a "storm flag" was flown over Fort McHenry. It was replaced early on the morning of September 14, 1814 with a large garrison American flag, signaling victory over the British in the defiant Battle of Baltimore.

Flags waving in a spirit of victory, I embraced my granddaughter Adeline Mae on Christmas Eve. I held her tightly. New life. New hope. Something **new** to live for. God is good!

23

"Which One of You Nuts Has Got Any Guts?"

Three geese in a flock.
One flew east, one flew west,
One flew over the cuckoo's nest.

—*MOTHER GOOSE FOLK SONG:*
VINTERY, MINTERY, CUTERY, CORN

"Man, when you lose your laugh, you lose your footing," wrote Ken Kesey, author of the iconic prize-winning, pioneering 1962 novel *One Flew Over the Cuckoo's Nest.*

Kesey never lost his footing in his finest work, writing of the misunderstood and the struggle against the system, adapting personal experiences from working the night shift in a psychiatric ward at a mental institution. Kesey never accepted that the patients were insane, but instead that the world had cast them out, given they did not meet conformist standards of behavior. Born in 1935, Kesey attended Stanford University, and was a paid volunteer for a U.S. Army experimental subject, administered mind-altering drugs and asked to report on their effects at a time when profound changes in the delivery of psychology and psychiatry were afoot, as noted in an assortment of summaries.

Cuckoo's Nest was adapted on Broadway and in 1975 in a film, starring a young Jack Nicholson, that won five Academy Awards. Eighteen years later the film was deemed "culturally, historically, or aesthetically significant" by the United States Library of Congress, and for preservation in the National Film Registry.

There are compelling parallels between *Cuckoo's Nest* and Alzheimer's disease—in how stereotyping and misunderstanding widen the rift between the observer and the afflicted, and how avoidance, intentional or otherwise, acerbates the delusion between the two, causing greater pain for the stricken.

In the movie, Nicholson's character, the rebellious Randall Patrick McMurphy, a swaying personality of a convict looking for an easy way out, becomes a symbol of freedom, instilling courage, confidence, and self-esteem in the patients around him. His insurgent conduct deeply annoys ward captain Nurse Ratched, a symbol of the system, who intimidates patients with demoralizing passive-aggressiveness. Her discipline heightens as McMurphy teaches patients to bet cigarettes playing cards, then steals a hospital bus, escaping with some patients for a fishing trip, then throws a surprise Christmas party on the ward. McMurphy becomes a role model to his diffident followers, among them: Billy Bibbit, a terrified thirty-one-year-old man with the mind of an adolescent; Scanlon, a patient with ruinous delusions; the playful, loveable Martini; and Chief Bromden, son of the chief of the Columbia Indians who leaves others with the impression that he cannot hear or speak.

"Which one of you nuts has got any guts?" McMurphy challenged them.

They all answered the call, as many do in disease.

My close friends in this disease, from all walks in life, have answered the call; they got great guts in educating and breaking down the stereotypes of Alzheimer's for those with the disease and family caregivers around the country. All are heroes, faces of the disease from every perspective of life, among them: Brian LeBlanc, former newspaper worker, radio host, and accountant; Presbyterian minister Rev. Cynthia Huling Hummel; senior telecommunications technician Mike Belleville; Boston financial analyst Ken Sullivan—all past or present contributing members of the national Alzheimer's Association Early Stage Advisory Group; native Puerto Rican Daisy Duarte; *Still Alice* producer Elizabeth Gelfand Sterns, a close associate of Maria Shriver in the fight against Alzheimer's and former member of the Alzheimer's Association national board of directors; 1960s civil rights activists Rob and Margaret Rice Moir; Dr. T. Berry Brazelton, world-renowned pediatrician, author, and founder of the Brazelton Touchpoints Center at Boston's Children's Hospital, a Harvard Medical School teaching hospital; Trish Vradenburg, co-founder of UsAgainstAlzheimer's, a powerful alliance in the fight; John Joe Vaughan of New Ross, County Wexford, Ireland, who's attacking his Alzheimer's as if it were pillaging eighth-century Vikings invading Éire; and finally, Bob Bertschy, a former catcher in the Los Angeles Dodgers organization, who pressed on with three strikes against him.

Kesey writes in *Cuckoo's Nest*: "You have to laugh at the things that hurt you just to keep yourself in balance, just to keep the world from running you plumb crazy."

Brian LeBlanc sees himself as a modern-day Randall Patrick Murphy in his struggle against Alzheimer's.

"I'm definitely Randle Patrick McMurphy, though in nonviolent ways," LeBlanc, diagnosed with early-onset Alzheimer's in 2014 and fully symptomatic, tells me in an interview from Pensacola, Florida, where he lives with his wife, Shannon. "I'm thinking I'm not crazy, but yes, to some extent I am. McMurphy witnessed how patients were being treated, and he wanted, in his own way, to see them have a better quality of life, rather than suffering. Makes me think of the stigmatization of dementia. Just because we have a terminal disease doesn't mean we can't have a good quality of life, doesn't mean we have to stop living."

Several months ago, he wasn't so sure. LeBlanc woke up on Super Bowl Sunday in February 2017, unable to speak, the apparent result of an Alzheimer's-induced brain hemorrhage. Loss of speech came on the heels of accelerated memory loss, hallucinations, loss of balance, greater rage, loss of smell and taste, diabetes, and other representative on-going daily symptoms of the disease.

"I woke up early that morning and my voice was silent," LeBlanc, 56, recalls, adding he passed notes to his wife to communicate. "I curled up like a ball and started crying."

Shannon took to her knees to pray, while doctors in vain searched for treatment. "For the first time in years, I prayed. I asked the Lord, 'Show me something,'" she said.

Hours later, she opened her mail to a promotion from Disneyworld in Orlando, Brian's "sweet zone," a place he has visited more than 25 times over the last 40 years, which brings him back to childhood, more and more now. So for their 10th-wedding anniversary, two and a half weeks later, she booked a trip. Brian was reluctant this time, but agreed to go, though the trip did not get off to a good start. Upon arriving, he lost his balance, tripped on a carpet, and fell down a flight of stairs.

On the night of February 19, watching a brilliant display of fireworks in front of Disney's Cinderella's Castle on Main Street, Brian looked up at the sky and avowed, "Oh my!"

"WHAT DID YOU SAY?!" Shannon exclaimed, tearing up.

"God, it's so beautiful!" Brian said, in awe.

The Lord works in mysterious ways. In an instant, with the boom of brilliant light, Brian's voice was returned. He calls it the Miracle on Main Street. "My doctors agree," he adds. "They say it was nothing short of a miracle."

Shannon and Brian now start each day with a prayer.

Still, his road is rife with twists and turns. Brian has lost his grandfather, his grandmother, and his mother to Alzheimer's, and his dad died of vascular dementia. Brian has two copies of the Alzheimer's marker gene APOE-4. His life, like the rest of us, has become a daily strategy session; sticky note reminders cover his desk at home like a patchwork quilt, and the markings on his calendar look like an old-school football chalkboard with X's, O's, and arrows, pointing in all directions, outlining the plays of the day. Finances are also a common and mounting issue. Brian can no longer work. His wife supports the family as a full-time operations manager at a Pensacola area HUD housing project. "The disease takes family finances down, and puts tremendous stress on a couple, changing the dynamic of a marriage," says Brian.

Then there is the rage many of us deal with.

"The rage," Brian says, "comes on when things that I was very familiar with I can no longer figure out, like the television remote. I only wish they made remotes out of rubber instead of plastic, so when I hurl it in anger at the brick fireplace, it doesn't smash into pieces."

When Brian got word of his diagnosis he says he went into "a rabbit hole" of dark depression, but then decided to get off the mat. "Then I asked myself, 'What the hell are you doing?'"

A pity party, Brian says, is a lonely place. "You're the only guest. I could have lain there like a baby, or try to do some good, dispel some of the many myths about Alzheimer's."

Brian is doing a lot of good these days. He's an advocate for Dementia Alliance International-Global; a keynote Alzheimer's speaker; a member of the Dementia Action Alliance in Falls Church, Virginia; an advocate and speaker for the Alzheimer's Association Alabama/Florida Panhandle Chapter; and served with me in 2015 as a member of the Alzheimer's Association Early Stage Advisory Group, based in Chicago, an incredible organization with a broad reach.

Recently, Brian and I, as well as others, lost a good friend to the disease who had served on the Early Stage Advisory Group, Ron Casola, diagnosed with early-onset Alzheimer's in 2011. Ron, who spent many years in Texas and Arizona, also served as a board member of the San Antonio Alzheimer's Association and was an Alzheimer's advocate in the Phoenix area. A man of great talent, who also pushed back stereotypes of the disease, Ron was extraordinarily talented in music and performed as a soloist with the Phoenix Symphony, with the San Diego Opera, and with the famed Boston Pops under the

290 On Pluto: Inside the Mind of Alzheimer's

direction of the late Doc Severinsen at Carnegie Hall. Ron also was gay, and spoke candidly about the trials in living with the disease.

"I wish people would be more open about Alzheimer's," he said shortly before his death. Ron, at first, was reluctant to talk about it, but after marshaling the courage to do so and after sensing the support, he began reaching out to others. "It inspired me to try to help others 'come out of the closet,' and get the help they need."

And that's what is required in this fight, to bring Alzheimer's out of the closet before millions more and their families are afflicted. While buoyant about a cure sometime in the future, those in the throes of the disease, like Brian, me, and others, look to the future in other ways. The cure won't come for us.

"Until one is able to get inside the mind of Alzheimer's, living with the disease, no one can fully understand it. In the past, we've allowed the experts, the doctors, and society all to speak for us. Now we're speaking for ourselves. To a large extent, we know better. We know what it's like to be inside the mind of Alzheimer's. It's open, honest, and raw."

In the meantime, Brian, the pragmatist, adds, "Do I want to live another twenty years with the progressions of this wicked disease? I don't think so..."

Easter in the Christian faith is a time of redemption.

On Easter Sunday, 2017, the Rev. Cynthia Huling Hummel stood in the pulpit of a Presbyterian church in upstate New York, delivering a carefully prepared homily on the resurrection. She did her holy best to describe the crucifixion and burial of Jesus, and was at the part of the sermon when Mary Magdalene arrived at the empty tomb of Jesus and was confronted by an angel—the defining moment of her homily.

Cynthia turned to the next page in her sermon, and it was blank. Just blank. As white as Roman guards witnessing a risen Christ. There were no following pages. Cynthia had either left the ending of her sermon at home, or never printed out the page. She panicked.

"You can't swear in church," she says with candor. "Particularly on Easter."

And so she looked to Heaven, and just rolled with it, edifying the congregation on how the angel, according to scripture, instructed Mary Magdalene: "Go and tell his disciples."

"Now who are you going to tell?" Cynthia said in conclusion to the sermon.

Recalling the moment of angst, she says the homily was "a bit shorter" than usual, but that she "stuck the landing" like a good gymnast, and had connected with the Almighty on the day of the Resurrection, up-front and personal: "OK, Lord," she prayed quietly, "you gotta help. I'm here doing the best I can."

Prayers were answered. But for Cynthia these days "the best I can" is a moving target. She has been diagnosed with Alzheimer's, a disease that took her mother. After an onset of symptoms—memory loss and forgetting familiar faces and places, including getting lost on her way to a burial with the family waiting for her at the cemetery— she resigned years ago as a full-time pastor, and now substitutes in the pulpit at various churches.

"I slough through old sermons," says Cynthia, 63, who grew up in street-smart central New Jersey. "I re-gift them, trying to remember where I've used the sermons before."

It's akin, as they say in Alzheimer's, to meeting new friends every day.

"I try to keep an elaborate system," she adds, "so I don't keep giving the same sermon in the same place."

A mother of two with a grandchild on the way, Cynthia earned her bachelor's degree at Rutgers, graduating in the first class to enroll women. Early on, she served in the Peace Corps in Jamaica in the West Indies as a special education teacher, and received a Master of Divinity in Ministry from New Brunswick Theological Seminary, adjacent to the Rutgers campus, and a Doctorate in Ministry from McCormick Theological Seminary in Chicago, where she began noticing symptoms. During preparations for her doctoral thesis, she could not recall course material or concepts she had been studying for years.

The warning signs continued in her ministry work, she said. "I was struggling to remember topics of earlier sermons and the names of parishioners. That's a problem when people are telling you their darkest secrets, then days later you don't know their names."

Cynthia tried to camouflage her difficulties with detailed notes and the support of friends, who ultimately encouraged her to see a doctor. In 2011, she was diagnosed with Mild Cognitive Impairment (MCI), a diagnosis that was changed in 2016 to Alzheimer's when a PET scan discovered abnormal amounts of tau protein in her brain, a sign of the disease.

Her diagnosis, at first, tested her faith, then her faith guided her journey.

"A woman at church one day told me, "God is scraping your plate, preparing room for you to do something else."

"REALLY?" Cynthia replied sarcastically.

She didn't want to hear it, but came around in trust. Now, she says, her ministry has taken on new direction, witnessing to those with Alzheimer's, through her ministry, the Alzheimer's Association, and singing in a band called "Country Magic," which has been inducted into the New York State Country Music Hall of Fame.

"I think the Lord has been preparing me for that all my life. Not that Alzheimer's is any greater plague than any other killer disease, but the sheer numbers of those who will be impacted by Alzheimer's and thus will struggle in their faiths give it a whole different perspective, a class in itself."

Asked if she were afraid to die, Cynthia says, "No. I know where I'm going." She pauses, then adds, "But before I go, I want to hold my grandbaby."

My friend Mike Belleville sees himself as the taciturn "Chief" in the ward with Randall Patrick McMurphy. But I see Belleville as the innocent, fun-loving, affable Martini, the caring, bear cub of a man in Cuckoo's Nest who loved just hanging out. Remember the scene in the hospital ward playing cards with McMurphy and the other patients:

Martini, after ripping cigarette in half: "I bet a nickel."
McMurphy: "Dime's the limit, Martini."
Martini, putting the two halves of the cigarette in the center of the table: "I bet a dime."
McMurphy: "This is not a dime!" *After showing Martini a full cigarette, adds,* "THIS is a dime!"
McMurphy: "If you break it in half, you don't get two nickels, you get shit. Try and smoke it. You understand?*
Martini: Yes.
McMurphy: You don't understand.

Belleville, like Martini, has had to put up with a lot of crap in his life, now more than ever. And yes, he does understand.

It was an ordeal getting his young grandchildren to understand at a recent Thanksgiving. Mike, 56, who lives with his wife, Cheryl, outside Boston, has been diagnosed with early-onset Alzheimer's. Noise is an intensifying issue for him. Simply put, he can't process noise, too thrashing for him. And thus he withdraws, acutely withdraws, as most of us do. Thanksgiving, a time of family, is a bruising time to withdraw. Mike knows that. He understands.

So Mike and Cheryl decided, in concert with their two grown daughters—Monika, who also lives outside Boston, and Krystal, who lives in Rhode Island, both married, with two children each—to have separate Thanksgivings a day apart, or Mike would have to withdraw, too much noise, too much disruption. It was painful for Mike, and wrenching for the grandkids who call him "Pappy," but that's what this disease does. It robs. A bifurcated Thanksgiving, a time of devotion to family. It's sad, but it's the art of compromise under the circumstances. Mike and Cheryl spent Thanksgiving with Krystal and her family in

Rhode Island on Thanksgiving Day, and with Monika and her family the day after.

"It tore me up, knowing it was all my fault," says Mike. "When we arrived at Krystal's, her children asked why their cousins were not coming for Thanksgiving; they wanted to spend the day with the entire family. Broke my heart. I'm supposed to be the father, the patriarch, and now I'm the guy who can't filter noise, who withdraws. It's disturbing to me. I don't want to take time away from them…yet I feel I'm robbing them of time."

Still, even with a separated Thanksgiving, Mike had to withdraw, heading outside alone for a break, or "wearing ear plugs."

Married for 36 years, Mike is now on disability. He stays at home, now a prisoner most days in his own house, while Cheryl works full-time; she's an administrative assistant for a firm that does data processing. At home, Mike thinks about the future, though the future holds little promise. "What scares me the most is that I will turn into someone who is not a pleasant person. The last thing I want to do is to hurt myself or someone else."

Active in the Alzheimer's Association Massachusetts/New Hampshire branch and a former member of the National Alzheimer's Association Early Stage Advisory Board, Mike is also wounded by the "drive-bys" in his grapple with this disease. He's angry.

"Drive me crazy," he says. "Bothers me tremendously! When those in Alzheimer's who can, fight, instead of lay down, people think we're fine. They don't have a clue, either because they can't get below the surface or perhaps out of fear, they can't. They don't have a clue. Sometimes in my personal rage, I want to slap them upside the head."

Asked if he ever thought earlier in life that he'd be on this journey, Mike replies, "This is the last thing in the world I expected, but it's the future for so many millions of us. Please see it. Alzheimer's is a four-letter word: Sucks!"

It is early spring on inner Hingham Harbor, just south of Boston, and one can hear the orderly slap of halyards against the tall aluminum masts of sailboats launched early in the season. A raw wind is blowing from the southeast, and the bump of vessels against the dock has the beat of war drums. The marina is protected from the north by a scattering of small islands and from the east by World's End peninsula, a 250-acre conservation park, proposed in 1945 as a site for the bourgeoning United Nations.

Inside the nearby rustic Trident Gallery and Raw Bar sits Ken Sullivan and his wife, Michelle Palomera, successful financial services and technology professionals in their own right. At first glance, they appear to be the impeccable couple. With apologies to them both, they have the look of "Ken and Barbie," perfectly formed Mattel dolls of the 1960s. Ken, 51, comes across as handsome, athletic-looking, and erudite, belied by his premature gray hair. Michelle, 49, is the picture of beauty and smarts, inside out. Yet the war drums are beating.

My buddy Ken is not on his game today. He was diagnosed with Alzheimer's at age 47, after an MRI and battery of neurological tests—at the time when daughters Abby and Leah were 8 and 6 respectively, further testimony to the fact that this is not your grandfather's disease. Still handsome, athletic-looking, and with the same disarming smile, Ken's acumen today stops there. His progressions have moved exceedingly quickly: loss of memory, loss of self, dislocation, inability to process noise, and other symptoms, all batting down yet another stereotype of the disease—predictability of the advance of Alzheimer's. In March 2016, at the age of 50, Ken was moved, on the recommendation of his doctors, into a caring assisted-living complex, Bridges by EPOCH, across from the Trident; the demons had chased him there from his stately home in Scituate, on the coast south of Boston. Home was no longer an option. Care for Ken would now cost $10,000 a month, plus other costs. In a wink, half of the family income was gone. Alzheimer's doesn't respect demographics of any sort.

"The decision was excruciating for me and the girls; Ken in his disease seemed good with it," says Michelle, outside her husband's earshot. "I felt terrible, confused, heartbroken, and angry, but I knew all along it was the best thing for him."

Coordinating with Ken's doctors, the decision was made in the dead of winter. "That weekend I was alone," she recalls. "I mean alone. The kids were out of town, and Ken was in the hospital recovering from efforts to adjust his medications. I had time by myself; it was cathartic, a moment to grieve and process what was happening to my husband in his prime. It was really hard."

She pauses.

"Still is…"

There were premonitions on the horizon. The year after Ken was diagnosed, he attended an Alzheimer's research event in Boston, still with the intuition of a bright analyst. He came away with a business card that he handed to his young wife; it was from the director of Bridges by EPOCH. "If and when the time ever comes," he told Michelle, unable to complete the sentence in his emotion. "I want you to check this place out, but I don't want to talk about it now…"

Now there's not much to talk about.

Ken and Michelle met at Fidelity Investments in Boston, where they worked many years ago. It was love at first glance, at least by Michelle's account. "I spotted him from across the room. He was a pretty hot guy. We worked at the time at Boston's Trade Center, then infiltrated with twentysomethings. Ken, with that trademark smile, used to call it the 'World Babe Center.'"

In time, they dated, married, and moved on to analyst jobs elsewhere in the Hub, joined at the hip forever. But over time, there were some troubling signs. Ken began having difficulty with the numbers; he began struggling at his job. The math, the executive left side of the brain, wasn't computing for him. He was feeling intense stress, confusion, anxiety, and wanted to pull back, sought to withdraw. And so, he was let go before his diagnosis. Who, in the moment, could understand? His employer after the fact was highly supportive and cooperative.

At age 47 with two young daughters, Ken searched for other work. There were no takers. No one was surprised, least of all Michelle, then

45 years old, a superstar of a woman, who became the sole provider and the caregiver. Lots of juggling with her husband and children, no complaining. Not the life she had imagined. Their income had been cut in half in a blink; the cost of care and ancillary, out-of-pocket expenses dug the hole deeper. Then there is saving for the girls' college. Alzheimer's respects no demographic, no stock portfolio, not a race, a color, a preference, or a gender. The disease is an equalizer.

In 2013, Ken was formally diagnosed after a series of neuropsychological tests and an MRI, the first in his family tree. "When we got the diagnosis, we were shell-shocked, freaked out. It's an isolating disease," Michelle, at the time, told *Boston Globe* reporter Bella English in a compelling story about Ken, who said in the moment, "My role is to tell my story."

And Ken did just that while he could—advocating as a member of the Alzheimer's Association Early Stage Advisory Group, speaking on Capitol Hill, enrolling in a clinical trial. His voice has gone silent for the most part now.

At the Trident Gallery and Raw Bar, the conversation today is just that: raw. "I'm so sad," says Michelle, tearing up, yet fighting off the sentiment, while dealing with her own depression and stress of caregiving. "There are so many layers to this disease, affecting individuals in so many different ways."

Adds Ken from the heart, "I've just had to let it go."

The upshot of letting it go required the help of others; among them, child psychologist Maria Trozzi, director of the nationally known Good Grief Program at Boston Medical Center. Trozzi, author of *Talking with Children about Loss*, has worked in crisis intervention in the aftermath of 911, the Boston Marathon bombing, the killings in Newtown, Connecticut, and other tragedies. Ken and Michelle met with Trozzi before telling their daughters about the diagnosis. She continues to counsel Michelle and the girls in their grief.

"I still feel blessed," says Michelle. "There are so many people who have it even worse. So I try to stay focused."

Ken reaches gently for Michelle's hand. "You ok, honey? I love you!" he says from the heart.

She smiles, the gaze of a loving, selfless partner. "I love you, too..."

Back at EPOCH around the corner from Trident, Ken shows me his room again. The first time I saw it, I cried; I cried for all of us in this disease. Walking through the lobby of the nursing home complex, Ken still turns heads, only now they are 80-year-olds'. He takes it all in stride, perhaps unaware of the variance in age. His room has a boyish look to it; sports memorabilia abounds: his baseball mitt; a prized National Hockey League stick signed by the Stanley Cup-winning Bruins team, led by Bobby Orr; a framed larger-than-life high school photo of Ken, a sturdy lineman, Number 73; watercolor paintings he has done at EPOCH to keep the flow of creative juices; and other sports memorabilia from his football and baseball days. He was an infielder, pitcher, and catcher.

"Catchers control the game," Michelle interjects, a reference to Ken's attempts to backstop Alzheimer's.

And then there's a framed front page of the *Boston Globe* celebrating the Boston Red Sox World Series championship, breaking an 86-year-old drought and putting the "Curse of the Bambino" to rest. Proudly, "Bad boy Ken," as Michelle calls him, caught a St. Louis Cardinal home run ball in the series, threw it back onto the field at Fenway Park, and was ejected from the park for bad behavior.

"I made the paper!" Ken exclaims.

There's a knock at Ken's door—Paul and Susan Boyce, longtime close friends, who have "adopted" Ken, Michelle, and the girls. Ken and Paul, who lost his grandmother and mother to Lewy Body Dementia, have known each other for fifteen years. Paul, born outside London and who sailed for Britain in the America's Cup Race of 1987 held off Australia, knows much about navigating hazardous currents. He tells me privately, "If you'd want anyone in your corner for this, it would be Michelle. There is a bottomless component to her. I haven't seen the bottom yet of her ability to deal with this disease, but I worry about it. She's a hero."

Paul, who has two girls of his own, has tremendous admiration for Ken's fight, and relates on so many personal levels to the sadness of Ken living outside the family. "I get to hug my two daughters in the morning, and Ken doesn't," Paul says in the simplest of contrasts. "That's not fair."

They used to talk about the "fairness" of Alzheimer's over a few beers at a local tavern after Ken's diagnosis when he was fully in the moment. Like the final scene in the movie *Charly*, adapted from the book *Flowers for Algernon*, they talked about the day when Ken will not recognize Paul.

"You won't see it coming," Paul told him. "But I will."

"I know," Ken replied. "I'll just be along for the ride…"

It's been a long ride for Puerto Rican native Daisy Duarte. She cares 24/7 for her mother, Sonia Cardona, also born in Puerto Rico and struggling with a rare, deadly hybrid of Alzheimer's from a gene mutation that advances at a fast pace and literally guarantees the disease before one is in their mid 60s. After her mom's diagnosis and great onset of symptoms, Daisy closed her sports bar and moved into her mother's home in Springfield, Missouri, trading a vibrant business for full-time caregiving. Daisy's father is deceased; she has two siblings, a sister and a brother, but Daisy is the sole day-to-day caregiver. The two live off her mother's meager $2,000-a-month teachers' pension at the poverty line, which must cover rent, food, rent, utilities, adult diapers for Sonia, and medications that are not completely covered by insurance.

Sonia, 61, at this point can only mumble, speaking a few words in blurts, and is confined to a wheelchair. She's down to 82 pounds. Daisy, 41, has a long ride ahead of her; she carries her mother's gene mutation. For now, she only has time to focus on her mom and to advocate for a cure. Daisy will be the sixth generation of her family inflicted with Alzheimer's. Her grandmother was one of eleven siblings, all of whom died from Alzheimer's.

"I'm trying not to think about it," says Daisy, featured with her mother in the PBS Alzheimer's documentary *Every Minute Counts*.

"My focus is my mother, though I'm not sure who she thinks I am. She calls me 'Mom.'"

Daisy, when time allows, has become a champion for the Washington, D.C.-based advocacy group UsAgainstAlzheimer's, speaking at forums and on Capitol Hill. "It's one of the best Alzheimer's advocacy groups in the nation, with an unremitting passion to find and fund a cure," she says.

With the encouragement of UsAgainstAlzheimer's, she is participating in a clinical trial, the "Diane Study," associated with Washington University in St. Louis. Daisy stands out in the Hispanic community, which to date has been reluctant to enroll in clinical trials. According to studies, Hispanics are 1.5 times more likely to develop Alzheimer's than Caucasians.

Daisy is fully engaged in the fight, and has the faith to sustain. Raised Catholic, Daisy goes to Mass every Sunday. "My faith keeps me going, gives me the courage," she says, noting she had decided against taking her mother to a nursing home. "My mother will die in my arms," Daisy says. "She's not going anywhere."

Still there are the dark moments, sitting home alone with her mother, holding her hand, watching the blur of daytime television with Sonia, both shut-ins. Fear plays games. "What happens if I start to show symptoms," she says. "Who's going to see it? How is anyone going to know when the demon is coming?"

Perhaps Judy Jaffe Gelfand saw the demon coming years ago after the disease stole her mother, but Judy never spoke about it. Alzheimer's pursues at a calculating pace, but such talk then was unmentionable. So Judy, as her mother had done previously, led by heroic example that inspired her family. Her example now inspires others nationwide to talk about this prowling demon that seems to be locked on to a gender, affecting women far more than men.

The numbers are numbing. To say that Alzheimer's disproportionately affects women is an understatement parallel to saying that Judy Jaffe Gelfand had the courage and heart of a legion of fighters.

A concert pianist, a remarkable music teacher, and a remarkable woman inside out, Judy Gelfand died in 2004 of Alzheimer's after close to decade-long battle with the disease—3,652 days, 87,658 minutes, 315,360,000 seconds, to be exact.

Alzheimer's never sleeps.

Observes Judy's daughter, Elizabeth Gelfand Stearns of Santa Monica, co-producer of the Oscar-winning film *Still Alice*, "As the smash Broadway musical *Rent* asks us to consider: 'How do you measure a year? In daylights, in sunsets, in midnights, in cups of coffee, in inches, in miles, in laughter, in strife.'"

Perhaps all of the above.

Like the fictional Harvard Professor Alice Howland in Lisa Genova's bestselling novel *Still Alice*, Judy Gelfand, a pianist at the Julliard School of Music, has become a face of Alzheimer's and a barometer of the tempest that is brewing. Women are at the epicenter of this disease. More to the point, says the Alzheimer's Association. Consider the following:

- Among the more than 5 million Americans diagnosed with Alzheimer's, two thirds are women age 65 and older.
- At 65, women have a one in six chance of developing Alzheimer's, compared with a one in eleven risk for men.
- Sixty-three percent of the 15 million unpaid Alzheimer's and dementia caregivers in the U.S. are women, sustaining high levels of stress and depressive symptoms.
- A woman in her 60s is twice as likely to develop Alzheimer's disease as she is to develop breast cancer.
- With 78 million baby boomers entering their later years, the cost of Alzheimer's care in the U.S. is expected to reach $20 trillion by 2050.

So do the math.

"As tragic as it is, Alzheimer's picked the right person in Judy Gelfand," says Elizabeth, a colleague and close friend. "We all stood by, watching her slowly fade, a heartbreaking train wreck for our family. Yet in spirit, my mother fights on."

It is the spirit of The Judy Fund that offers great promise, igniting awareness of the staggering number of women afflicted with Alzheimer's. Since its establishment 14 years ago, The Judy Fund has raised more than $8 million to support Alzheimer's research and advocacy in partnership with the Alzheimer's Association.

"The Judy Fund is a wonderful example of how one family chose to transform loss into action, honoring Judy, while also working to change the future for millions," says Angela Geiger, former Alzheimer's Association chief strategy officer. "Over the years, The Judy Fund has contributed to Alzheimer's Association mission activities including research, care, and advocacy, and most recently the focus has been on raising awareness and learning why women are disproportionately impacted by Alzheimer's disease," says Geiger.

This donor-advised fund at the Alzheimer's Association was created by Judy's husband, Marshall Gelfand, of Palm Springs, a founding partner of Gelfand, Rennert & Feldman L.L.P., a leading entertainment business management firm. The Judy Fund is managed by Elizabeth, who left her post in 2004 as senior vice president of strategic marketing at Universal Pictures. Elizabeth, the fund's chairman, also previously served on the board of directors of the national Alzheimer's Association. The Judy Fund is the fastest-growing family fund in the history of the Alzheimer's Association.

"The gifts of my mother continue to flow," says Elizabeth. "She is present in our family's lives, a role model to strive for. She was a beautiful woman physically and at heart until her last breath. In Alzheimer's, she had incredible capacity to still be Judy, even in her silence. That's also the power of the message of *Still Alice.*

"There needs to be a much better plan in place today than there was for my mother and my grandmother," says Elizabeth. "The tragedy for them, is that there was no plan in place. We've never really taken the time to figure out why. Science and trial studies have ignored women."

Most of the research studies to date have been done on men. Surprisingly, with the higher incidence of Alzheimer's among women, a gender under siege, there has never been a comprehensive study completed of women's brains and Alzheimer's. Of particular concern, says Elizabeth, is the fact that 66% of the Alzheimer's population here in the U.S. are women, and those women share another biological fact—the loss of estrogen through menopause. When studied, this estrogen loss may be a factor that leads to deficits in brain metabolism that could lead to Alzheimer's. While women live longer than men, the estrogen impact could be significant. In short, the manner in which women's brains change later in life could put them at higher risk for Alzheimer's or a decline in cognitive function.

Does Elizabeth, a mother of three, and her husband, Richard, worry about her future, about a genetic hand-me-down?

"Am I afraid? Of course I'm afraid," she says. "I'm a face of this disease. But I've decided there's a lot I can do. There's a lot we can all do to stop Alzheimer's. That trumps my fears. I don't want this disease. We can make a plan, and do far more in funding and research for a cure. We can do it in our lifetime. The fear of Alzheimer's drives me. There's no way I'm going to just sit back and allow this disease to keep going. Not happening. No way!"

Judy Jaffe Gelfand is smiling. Her daughter makes her proud.

Rob Moir fit the bill for his generation, a 1960s activist— advocating for civil rights, the rights of farm workers, and protesting the Vietnam War. As a veteran history teacher for almost 40 years and president of the teachers' union at the Rumson/Fair Haven Regional High School in Rumson, New Jersey, Rob put his principles on the line; he was a truth teller, and thus often the object of criticism and ridicule in this fertile suburb, not far from the Manhattan skyline.

Legend has it that the town got its name from early settlers who purchased the land from Native Americans for some rum. The merriment ends here. Rumson, dotted with sprawling nineteenth-century estates along the Navesink and Shrewsbury rivers, was no place for activism or opposition politics. As an activist teacher, Rob stood out, a product of the "progressive Catholic left movement," as he calls it, a movement that shaped him.

"I was always under attack," says Rob, who reminds me in some ways of Dale Harding in *Cuckoo's Nest*, president of the patients' council and the most educated in the institution. Harding sagely observes in *Cuckoo's Nest*: "Never before did I realize that mental illness could have the aspect of power."

Rob notes that he was able to survive—an instinct that carries him today. "Somehow I was able to survive the attacks and thrive supporting issues of people's rights and social justice."

Rob met his wife, Margaret, when he came to speak about the rights of United Farmworkers at nearby Monmouth University, where she was attending school. "I thought, 'This guy is unbelievable,'" she recalls. "'I'm going to pretend I'm really interested in farmworkers.'"

The strategy worked. Soon Margaret, a teacher herself, was involved with Rob and the plight of farmworkers, and never looked back. "I was hooked."

Today, the couple looks back, but with different eyes. About eight years ago, Rob, a marathoner and a good one, began to lose his gait, not so much as a runner, but in cognition. Sparks were flying, but missing their mark, causing symptomatic confusion, loss of memory, and loss of place. A gentle, yet vigorous man, Rob was slowly becoming a study of slow motion, unnoticed at first, then apparent to all. The transition scared Margaret. In 2012, Rob was diagnosed with Mild Cognitive Impairment (MCI), then in 2015 with Alzheimer's.

"You can't roll up in a ball," Rob says over coffee at a funky coffee shop on Cape Cod, the Chocolate Sparrow, that captures his persona. They've retired to the Cape to complete their journey. "I'm going to fight this, I'm going to fight it as long as I can, but I clearly know that something is terribly wrong."

So did Margaret, who at first thought the symptoms were the indication of marital difficulties. The two sought marriage counseling. "Rob was withdrawing, from me and from others," she says. "He didn't seem connected."

It worsened.

"I would ask him to call the doctor, and he'd just stand in front of the phone," she says. "It made me crazy. I thought he just didn't want to call, but he was actually confused about how to call. Another sign was that he would drop me off at meetings, and then go off in the wrong direction. The confusion made him more anxious. Not fully understanding the cause of his angst, I was getting enraged, more and more, as well. I knew something was seriously awry. One day, Rob got lost on his way to the doctor's office, despite the use of a GPS. He called me, broke down and cried. He was upset and disorientated. It clearly frightened him."

Their journey, following the characteristic course of the disease, has been a meandering, unpredictable one, as Rob continues to slip slowly into the void of Alzheimer's, trying to fight every inch of the way, and yet delighting in moments of joy, in being in the moment. He also has prostate cancer, which he is not treating—an end-game strategy. Rob still works out daily at the gym to recharge his brain, often next to me on the treadmill. I tell him not to get lost, or we'll both be screwed. I'll have to look for him and we'll both be lost.

Rob is gradually withdrawing more and more, socially and cerebrally. Margaret, as in love with Rob now as when she first heard him speak, has stepped up as a self-sacrificing caregiver, representative of caregivers in this disease. She often speaks for him now.

"Rob is accepting of the disease; this is his path and he is determined to walk in grace," she says. "I'm the one now who fights for Rob because I want for him a life that is as full as possible, still powerful and good. I'm grateful for the years we've had together. I love my life now and I love Rob very much, but there will be a time when I want my life back. There is purpose in what I'm doing. On this path, I am strengthened by the depths of relationships with others in this disease. Alzheimer's strips away the minutia of life and leaves one with true richness, if one is willing to seize it. There is always conflict, but there is joy in the moment. Margaret now has taken to writing, poetic observations of their plight.

"Imagine watching a loved one begin to unravel before your eyes," she writes. "Imagine it starts so slowly that you think you're imagining things. But then you find yourself starting to get impatient, soon uneasy. And at some point you are very afraid. Afraid that this disease, the dreaded 'A' word has now come for the one you love—the partner you built your dreams with.

"The moments of each day now are heightened by the whisper of angel wings, waiting in the shadows. For myself, it is often hard to fully understand all that I'm feeling, all that I'm experiencing. I find myself at times both an observer and an actor in a play that is unfolding around me, my new life."

If anyone knows the journey from the cradle to the grave, it is Dr. T. Berry Brazelton, personification in so many ways of the Baby Boom Generation. At age 99, Brazelton—raised in rural Waco, Texas; a Princeton, Columbia, and Harvard graduate—is still considered among the world's foremost experts on pediatrics and child development. His brilliant scientific research—which began in the 1950s and has spanned six decades, reshaping worldwide early child development and the practice of pediatrics—gave voice to infants at a time when babies were considered a blank slate, "tabula rasa," without inherent capacities.

I'm blessed to call him a friend for four decades.

Brazelton, who has testified on medical issues before numerous key Congressional Committees, is a Professor of Pediatrics Emeritus at Harvard, former child specialist at Boston's Massachusetts General Hospital (MGH), former fellow at Harvard's Center for Cognitive Studies, founder of Boston's elite Child Development Unit at Children's Hospital where he still holds court, and was founder in 1996 of the Brazelton Touchpoints Center (www.brazeltontouchpoints.org) that gives new dimension to age, ensuring that what experts learn in observations of children and families are conveyed into practice and policy, as its mission states. The Brazelton Touchpoints Center in Boston seeks to establish scalable and sustainable, low-cost, low-tech interventions that propel children's healthy development and strengthen the collaborative relationships among families, parents, caregivers, providers, and communities.

The author of 30 books, translated into 20 foreign languages, and more than 200 scholarly papers, Brazelton has been a leading force "behind the pediatric healthcare revolution that has opened hospital doors to parents and empowered them to become active participants in their children's care," his biography notes. In 2013, on the eve of his 95th birthday, he received the Presidential Citizens Medal, the nation's second-highest civilian award.

But who's counting?

Brazelton continues harnessing his infinite energies into guiding Baby Boomers, whom he coached as parents, as they glide into their senior years. He takes aging personally. In 2015, he lost the love of his life to complications from dementia—his beautiful wife, Christina "Chrissy" Lowell Brazelton, whose ancestors arrived on the *Mayflower*, a Who's Who of American history that traces back to: John Lowell, a member of the Continental Congress that governed the colonies during the American Revolution, and who was appointed to the federal bench by President George Washington; Francis Cabot Lowell, founder of the nation's Industrial Revolution; Pulitzer Prize-winning poets Robert Lowell and Amy Lowell; noted nineteenth-century poet and ambassador to Spain and England James Russell Lowell; famed author, mathematician, and astronomer Percival Lowell, founder of the distinguished Lowell Observatory in Flagstaff, Arizona, and who first fueled speculation that were there canals on Mars and was instrumental in efforts that led to the discovery of Pluto; playwright Tennessee Williams, author of *The Glass Menagerie*, *A Streetcar Named Desire*, and *Cat on a Hot Tin Roof*; renowned poet and essayist T.S. Eliot; irreproachable former U.S. Attorney General Elliot Richardson, fired by President Richard Nixon in the "Watergate Saturday Night Massacre," to name just a few of the notables of the family tree, as well as trusted advisors to several U.S. presidents.

The stature of such Boston Brahmins was embroidered in the doggerel "Boston Toast" by John Collins Bossily in the early 1900s:

> *"And this is good old Boston,*
> *The home of the bean and the cod.*
> *Where the Lowells talk only to Cabots,*
> *And the Cabots talk only to God..."*

If anyone knows the journey from the cradle to the grave and how to find one's way, it is Dr. T. Berry Brazelton.

The sturdy oak door to the prestigious Hyannis Yacht Club, overlooking Lewis Bay off Nantucket Sound, just around the corner from the Kennedy Compound, requires a code. I felt on this splendid spring day—having been invited by Dr. Brazelton for lunch with Mary Catherine—as if the Boston Irish diaspora was still in play: Gaelic need not apply. All I required was the code.

No dice. We had arrived early before Dr. Brazelton and his caring attendant. So I spotted a young guy at the door, a sentry with red hair, and he dutifully escorted us in, upon the promise that we were part of the Brazelton party. Promise. Within fifteen minutes, I heard a familiar thumping on the floor—the cadence of Dr. Brazelton's trusted walker, with spliced tennis balls at the base for smoother flow.

"Greeeg," he said in his soft Texan drawl. "I've joined the club to meet new friends!"

Brazelton has been meeting new friends on Cape Cod since 1954, summering at a historic family home on a hill overlooking the bay in Barnstable, formerly owned by the Dillingham family, one of the Cape's early settlers in the 1600s—an easy weekend commute from the Brazelton house in Cambridge.

Overlooking placid Lewis Bay, it is eminently clear that his wife Chrissy is never far from his memory. He talks openly and often about her, echoing today folklore about Christina, retold in a fine *Boston Globe* obituary written by J.M. Lawrence: Christina in the 1950s was about to be introduced in New York City to the Duke and Duchess of Windsor—the former king of England, Edward VII, who abdicated in 1936 the throne to marry American socialite and twice-divorcée Wallis Simpson of Maryland. As the story goes, Chrissy's brother-in-law, who knew the former king, advised her to curtsey before Simpson, to which Chrissy instantly replied, *"Boston bow to Baltimore? Not on your life!"*

Says Brazelton, "That's what I loved about Chrissy. She always spoke up. We argued for sixty-six years, and I always let her win. It kept everything alive. I could never have done what I did without her."

Yet, the introduction didn't go so well, Brazelton adds, recalling that as a young man training at Children's Hospital he was invited through a roommate to dine with the famed Lowells. He was seated next to Chrissy, who barely spoke, leaving Brazelton to conclude that she was a snob, only to find out later that Chrissy had been horribly ill that night. On the counsel of friends, he persisted, soon to realize that while Chrissy was shy, she was also never hesitant to speak her mind and in ways, at times, that could cut through cinderblocks.

"I loved her sharp-witted intellect, and she was so sweet and so beautiful that I asked her to marry me on our third date," Brazelton says over fried fresh fish and chips, taking in the panorama of the harbor. "She always insisted, though, that she never accepted my proposal, but we ended up having four children."

Chrissy, who grew up on Boston's dignified Beacon Hill, was a graduate of Radcliff College, an art lover who started and operated a gallery in Cambridge, and served on several Boston nonprofit boards, including the Home for Little Wanderers and the Institute of Contemporary Art. And when it came to raising children, Chrissy dismissed all theories, including those of her husband, a budding international all-star in the field. "I don't need any advice from you," she often told him.

Brazelton still laughs at the comment, and relishes the story of publication of one of his first books in 1969, *Infants and Mothers: Differences in Development.* When a *New York Times* book reviewer called to tell him it was one of the finest books she had ever read on the subject, Brazelton replied over the phone, "I can't hear you. Could you speak up louder?" He then motioned to his wife to come to the phone to hear the exclamation from the venerable *New York Times.*

Chrissy listened, rolled her eyes, then told her husband bluntly, "What do they know..."

It was the fight in Chrissy that helped in her battle with dementia in later years, along with the unflinching, resolute love of Brazelton, who devotedly tended to his wife until she passed away at age 94. The couple moved from the sprawling house on the hill in Barnstable to a nearby smaller, one-story home to better care for Chrissy and ease her confusion. Her children later wrote in a eulogy: "Even as dementia weakened her understanding, there were moments of brilliant insight, seemingly accidental, but they weren't. It will take her family a long time to recover their forward motion without her. But the challenge of getting underway again offers the opportunity to learn that her impact is permanent and that her leadership lives on inside each heart and mind that knew and loved her well."

Chrissy always spoke from the heart, teaching about touchpoints up until the end. Two days before her death, after she had been unable to utter a word for some time, Brazelton asked a close friend, an extended family member named Seth, to play the banjo for her that she had always loved to hear.

Chrissy came alive with the music. "Seth," she said distinctly, "that's beautiful!"

Chrissy Lowell Brazelton is a study in determination, courage, and beauty. Her legacy heartens her husband every day and guides him to seek new horizons. Writes Brazelton in a draft of a new book about aging, Alzheimer's and dementia, loneliness, last touchpoints, the road to acceptance, faith in a higher being, and railing against the end of life: "As I watched my wife of sixty-six years begin to deteriorate with dementia, it was the first serious trauma I had faced since losing my parents. After her death, I realized that I had to face living alone, as well as retiring from my work, selling my house in order to pay for my wife's illness and the cost of aides that were necessary to keep her home. As I result, I had to move away from friends and colleagues, and ultimately to live alone... But I'm also aware of how lucky I am. I am particularly grateful to have had a partner in my wife, a person who believed in what I was doing and was able to put up with my manic devotion to my career. Our four children have supported me all along, and are now even more important as they help through my final years, my Last Touchpoint."

Touchpoints, Brazelton says, are opportunities for learning that precede a leap in physical, emotional, or cognitive growth, and in the aging process, in the decline.

"Memory changes are inevitable as we age," he writes, "but simple prompts, like making lists, posting reminders for ourselves, or setting up deliberate routines, can decrease the impact of these changes… Alzheimer's disease and other dementias offer quite a different scenario for the 'Last Touchpoint.' In the early stages of the disease, we may be aware that we are declining, but quickly one is robbed of the most precious memories, like the names of a spouse, children, or other loved ones, and the history of their life… By embracing this Last Touchpoint in life we have the chance to see ourselves through our final developmental stage in keeping with our beliefs and desires, and to feel a sense of satisfaction and pride in a life well-lived…and well-ended."

As Brazelton carefully guides his walker from the Hyannis Yacht Club at the end of lunch on this brilliant spring afternoon—a day meant for me as a time of reflection as much as a moment with a close friend—I sense the spirit of Chrissy upon him as he walks assuredly with a sense of satisfaction and peace in a life well-lived.

In the fight against Alzheimer's, there are foot soldiers, field commanders, and victims. The consummate caregiver, Trish Lerner Vradenburg was a fearless commander, a face of the resistance who became a victim at heart. Trish's life is a word picture of commitment, determination, and devotion to the cause—part of the patchwork, a primary fabric, of the war against dementia, and an inspiring portrait of creativity and versatility. She wrote early on for various television shows, including *Designing Women, Family Ties,* and *Kate and Allie.*

Her novel, *Liberated Lady*, was chosen as Literary Guild and Doubleday Book Club selections, and was translated into three foreign languages. She also wrote often for the *New York Daily News, The Boston Globe, The Washington Post, Ladies' Home Journal, Huffington Post,* and *Women's Day.* Her autobiographical play, *Surviving Grace,* about her love of her mother and the trials of caregiving, was produced at the Kennedy Center in Washington, D.C. and Off Broadway at the Union Square Theater. It has been performed at various community theaters throughout the country and in Portuguese in Brazil.

Trish came from great stock. Her mother, Bea Lerner, was a stylish and forceful Democratic party activist, who in 1960 delivered the State of New Jersey to help John F. Kennedy win the presidency. Trish herself was a fearless political advocate, and her husband, George, served in senior executive and legal positions at CBS, FOX, and AOL/Time Warner, and is a member of the Council on Foreign Relations. The Vradenburgs were a Washington, D.C. "power couple," but dementia respects no boundaries. After Trish's mother began experiencing frightening symptoms of Alzheimer's, Trish and George put their lives on hold to care for her. Bea died in 1992 after a valiantly fighting off complications of the disease.

"My early up-close-and-personal experience with Alzheimer's," says George, "was when my mother-in-law Bea called at 3 a.m. one day to complain about a strange man in her house. My wife and life-partner, Trish, and I immediately went there to find only one man in the house, her husband. When asked about a strange man, Bea pulled us aside and carefully pointed to her husband, saying 'that's the strange man; he's nice, but I don't know him.' After that, the powerful pull of the Alzheimer's downward spiraling trajectory never let up. Years later, Bea died in a nursing home, unable to speak, to move, to recognize her daughter. This disease is a cruel monster."

So George and Trish flexed their substantial financial, creative, and activist muscles to create UsAgainstAlzheimer's, a powerful D.C.-based national and international force committed to ending Alzheimer's as soon as humanly possible. Driven by the suffering of millions of families, the organization takes no prisoners in pushing for greater urgency from government, industry, and the scientific community in funding and finding a cure. Often walking the halls of Congress and seats of power around the world with the stamina of long-distance runners, the Vradenburgs raised millions of dollars, and roused their political, corporate, and show-business connections to create—as the UsAgainstAlzheimer's mission states—"a national will to prevent and treat Alzheimer's by pressuring our political, business, and civic leaders to devote the necessary resources to outcomes-oriented research and to reform the drug development systems that currently slow the development and availability of promising treatments."

All the while, Trish herself feared she was genetically predisposed to Alzheimer's, watching carefully for signs, still pressing on. Such pressures, the trepidations, the work flow, the heartbreaks along the path, slowly wore her down. In April 2017, she died of a heart attack, a victim at heart.

"A piece of light in the universe has gone out," George said upon her passing. "There is a brightness that will be dimmed."

On the floor of Congress, Senator Ed Markey of Massachusetts, a close friend of the Vradenburgs and a key UsAgainstAlzheimer's champion on the Hill, spoke of Trish's contributions and the need for such steadfast determination in the fight against dementia.

"Trish was a multidimensional force of nature—creative, caring, and compassionate," said Markey, a member of the U.S. Senate Foreign Relations Committee. "Trish was a master communicator and humorist. She did not mince words and knew how to convey a message. This was a great woman whom we have just lost, a champion for finding a cure for Alzheimer's disease, and I am so honored to be able to speak in the U.S. Senate to tell the nation of the work of this great woman."

Markey, who lost his mother many years ago to Alzheimer's, knows well about the pluck needed to win a fight. As a young state representative on Beacon Hill, he oversaw passage of the most sweeping judicial reform legislation in Massachusetts history. Commanding interests that ruled the State House at the time moved his desk out into the hallway. The message fell on deaf ears.

Like Markey, Trish never took "no" for an answer. Her unswerving perseverance was a cornerstone of her life. Indeed, we have lost a hero, a fighter, a crusader, a saint, a poet of a writer, and one extraordinary, brilliant woman in Trish Vradenburg. In so many ways, she was the embodiment of her mother, in her selfless love and ceaseless caring. Trish once wrote of her mom, "My mother was larger than life. She embraced life with style and grace and passion. She could capture a room just by entering it…There was no one who loved me more unconditionally. That's what mothers do. And nobody did it better than she. I then watched helplessly as her mind, her dignity, her soul, and finally her body succumbed to this killer."

In the fall of 2016, I was honored, humbled, that Trish and George named me as the first recipient of the annual Bea Learner Award for courage in Alzheimer's. Ceremonies were held appropriately at the Reagan Building in D.C., a non-partisan event with former First Lady Laura Bush and House Minority Leader Nancy Pelosi on stage. Speaking before more than 500 of Washington's elite, at the request of Trish and George, I felt again like the Scarecrow in *The Wizard of Oz*.

It's been said that when one has Alzheimer's, the entire family is afflicted. And thus when a loved-one passes, we all die a bit.

George, and all of us, have died a bit with Trish's passing. But as Trish often braced high-ranking members of Congress in the push for a cure for Alzheimer's: "We will go away when Alzheimer's goes away."

Trish hasn't gone away yet…

I myself came full circle a few years ago on the Irish Sea. By hook or by crook, I was destined to connect in Ireland with John Joe Vaughan—two brash Irishmen separated by a sea of blue, roiling waters rushing to a horizon where water flushes up against the sky. It was God-ordained.

I had met John Joe earlier at Logan Airport upon my return to Boston from Dublin, an annual pilgrimage to Éire. He had just arrived himself with family to visit his daughter Rena, who now lives in New Hampshire. While I was on the cell phone responding to a queue of backlogged voicemails, Rena began waving at me. She recognized me from a photo in *On Pluto.*

"I want you to meet my father," she said, noting that her dad had been diagnosed with Alzheimer's, and was reticent to talk about it until reading *On Pluto.* She had given him a copy.

I was humbled, but that was just the beginning.

The Lord works in mysterious ways.

John Joe, 79, of New Ross in County Wexford, ancestral home of the Kennedys, has a smile that would light the River Liffey and the handshake of a heavyweight champion. He embraced me, eyeball to eyeball, and I saw the tears streaming down the side of his creased, righteous face, the two of us in a fight against a demon of a disease.

I cried, too.

"I know how it feels," he said to me. "We fight together now as brothers, right?"

"Right!"

And so we are brothers, joined now in a worldwide fight against Alzheimer's, from Cape Cod to the Irish Sea. On the lip of Worldwide Alzheimer's Day, September 21, marking a month-long international awareness campaign, the fight is fully engaged.

And if the tag-team, rope-a-dope of John Joe and I are any indication, Alzheimer's, in time to come, could be down for a hand count, if lawmakers worldwide, various committed parties, caregivers, and those with the disease join forces around the planet.

This was no brief encounter with John Joe—a father of eight with his devoted wife, Peggy; grandfather of seventeen; a retired teacher and school principal, raised in rural Marshalstown without electricity and paved roads. He invited me to spend a week in late July writing and just hanging with him over a few pints at his family's summer cottage on the Irish Sea in the fishing village of Duncannon, out on a peninsula at the mouth of rivers Barrow, Nore, and Suir, overlooking the majestic 800-year-old Hook Head Lighthouse. It's one of the oldest working lighthouses in the world where legend has it that monks from the nearby Dubhan monastery lit fires in the fifth century to warn ships from the treacherous rocks. Today, the Fresnel lens flashes every three seconds; I counted the blinks in my bedroom each night as I tried to sleep, captivated by the night sky flecked with infinite specks of white, reflecting on the lighthouse and the craggy peninsula just across from the narrow strait called Crooke. It is a place where in the mid-1600s British military tactician Oliver Cromwell, charged with defeating the rebellious Confederate Coalition in Ireland, declared that he would take the country "By Hook or by Crooke," a declaration that would last in the vernacular.

And so John Joe and I met by Hook or by Crooke, in County Wexford, where my mother's family hailed. John Joe's mother also died of Alzheimer's and his older brother is stricken with the disease, and now doesn't recognize John Joe, a journey that awaits him, he fears.

The Lord works in mysterious ways.

Over a pint in Wexford Town, John Joe, named for his uncle John and his father Joseph, talked for one of the first times about the horrors of Alzheimer's that is consuming a generation worldwide, one diagnosis of dementia about every minute. "I'm emotional about this," says John Joe. "I can't control that. It's the card I was dealt. What can you do about it? I refuse to give in. So I fight on. I retreat into myself and fight on. It makes me nervous, the progression I have to face."

Once quick-witted and gifted with the Irish natter, John Joe is now slower to the draw, yet he uses humor to make fun of the fact that he can't remember. As we say in Alzheimer's, he makes new friends every day. A remarkable man, an incredible teacher—to his children, his students, and to me—John Joe has always had a fascination with the world beyond him. He encouraged everyone around him to open their minds to broader horizons. Now his world is shrinking in disturbing ways, but he presses on in muscle memory, indelible images, analogous to a palate of oil colors ready to paint a canvas.

John Joe has always been a fighter, yet he has an artistic soft side, a thriving right brain that is guiding him back to his love of art, a self-healing therapy from the ravages of a disease that robs a sense of self. He spends hours now painting in oils; it's a passion and yet a challenge to remember what colors to use. So he has devised a scheme of selecting the proper oil colors, somewhat similar to a carpet swatch display where John Joe has laminated and labeled the colors to choose the right ones. And he does.

Art—whether painting, music, or writing—stimulates the brain, stirs memories, and reduces agitation caused by Alzheimer's. Where I run, John Joe paints. By his own admission, he is no Michelangelo, yet his work is inspiring in so many ways. Upon my visit to Duncannon, he presented me with an impressive painting of Hook Head Light. It hangs now in my family room.

"What scares me about this disease," he says over another sip of his pint, "is the loss of memory and the inability to carry a conversation. The brain just isn't processing; it's stalled. It's embarrassing. So I often avoid conversation. I retreat into myself, and at times deal with rage. People who know me say, 'He's changed a lot.'"

I understand. I tell him about my daughter's wedding two summers ago when I had to detach myself several times from family and friends to retreat in solitude and restart the brain. "I used to hold court at such gatherings," I tell him. "I thrived on it. My nickname among friends was the 'Senator from Cape Cod.' No longer. I've left office. Things have changed."

What hasn't changed about John Joe is his heart and his gut Irish humor. Alzheimer's drives one from the mind to the place of the heart, the soul. "I may have tears in my eyes," he says, "but I'm not crying out of sorrow. It's part of what I've been handed. I was blessed with a good family that gives me strength. I have no cause for complaint.

"I laugh, like you, at how long it takes me to remember."

I draw the analogy with John Joe, one he relates with, of comparing Alzheimer's with the basement of a house. "Ever been in a basement doing laundry at night when someone in the kitchen turns the cellar light out?" I ask him. "You scream, right, and you throw a few 'F' bombs until someone upstairs turn the light back on. That's

Alzheimer's. A light goes off, and one goes into rage because it's dark. At some point, the light goes off forever."

John Joe laughs, the kind of gurgle one would expect from a leprechaun. I'm looking for the rainbow now. He's on a roll. "If a cure comes," he says, "it will likely come from America. I hope you call me up some day and say, 'John Joe, I have a little pill for you...'"

"You'll get the first call," I tell him.

Two Irish guys in a pub at sunset, full circle near the Irish Sea, separated by 2,992 miles, connected for a lifetime by a disease that will take their lives. In some ways, doesn't get any better...

The Old Testament book of Ecclesiastes, chapter three, invokes: "to everything there is a season." The storied folk rock group, the Byrds, got religion in the mid 1960s and sung about Ecclesiastes— an anthem for the Baby Boom generation—in their hit "Turn! Turn! Turn!"

> *To everything there is a season, and a time to every purpose under the heaven:*
> *A time to be born, and a time to die; a time to plant, and a time to pluck up that which is planted;*
> *A time to kill, and a time to heal; a time to break down, and a time to build up;*
> *A time to weep, and a time to laugh; a time to mourn, and a time to dance...*

Today is a time of weeping.

At 78, there are a lot of miles on Bob Bertschy, who, as a lanky young ballplayer, crouched behind home plate, wearing the "tools of ignorance," as a catcher with the Los Angeles Dodgers organization.

The term—coined by either Muddy Ruel, who caught for the New York Yankees and the Boston Red Sox in the 1920s, or Yankee Hall of Fame catcher Bill Dickey, who played with Babe Ruth and Lou

Gehrig—implies that smart people would never don such apparatus and play such a precarious position as catcher, with baseballs thrown at them at hurricane speeds. Yet the intelligence required to handle duties behind the plate, directing play as a field general while bumbling with the tools of ignorance, is a disconnect of remarkable proportions.

We catchers stick together, a fraternal body of friendship. On several occasions, Bob and I have talked about our early years behind the plate. Something that still distresses us, clearly not over it yet, is that catchers in the days before batting cages generally never got to hit in batting practice. We were too busy digging balls out of the dirt. No wonder our batting averages were lower. For hours, we patiently backstopped the practice lobs, looping curves, and fastballs to the team roster, then the coach summarily called it quits. Pissed all us catchers off. Behind the plate, we were always on defense, never on offense. In the Dodgers organization, Bob, in fact, one day pleaded as a brash 19-year-old to hit at the end of batting practice, saying he'd even wear his bulky catcher's equipment to the batters' box to save time. Rebuffed and frustrated by the system, he tells me, he dropped an expletive here and there. I tell Bob about the time playing catcher at Fairfield University when the umpire was calling a horrible game; he didn't like my pitcher. So I told my buddy on the mound to throw one in the dirt. I dropped to my knees, pretending to block the ball, then skirted to my left, so the ball bounced up and hit the umpire in the groin. Ouch! The ump bent over in pain. I looked him in the eye, and said, "Play ball!" We had no trouble after that. Shame on me, I suppose...

Bob laughs his ass off at the account.

Bob and I are close friends, and we still are wearing tools of ignorance, but of a different kind—still on defense, not offense, both of us fighting Alzheimer's. Bob also suffers from Parkinson's and Lewy Body disease, another form of progressive dementia with symptoms that include fluctuations in alertness, hallucinations, slowness of movement, trouble walking, mood changes, depression, and more. We know the infield baseline of dementia, having picked off in our day many a base runner leaning the wrong way. But extra innings don't bode well now for either of us. Lots of passed balls.

Bob was born in Dover, Massachusetts, in the working stiff "chicken coop" section of town; his mom used to stitch together Little League uniforms for his neighborhood team. The son of a school superintendent and a librarian, Bob, a Boston University graduate with a PhD in business management, was always a fighter, but there is a tender side to him, too. For many years, he taught chemistry and performing arts at the Hyde School in Bath, Maine, a private college prep boarding school that instills in its students courage, integrity, leadership, curiosity, and concern for one another. At the Hyde School, Bob also coached football, basketball, soccer, lacrosse, and tennis, and choreographed dances with his Hyde students, which they performed on Broadway and at the Kennedy Center. Always striving, Bob in his 40s began painting stunning oils and watercolors, and at age 62, he took up the violin, forever encouraging those around him to persevere. Bob saved lives at the Hyde School, and now his students are trying to save him. That could be a reach; sadly, he's fading out to Pluto.

A man of strong faith, Bob straddles this life and the next, seeing things beyond the view of others, oftentimes seeing things that aren't there. Frequently, he notices strangers lurking in the house—illusions from the disease. Then he'll spot his golf bag in the corner with thick wool head covers for his drivers. One day, having one of his hallucinations, he yelled at his wife, Pat, saying, "There are a bunch of midgets over there staring at me! What the hell are they doing here?" demanded Bob, a guy who used to call his errant golf ball "Mr. Peckerhead," until he started playing with members of Brewster Baptist Church, then changed the name to "Mr. Pee."

Removing the head covers, Pat gently reassured Bob that the "midgets" were his golf drivers. He settled down in the moment, until more strangers appeared.

Another interloper arrived weeks ago in the form of stage 4 terminal stomach cancer, with Bob's body continuing to break down from an onslaught of diseases. The inoperable tumor has enveloped most of his stomach, and has crept into his esophagus. His pain on a scale of one-to-ten is at a twenty. Doctors at first sought to shrink the tumor with palliative radiation so Bob could swallow. Bob, reaching deep into the soul, rejected stutter-step treatment, pending recommendations from Boston's finest cancer doctors. Catchers control the game, until the game is over. Death is the only other option now. Bob is on hospice and on morphine to ease the journey beyond.

Alzheimer's in later stages poses its own difficulties in swallowing, called dysphagia. In Alzheimer's, the coordination and control needed to chew and swallow is wholly compromised. An individual may cough or choke when swallowing, or refuse to try to swallow, part of the end-stage Alzheimer's process of the body gradually shutting down.

Add to this a tumor inching into the esophagus and one has an idea of what hell looks like.

The latest health crisis comes off the heels of two vascular strokes, likely a dementia complication from specks of blood in the brain resulting from vessel damage and leaky blood vessels, the result in some cases of head trauma. Bob and I have had our bell rung many times over the years. The brain, one of the body's most fertile networks of blood flow, is vulnerable in Alzheimer's, leading to strokes or what doctors call TIAs, transient ischemic attacks—mini-strokes. I've had two of them myself; my mother, who died of Alzheimer's, had them as well.

Bob has fought on; the Lord has blessed him with great courage. Unlike other characters in *Cuckoo's Nest*, introspective Bob is Ken Kesey, cerebral in another dimension. His time now is short, and he knows it. We met for coffee the other day, and talked about his fears of the present and the peace of the future. The challenge, he said, is getting from the fear to the peace, a trial we all face in this journey from the cradle to the grave. Bob now seems more open with me than others in talking about the fears. Perhaps it's because we're on the same train. The other day, I tell him, I couldn't figure out how to put my shirt on, a black pullover with no buttons to wrestle. I stuck my head in the right sleeve, looked like a bank robber, then yelled, no, screamed, for my wife. Days later, I tell him, I reached for my razor to brush my teeth; my heart told me it wasn't a good idea. I fear the day when I think it is. Bob winced. Watching him today is ripping me up, sitting in the caboose, knowing Bob is in the engine room. Yet Bob doesn't feel sorry for himself; he's just worried about his wife and family. He's realistic, sad, scared, thankful, and loving all at once—attributes critical in the fight against Alzheimer's.

Reserved in so many fundamental ways, Bob is reaching out in these final moments to close male friends to tell them that he loves them, something he was averse to do in the past. Not bad for a guy who once wore, with pride, the tools of ignorance.

"I love you," Bob tells them from the heart, still feeling a bit discomfited at the invocation, a little awkward, but he knows in his soul it's the right course.

He confided in me in his confusion on this the other day. Catchers stick together.

"Do you think I'm gay now?" he asked.

"Yes, Bob," I replied. "We're all gay in the full reaches of love and faith. And that's the way it should be, the freedom to love…"

Alzheimer's teaches perfect love. In Heaven, you leave the stereotypes at the door.

One dark day, I received an email from Pat, sent to all family members and close friends after Bob had seen specialists in Boston. She said Bob's neurologist, knowing the end game, stressed that he didn't think radiation would work in shrinking part of the tumor to help Bob swallow, that it wouldn't be successful enough to warrant the pain it would cause. "The doctor told Bob that if it were him, he would go home and enjoy the time he has, watch more sunsets… listen to music and be at peace. The neurologist told Bob, "You have earned the right to enjoy your days without more pain." Bob agreed. Days and a few sunsets later, Bob died peacefully in great courage, sitting next to Pat, holding hands. It was the way Bob wanted to go. They were the perfect battery—pitcher and catcher. Bob caught his final game with great distinction, protecting the plate, protecting his family, and in Heaven, he now has retired the tools of ignorance…

Perfect love comes in many ways. I saw Bob for the last time shortly before he died. We both knew what lay ahead. The elephant in the room was speaking; always best, he said, to say goodbye before the fact. We hugged in a way that reinforced it was the last time. I knew he expected a final smile from me. "Bob," I said after he sat back down on the couch. "Why don't you pick me up tonight, and we'll go dancing and have a few beers!"

He smiled back broadly, then slowly raised the index finger of his right hand. Bob gave me the finger on the way out. Perfect love, from the heart in all ways. So cool. I knew he'd be fine up in Heaven. Us catchers stick together...

Yet today is a time of weeping. To everything, there is a season...

Early in the morning near Cape Cod Bay, the sun spills off Paine's Creek Marsh in West Brewster in a reflection of grace. The marsh envelops nearby historic Wing Island, a 140-acre pristine preserve that rises above the marsh, thick with salt meadow hay, spike grass, bulrushes, black grass, and seaside goldenrod. Named after the town's first English settler, John Wing, the island is traversed by a one-mile trail that leads across the island to the bay, past patches of highbush blueberry, chokeberry, sea lavender, beach plum, wild raspberries, and arrowwood, whose long straight shoots were once used by native peoples to fashion spears and arrows. The island has yielded artifacts as old as 8,000 years, near the time when native peoples first occupied the region.

At a table in a local coffee shop, near a rolling bend in the road, "Betty's Curve," I sit with Bob Bertschy's widow, Pat, just days after his passing. God, how I hate the word "widow." Scripture instructs us to care for widows, but today Pat is caring for me.

"How are you doing?" she asks.

"Not good," I reply. "Can't imagine the grief, the loss, the pain, that you're feeling."

Her tears flow like currents in the creek.

And so it is with caregivers in this disease. They put life on the line, only to feel the pull of loss far beyond Pluto. In the end, their identity—as guardian, defender, advocate—vanishes in a breath. The stinging loneliness of Alzheimer's replays like a loop tape in the mind of caregivers. One can't stop the reprise. What next? What next? There are no decorations or honors bestowed upon them, just intense isolation. Their mission has come to an end, yet they never forget. Caregivers are the heroes of this war.

We talk today about Bob's fear of death and his courage to accept the curtain call. She reaches for my hand, thanking me for preparing Bob for new horizons, along with counsel from our pastor Doug Scalise, and others. There is a guilt about being left behind. I, too, am feeling painfully guilty this morning. Pat senses this.

"I understand now," she tells me, noting she's schooled in Kesey's *Cuckoo's Nest*. "I understand your role, I do…You've been called to open the doors for others, to kick out the windows, to free souls."

"You're the Chief!"

The analogy seeps in, as we talk.

In Kesey's work, Chief Bromden in *Cuckoo's Nest*, the soaring Native American in the ward, has been in the institution the longest. At first, he chooses not to speak, mostly out of fear and intimidation. Bromden uses this as a tactic to deflect—a tactic I first employed as family caregiver for my mother and father, then as victim myself. Ultimately, Bromden, the narrator in *Cuckoo's Nest*, becomes the path to freedom. Kesey's book takes its title from a nursery rhyme the Chief was read as a boy.

When the Chief regains his voice, he declares, "I felt like I was flying. Free. I've been away a long time…"

"You are flying free now yourself," Pat reassures.

In Kesey's work, the Chief fights off hallucinations that he calls a "fog machine," and refuses to take Nurse Ratched's "little red pills," sedations to anesthetize the patients. I tell Pat that, right or wrong, I've declined heavier doses of antidepressants and other medications to chill me out—"stun pills," as I call them, to better control the despair and rage of Alzheimer's.

I tell Pat more about my own "fog machine." On a recent night, I tell her, that sleeping on the couch in the family room, anesthetized by watching wacky news of the world, I fell asleep, only to wake up hours later to witness another demon—this time sitting on the edge of a coffee table near the couch. "It was small, green, frightening," I tell Pat. She nods, having heard other stories of hallucinations in this disease.

Pat is distressed, I can tell, but has the presence of mind at the end of her husband Bob's journey to reflect that a central theme in Kesey's book is the importance of rational choices while one has the facility for it, fighting every way possible to stay in the moment. She reminds me that the Chief, after freeing fellow patients in ways that instill a measure of self-esteem, normalcy to the extent possible, escapes himself. In the dark of night in a remote section of the ward, he reaches for a heavy granite control panel that he rips from the floor, then races across the room with the panel hoisted high above his head and smashes it through a large window. To the applause of others in the ward, the Chief escapes into the night.

I often think about such escapes, leaving this planet for Pluto—searching, like the spacecraft *New Horizons*, for the light at the end of the tunnel. A fantasy of mine is a swan song off the Cliffs of Moher, which rise in splendor 390 feet above the Atlantic at the southwest edge of County Clare, Ireland. A heavenly view from the summit, one breathes in the taste of salt air, the rush of wind, the damp of fog rising above the ancient rocks, nature in its purest, rawest form.

Just to the north of the peak is O'Brien's Tower, a Doric, stone column topped by an urn. It was built by an ancestor, Sir Cornelius O'Brien, born in 1782—an Irish politician, member of Parliament, and County Clare landowner.

What a place for a farewell. In my office, there is a brilliant framed photo of the Cliffs of Moher. I stare at it every day. Wrote Kesey, "You had a choice: you could either strain and look at things that appeared in front of you in the fog, painful as it might be, or you could relax and lose yourself."

But not my time, not the moment to lose myself, the angels, the Almighty, and the universe tells me. And besides, my first granddaughter Sweet Adeline would have nothing to do with this. And so for now, while Pluto awaits, I fight on, carrying a torch for Bob Bertschy, Trish Vradenburg, Bea Lerner, Ken Sullivan, Brian LeBlanc, Mike Belleville, Rob Moir, Chrissy Brazelton, Judy Jaffe Gelfand, the Rev. Cynthia Huling Hummel, Sonia Duarte, John Joe Vaughan, and millions of others.

Time is fleeting. Far more torchbearers are needed to curse the darkness, to generate far more funding for better care and a cure. Will you fight with and for us, for your children and for grandchildren? Please fight!

"Which one of you nuts has got any guts?"

PART THREE

REFLECTIONS
of the Family

24

"Miles from Nowhere"

Mary Catherine McGeorge O'Brien

Twenty-seven hundred and fifteen miles is a long way from home, particularly when you grow up on a rustic 1,120-acre ranch about 20 miles outside Phoenix in the 1950s, as far flung from Boston as the north rim of the Grand Canyon.

Moving to Boston with my world-beating journalist husband in 1979 after his tenure as an investigative reporter at the *Arizona Republic*, covering white-collar crime, the Mexican Mafia, and the Aryan Brotherhood, I clearly discerned we were on new ground. It snows here, is biting cold in winter, and rains often; spring is a day in early June, and summer is the bliss of all. But don't hold your breath. Early on, Greg lived in my world; now I live in his, and it's getting far more complicated now.

When I moved East, somewhat guardedly with Greg, paying homage to marriage vows, I was entering the forbidden city, land far east of the Mississippi—the dividing line, my rancher father had taught me, between "real people" and the Eastern Establishment. If you haven't guessed, my husband and I were born on different planets. He grew up in Rye, Westchester County, a short train ride from Manhattan. We have always agreed on child rearing, faith, hope, and charity, but when it came to geography, we are the inverse of simpatico.

Just sayin', as my husband likes to quote.

I dream of returning one day to Phoenix, to my family, six supportive, loving brothers and sisters, their children, and extended family, in the valley of paradise—particularly now as my husband, of 40 years of marriage, declines in Alzheimer's, a black hole now slowly sucking him in, often beyond the notice of others. Yet Phoenix is not in the cards for the moment. Likely, I will not return until my husband is in a nursing home, or writing in Heaven for the *Daily Amen!* The life of a caregiver is fraught with the unknown. For better or for worse...

What's a nice girl like me doing in a place like this?

Like the probing Cat Stevens song of 1970, I feel, as a caregiver in the throes of Alzheimer's, that I'm "Miles from Nowhere." Some tea for the tillerman might be nice. The family tiller has now been handed to me, and there's no land in sight.

The rugged White Tank mountains, 20 miles northwest of Phoenix, frame Litchfield Park like a Frederic Remington painting. Litchfield Park is an anchor to the McGeorge family. In 1923, Col. Dale Bumstead, a World War I hero, and his wife, Eva, purchased about 1,100 acres of failing citrus gardens and date groves just outside Litchfield Park with a vision for a ranch of international renown. Col. Bumstead named the ranch Tal-Wi-Wi, Hopi Native American that translates to: "Where the sun first shines upon the fertile earth." In time, the name would have new meaning for me.

Visionary Col. Bumstead didn't have much to work with from the start. Yet fast forward to 1946 when he hired my father, Ken, another war hero, a Lt. Colonel who served in World War II under Gen. George Patton. It was Dad's first job out of the Army, employed on the recommendation of his father, William, a close friend of Col. Bumstead, and at the time a noted agricultural chemist at the

University of Arizona Agricultural Chemistry and Soils Department. My dad had no previous farming experience, but Col. Bumstead wanted a hard-working war veteran who wanted to get his hands dirty. And he got one!

And so I was raised on magnificent Tal-Wi-Wi, with my devoted mother, Mary Ellen, a saint of a woman, and six siblings: Martha, Tommy, Louie, Barbara Ann, Nancy, and Robert. I was fourth in line in this magical oasis in the middle of the desert that defines Phoenix. We were surrounded by vineyards and sweet orchards of oranges, grapefruits, and tangerines, where we could pick our lunch before school. The entrance to the ranch welcomed with giant date palms and beautiful eucalyptus trees that lined the perimeter. We had rose gardens and gardens filled with snapdragons, gardenias, camellias, and every other variety of flower that could greet the dry Arizona sunshine.

Tal-Wi-Wi, over time, attracted worldwide attention for its incredible fruit, prize-winning Hereford cattle, dates, and grapevines, including the first commercial production in the world of the prized cardinal grape, a transcendent cross between the flame seedless and ribier table grapes. The New York markets were agog. Little did I realize as a young upright girl on a farm in rural Arizona that my future one day would be Back East, Miles from Nowhere.

As Tal-Wi-Wi grew in stature, it attracted notoriety around the world, among them, many years ago, the Crown Prince of Arabia, his royal highness Saud Al Saud, and on December 2, 1949, the Shah of Iran, a young, handsome 30-year-old Mohammed Reza Pahlevi, a Middle East strongman who in 1967 took the title of Shāhanshāh ("Emperor" or "King of Kings") and was overthrown by the Islamic Revolution of 1979. At Tal-Wi-Wi that day, the Shah was sovereign. He had come here at the invitation of President Harry Truman to witness the miracle of transforming arid desert to productive land through irrigation. Truman, a Missouri boy from Independence, had known my grandmother, Catherine McGee Soden from Kansas City; they were friends. Family lore has it that after Truman recognized the State of Israel in 1948, my grandmother, a devoted Irish Catholic, congratulated him, having recently visited Israel herself, proclaiming, "Mr. President, they think you're Jesus Christ over there!"

"Now, Catherine," Truman is said to have invoked, "You know they don't believe in a divine Jesus!"

The Shah that day on Tal-Wi-Wi was feted with Arabian dishes, as well as elk venison, wild turkey, and antelope broiled over an open fire. Col. Bumstead, we're told, had bagged the game in a hunting trip. It was a feast fit for a king. My pretty sister, Martha, three years old at the time, was on hand for the occasion. Reported a local periodical, "When she (Martha) presented a large rose to the Shah, she was lifted into his arms for a big hug by the world's most eligible bachelor."

Did I tell you that my husband and I are from different planets?

Like many mixed marriages, Greg and I have hit for the cycle: first attraction, then marriage, children, and yes, along the way, plenty of private intimacy. Given that I studied journalism at the University of Arizona, I was attracted to Greg because he was a writer, and a good one; he was also good-looking. He isn't particularly romantic, but he is smart and easy on the eyes. The two seemed to go together for me. There's nothing romantic about living with a journalist; there have been times I wished I had listened to my mother.

She once asked me at the start of the relationship, "What does Greg do for a living?"

"He's a writer," I said.

"I know," my mother replied in great wisdom, coming from some family wealth, "but how does he make his money?"

Still, the two of us made for loving parents. But as the kids grew, and took up lives of their own, we began to drift, just as Greg's parents had years earlier. It was obvious to the children. It was no one's fault. Over time, there were the predictable hostile exchanges of marriage, penetrating moments of silence, perhaps even thoughts of separation, as we tried to discern the new "us," life after parenting. The intimacy was gone; Greg often slept on the couch. Alone in our bed, I often dreamt of Tal-Wi-Wi.

Years ago, it got worse as Greg's mother drifted deeper into Alzheimer's, and we became family caregivers. I saw firsthand the terrifying, disconnected, debilitating, hostile nature of this disease. Then to my horror, I began to see it in my husband; *Invasion of the Body Snatchers,* as Greg calls Alzheimer's, slow at first, then a quickening pace. The explosions, the rage, the drifting, the ceaseless short-term memory loss, absence of filter and judgment, absence of balance at times, repeating himself, asking the same damn questions. I was out of my mind. I was in denial, thinking he was just becoming more of a perfect asshole; Greg has always sought perfection. In time, the evidence was overwhelming, particularly after Greg's parents had died, and he was no longer consumed with caring for them. He was privately consumed then with fighting his own demons.

Yet before Greg's parents' death, I began noticing a change in them, a softening in their relationship. More and more, they depended on one another. They were both fighting off progressing dementia, and Greg's dad in addition had cancer and circulation disease that ultimately placed him in a wheelchair. More and more, they became one, completing a life circle. It was stunning to watch. They needed each other again. Alzheimer's had begun healing their marriage.

British novelist E.M. Forster once wrote, "You must be willing to let go of the life we have planned, so as to have the life that is waiting for us."

The life waiting for me is more and more a nightmare. I didn't sign up for this. When we received Greg's diagnosis at his neurologist's office, after a battery of tests, brains scans, and a gene test, I had very little information about Alzheimer's except through the experience with his parents, which was mostly destructive. Greg's mom, for example, was particularly nasty and made derogatory remarks to him, her main family caregiver. I didn't know at the time that this is part of the disease. Now it's my turn, and I am the receiver of that unbearable behavior. At least I can TRY to shove it off to Alzheimer's, but it is never easy. I had no sense of where to turn for help, support, or even how to express the diagnosis with family, friends, or co-workers. I was lost, and crept further inward. There is no single handbook one can read to prepare; each journey is different, each course of the disease takes different, meandering turns—no two are alike, the experts will tell you, an observation that is clearly numbing in so many ways, as best-selling authors and close friends of ours, David Shenk and Meryl Comer, write in their respective books, *The Forgetting* and *Slow Dancing with a Stranger*. Must-reads!

My family in Phoenix was first to respond. My loving siblings, who have known Greg since his 20s, were supportive and reached out to me in ways that told me I wasn't alone. Still, they were close to 3,000 miles away. Greg's siblings, in contrast, while far closer in geography, were generally more restrained in outreach. Understandably, denial is a survival instinct when a disease cruises through a family. As Henry David Thoreau calls Cape Cod the "bare and bended" arm of Massachusetts, I felt bare and bended.

It wasn't until legendary filmmaker Steve James (*Hoop Dreams, Life Itself*, and other award-winning films) produced a short documentary about our family's journey, *A Place Called Pluto*, part of Cure Alzheimer's Fund initiative, Living With Alzheimer's—documenting the various stages of Alzheimer's (livingwithalz.org)—that word got out. The film played at notable film festivals across the country, including Tribeca in New York, Washington, D.C., out West, and a preview at the Museum of Modern Art (MoMA) in midtown Manhattan.

But still, I wasn't ready to deal fully with it, having just come off the cliff of Greg's mother. I was in denial, didn't want help, and was not emotionally prepared for it, in spite of numerous supportive outreaches from close friends on the Cape and Boston. Caring friends Leslie and Paul Durgin in Milton outside Boston hosted an unsung heroes cookout at their home, in support for two close women with breast cancer, Becky Smith and Nancy Souder from Cape Cod, and for me, the caregiver. It was awkward in its own way, but healing. Thank you, Durgins!

However, it wasn't until a Boston television show, WCBV-TV's *Chronicle*, produced with host Anthony Everett, did an incredible half-hour segment on our family—one that won an Emmy and a National Headliner First Place Award—that the story hit hard at home. I, for one, watch *Chronicle* every night, the best news magazine in the nation. I'm a big fan, but I never imagined the wide viewing it would get in my small little world on Cape Cod. Host Everett's father, I learned later, died of Alzheimer's. The segment, I'm told, had hundreds of thousands of hits on *Chronicle*'s website. When I arrived the following morning at my teaching assistant job at Nauset Regional Middle School in Orleans, I was greeted with scores of tearful hugs, encouragement, flowers, and generous offers from our three caring guidance counselors that "their door is always open." Oh well, thanks to *Chronicle* and Anthony Everett, everyone on Cape Cod knew, and I needed now to accept the disease as well.

Months later, after having read Ptolemy Tompkins and Tyler Beddoes's inspiring book, *Proof of Angels*, an angel came knocking at the door in the form of Frank Connell, a local painter and a saint of a man. I had asked him for an estimate to repaint a master bedroom with a high cathedral ceiling, a master bathroom, a stairwell, and hallway—work expected to cost thousands of dollars by today's standards.

Connell inspected the areas then asked, "When do you want me to start? I didn't know whose house this was until I drove up." Frank had just buried his mother after her bout with Alzheimer's, and had seen the *Chronicle* piece.

"Frank, I can't go forward until I have an estimate," I said, knowing our bank account was draining toward empty.

"Oh," Frank interrupted. "There's no charge for this. I'm doing it for free!"

I started crying. "No, you can't do that," I said.

Frank hugged me and replied, "This isn't something you need to cry about. You have plenty of crying ahead of you. It's your turn to be taken care of..."

On Pluto: Inside the Mind of Alzheimer's

I kept crying; my husband did as well when I told him later of the exchange.

Weeks later, when Greg and I were speaking in Phoenix and Tucson before the Literary Society of the Southwest, Frank and his crew of six performed a miracle. Proof of angels. There were more angels to come. To mention a few: our chimney sweep, Judd Berg, an old friend of Greg's, cleaned the wood stove chimney in the family room; landscaper Lindsay Strode cut the lawn when Greg's sitdown broke and he couldn't afford to fix it; childhood friend Mark Mathison replaced rotted siding; neighbor Charlie Sumner, retired "Mayor" of Brewster, loans Greg every home tool imaginable, then shows him how to use it; close friend Brewster Police Chief Dick Koch, a guardian angel in so many ways, along with Paul and Leslie Durgin of Milton; mentor Peter Polhemus, who guides Greg financially and tries to laugh at his sick jokes; and Boston attorney John Twohig, a surrogate brother to Greg, put us up on Nantucket for a long weekend getaway at the elegant White Elephant on Nantucket Harbor, and paid for our fine meal. And there were scores of other acts of kindness from organizations, noted in the Epilogue, like the Washington, D.C.-based UsAgainstAlzheimer's (UsAgainstAlzheimers.org), the Chicago-based Alzheimer's Association (alz.org) and the association's Massachusetts/New Hampshire branch, the Boston-based Cure Alzheimer's Fund (curealz.org), the Cape Cod-based Hope Health: Hope Dementia & Alzheimer's Services (hopehealthco.org), and the Brewster-based Alzheimer's Family Support Center of Cape Cod (alzheimerscapecod.com), run by our close friends Molly Purdue and Melanie Braverman. Molly talks about our family's journey in "The Nun Story" in this On Pluto expanded edition.

Today, I read a lot of Christian author C. S. Lewis. He also speaks to my heart. "It's not the load you carry that breaks you," Lewis writes, "it's the way you carry the load."

I first needed to learn how to carry the load, then I needed to learn that I was being carried. The heavy lifting took me back to scripture. A verse in Matthew 11:29-30 has new meaning for me. Jesus said, "Take my yoke upon you…for my yoke is easy to bear, and the burden I give you light…"

Light shines in all ways. One of the blessings and challenges of this journey with Greg is that through persevering, courageous, hard work he has attained national and international respect as a person living with Alzheimer's. At first, I felt left behind. Greg was getting the well-deserved attention, and I was cleaning up the mess, particularly difficult with his loss of continence at times.

"How's Greg doing?" I'm asked all the time.

I have to admit that at times it's personally distressing, the "drive-bys," as Greg calls them. But what about me, and what about all the other caregivers, who selflessly care for their loved ones, many of them in stages of dementia now deeper than my husband's? We deal with symptoms, we deal with terrible depression, our immune systems are breaking down. We are on the edge! How about us?

Greg is a cartoon guy and also loves watching black-and-white reruns of *The Three Stooges*. There's a *Bugs Bunny* cartoon that Greg loves where Bugs pipes up, "How about me, boss? How about me?"

Well, how about me, boss, and how about all the other caregivers?

I do think the focus is changing, collectively a better understanding as noted above, that when one person has Alzheimer's, the entire family gets it. I was shocked at a recent international Alzheimer's conference in Lausanne, Switzerland, when host George Vradenburg, head of UsAgainstAlzheimer's, asked me after Greg's speech: "I want to know how Mary Catherine feels?" Wow! So I told them of the paralyzing isolation, anger, and fear. Those in Alzheimer's are alone; so are the caregivers, as if one of Pluto's moons, perhaps Charon, the largest and locked into the ebb and flow of Pluto that the two in some scientific circles are considered a "double dwarf planet." My husband and I fear the same things in parallel emotions, searching for ways to vent. Like Greg, I cry, yell, feel numb in the head. Often we collide in our orbits.

The same happened at an Alzheimer's Association conference in Tucson, Arizona. It brought me to tears as I sat on a stage in front of about 500 people. I'm not a person who wears my heart on my sleeve, so this was difficult, but it was also very moving. People care....

"So, what are you going to do?" I'm asked all the time. This question is the most exasperating. How can I know what I am going to do when I don't know what the changes next week will bring? As one caregiver, a friend of mine said, "I lose a little bit of him every day."

If finances weren't a huge, distracting concern for us, this question could glean more answers. Greg, who can't make the money he once earned, has gone through all of his retirement funds, not that there was much to begin with, and with both of us from large families, there is no inheritance, other than some walking-around money. We face bankruptcy in years to come. So when your financial future has no future, the answer to the question "what are you going to do?" can be a walk off the plank. Yet angels abound, and this gets back to accepting the life I had not anticipated. Or as my husband likes to joke, "We got plenty of money; it's just tied up in debt!"

Let me vent a bit, if that's okay with you. I am a checklist lady—by the day, the month, the year. I love crossing all those "have done" off my list! With Alzheimer's, my checklist never ends, and never gets checked off. Frustration for a checklist lady. Enter more faith in striving to accept the unknown. Back to the marriage vows: "For better or for worse...til death do us part."

I'm heading into the worst part now. We are going on 40 years of marriage and memories together, but they are slowly fading for Greg. I've spent 40 years of my 60-plus years of life with someone who won't remember that we honeymooned in Hawaii or met in college, or traveled to Ireland. I will be left alone with those memories as I grow old. That is scary and sad for any caregiver. Sure, there are memories that I want him to forget; we've discussed that, so I have to be grateful to some extent! But to grow old and not share the more significant part of your life is more than disconcerting. I ask more and more "do you remember" questions, and he doesn't. It gets increasingly sad. The anger, now with both of us, escalates.

Kindness with Alzheimer's can go out the door. You have to become comfortable with a less-than-perfect relationship. Greg exudes kindness and softness and humor when he's outside the house, an effort that saps him. At home, he lets his guard down and is easily angered. For example, he gives me a list of what he wants me to get at the store for him. I come home with his three boxes of frozen fruit bars, Cracker Barrel cheddar cheese, salad, Bumble Bee tuna (he's addicted to that), but I forgot the chunky peanut butter. Not good—he is pissed and angry. The perfect asshole. Did I tell you about that?

When I forget something he screams, "WE talked about this!" But I have to listen to things over and over and over. Greg yells not just at me, but to his poor Mac laptop, but I believe the Mac is more resilient than I am. If only I could just be a technology source and not feel so embattled.

Technology has become Greg's friend now—his laptop, his iPhone, and last Christmas I gave him Google Home, a calming device that can help in his frustrations when he's writing and can't remember a word or what it means, or when he yells at me: "I don't understand; I'm confused."

"Okay, Google," you ask a white cone-shaped cylinder, and Google responds.

You heard he threw a shoe at me at the airport, absorbing confusion and rage. He feels badly about that. I made sure of it. In jest and in repentance, he asked Google Home recently if it was okay to throw a shoe at your wife. "That's not normal human behavior!" Google replied. Google is now my new best friend.

Then there's the time recently when he misplaced his phone for the 40th time that day. He's yelling and screaming at me and Conor, though I understand he's upset about losing memory. I worry sometimes in his anger that he will hurt himself. Conor in the moment told Greg to check in the car, that he would call the cell phone. In the car by himself, Greg could hear the phone ringing, but could not discern where the sound was coming from. His brain couldn't pinpoint; the ringing, the noise to him appeared throughout the car, on the floor, in the front seat, in the back seat…

Like a blind man, he told me later, Greg began checking for phone vibrations. Finally, he found the lost phone. You'd think he'd be happy. He was in such rage about losing his phone so many times that day that literally he had to hurt something. So he grabbed a coffee cup on the floor of the car, a souvenir of a memorable weekend trip to Manhattan with our daughter, Colleen. It had become my favorite, a Starbucks New York City cup with a yellow cab imprint. In rank anger, Greg hurled it against a nearby stone wall, a perfect strike fast ball with his left hand, though he's right-handed. I was in the front yard at the time. Greg looked up to the sky and yelled expletives. "If you want me, you can take me now," he yelled to Alzheimer's, then walked by me, slamming the door behind me. Seconds later, he sensed what had happened and opened the door. I was outside crying, and walked in. I hugged him, saying, "I know it's not you, it's the disease."

Greg then told me that he'd be right back. He went outside again, looking up to the sky, spewing expletives again. "You can't have me today, Alzheimer's," he told me he screamed.

Ironically, Alzheimer's now is starting to heal our marriage, as it did with Greg's parents, drawing us closer together, letting go of the past, holding on to the future.

I find myself relating more today to caregivers fighting the disease. They seem more real to me than others. There are no "drive-bys" with this group. One woman I've come to know and love is Margaret Rice Moir, a beautiful writer whose husband Rob is struggling with Alzheimer's, as Greg noted earlier. They live just a few blocks away from us. I find peace and strength in Margaret's writing about this disease.

"Many of us know the evolution of Alzheimer's," she writes. "We know the bone-chilling fear when you wake up in the middle of the night, worrying about what's to come, the financial hurdles, the shifting roles. Life surely changes after a diagnosis. It does for the patient. It does for the caregiver. Love becomes more complicated, intimacy more challenging, patience more ephemeral....We know the time we have now is precious. The good and the bad, it's all we have. So, lover, mother, nursemaid, nag, we caregivers are lost somewhere, floating in and out among our many, often conflicting, roles....While love can be ever so much more challenging in these times, it can also be richer, deeper, and more mature. And in our best moments, there is joy in that. Touch becomes the language between us."

As I often lay awake at night when sleep is robbed, I reflect back to the serene, innocent days on Tal-Wi-Wi when life and promise were ahead of me. The land "where the sun first shines upon the fertile earth" still embraces me. I used to watch in awe as the sun rose above the resplendent Arizona mountains. Now I watch the sun rise at first light over bountiful Nauset Beach and brilliant sunsets on Cape Cod Bay. Observing this inspiring earthy phenomenon has always been a soul-searching encounter for me. But "sundowning" now takes on a new meaning. As the sun sets and the light goes dim, Greg's confusion increases, his mood worsens, and his patience and reasoning ebb, generally followed by language unacceptable in polite circles.

I cringe. A favorite time of day is now a worst fear. Yet my friend Margaret is correct when she writes, "It's no one's fault. It's just the disease. Once my husband saved me; today I'm saving him."

Miles from nowhere...

(Postscript: A journalism major years ago at the University of Arizona, I wrote this with some assistance from my editor husband, Greg. It took many months to dig deep. The words are from my heart, my feelings, my soul, for better or for worse. We complete each other's sentences today...)

25

The Good and the Bad

Conor Michael O'Brien

Those with Alzheimer's are not the only ones who forget. We all forget. And more than not, we all want to forget.

When I was a baby, I had a bad bout with colic, my dad told me. He fought colic himself as an infant. Twenty-seven years ago, he wrote an expressive piece in *Boston Magazine* about it. Looking back, he calls the piece humorous.

I read it for the first time recently, and was immediately devastated, thinking of what he and my mother must have gone through day and night with a constant ringing in their ears from my deafening cries. I was in tears reading the piece, imagining my dad, almost three decades ago, trying to get through the work day with my ear-splitting screams screwing up his routine. The column, of course, was well-written—a similar style of writing he has today, and thank God he hasn't lost a step in that regard, though he struggles desperately in so many other areas. I've now apologized with a sarcastic smile on my face for the terror that my newborn-self caused them, then realized that that short chapter in Dad's life was a cakewalk compared to his challenging walk today. Witnessing firsthand his gut-will to fight against the weighty burden he carries is inspiring.

As Dad notes in his *Boston Magazine* piece, I fussed, actually cried, many hours a day, as millions of colicky babies do, a common phenomenon. My pediatrician, according to the column, told my parents at the time that infants "are nothing more than potatoes with a bunch of unconnected nerves."

Apparently, the colic got to the point where one day in his upstairs office in *The Cape Codder* newsroom, my dad heard a baby crying in the lobby. He panicked. "Oh, my God," he wrote in the piece. "Conor has tracked me down. He knows where I work!"

So Dad reached for the phone, calling a *Boston Magazine* editor, asking if he could write a column about colic, and interview one of the world's top baby experts, Dr. T. Berry Brazelton, the "Dr. Spock of the 80s," as Dad calls him. Dr. Brazelton, in an interview, reassured my father that colic was normal, that he and my mom should stop "fussing over it," that follow-up studies on colicky babies indicate that they "grow up to be extremely intelligent, alert children."

I feel good about that, and about my relationship with my dad today. We have much in common—physically, emotionally, and in how we often think. In some ways, we are a carbon copy of one another, and I am proud of that. Over the years, my dad has sacrificed, as all good fathers, to care for me, my brother, Brendan, and my sister, Colleen. He never ceases to amaze me in all facets of his life, trying to focus on whatever task is at hand and always delivering on it— even with a screaming newborn in the background. That's impressive enough at the prime of life; now what he's able to accomplish in his battle with Alzheimer's is truly astonishing.

A few years ago, when Dad told us about his diagnosis, we all feared the worst, but deep inside we all knew that he was going to put up a fight and rise above the disease as best he could. We were a close family before; we would be even closer now. So I signed up for duty. As it is with the New England Patriots and Coach Belichick when someone is down, *"Next Man Up!"* After Dad had cared for me all these years, the mantle had been passed, and I was to care for him now. I became his day-to-day associate, the family caregiver who assists with his work, does much of his research, helps in editing, participates at times in speeches and interviews, drives and travels with him, and finds his phone, laptop, and car keys scores of times a day when he loses them. My job, as we joke, is to try to make sure Dad "doesn't lose his shit."

My dad and I have grown through the process, learned more about each other, have become much closer. Looking back, I realize this is a blessing—on the road with Dad, across the country and parts of the world, in interviews with NPR, PBS/NOVA, Fox News, and scores of newspaper, radio, and television stations, in speeches to groups as large as a thousand, and as intimate as a gathering at a nursing home. There are a lot of ups and downs now. Dad's bad episodes now outweigh the good ones, but I cherish each time I see that he's having a good day for whatever reason. A smile goes a long way.

Dad could always light up a room with his smile, charm, humor, and presence; still does. It's muscle memory for him. He can captivate a room in an instant with his charisma, and simply his words. He can draw in an audience at the drop of a hat. Bad days now for him are as common as the sun rising in the morning. His ability to adjust, put a smile on, and strive on is as courageous as it gets.

But there has been a steep learning curve for both of us, so many twists and turns. There was a time not long ago when Dad and I were in Washington, D.C. for an UsAgainstAlzheimer's annual summit; Dad was speaking at the Capitol Hill event. The day before the speech I worked out in a fitness center at the downtown hotel where we were staying. Dad remained in the room, saying he was feeling a bit foggy. He wanted to rest. When I returned about an hour and a half later, he was on Pluto. He didn't know where he was, and in the moment, who I was. Freaked me out. I've witnessed these trips to Pluto before, but this one was more intense. It could have been a minor stroke, Dad was told later, a "TIA," a transient ischemic attack, as doctors call them, common in Alzheimer's and other forms of dementias. I had to look this up. A TIA, the experts say, starts as a brain stroke, but then lessens, leaving no noticeable symptoms or additional damage, other than a warning sign that the person is at risk for more serious and debilitating strokes. Upon Dad's return from Pluto we spoke about it; he said it had happened before. He didn't want to talk much about it.

More recently, I experienced yet another out-of-body Dad encounter—this one far more vocal, along the line of scores of Alzheimer's outbursts I have witnessed. My parents had been asked to speak at a special Alzheimer's panel at WGBH-TV in Boston. The forum was held after a special screening of the powerful PBS Alzheimer's documentary, *Every Minute Counts*. Traveling to the television station with my parents in a cab from our Boston hotel, Dad had another outrageous disconnect. This one was likely caused by paranoia from this disease. We were on track, on time, for the event. I was charting the course on my iPhone. The cabbie, though, took a wrong turn close to the station. Dad instantly was uncontrollable, yelling and loudly cursing in ways that would shave the hairs off a nun's neck. We couldn't control him. The paranoia of dementia was in full force. The cabbie, Dad thought, was intentionally trying to deceive him, or perhaps even take him prisoner. It was as if some alien force had taken control of him. With a few quick right turns, we were back on track. After multiple apologies to the cabbie from my mother and me, we got out of the car. Dad was still in such rage that he stormed across a busy Boston street toward the station, not caring if he was hit by a car. Angels must have sheltered him.

Once inside the station, Dad calmed down after a few minutes. An hour later, he was an all-star on the panel before an audience of several hundred. No one knew what had transpired earlier, until he turned to my mom after being asked a question about the rage of the disease. He reached for her hand, told he loved her, and started to cry. It was pretty moving.

Months later, Dad had a similar explosion in Manhattan with another cabbie on our way to stay at the Broadway Plaza Hotel, the day before an Alzheimer's podcast recording with author David Shenk at Argot Studios on West 26th Street. The cab driver, who spoke broken English, was having great difficulty maneuvering down Broadway, now a zigzag of a street, and my dad assumed the cabbie was lost, or worse yet, "taking us hostage." I know this sounds horrible. My dad is not a horrible man, but in Alzheimer's, I've found, paranoia often overtakes reality. Dad again began yelling swears at the driver. It got worse. He was out of his mind. Literally.

"Do you know where the (expletive) you're going?" he screamed at the cabbie. "This is bullshit…Where the hell are you taking us? Pull over, dammit, just pull over now!"

In full rage, Dad bolted from the cab. I followed. The driver, sensing my father was in the throes of an emotional issue, tried to calm him down. It worked to some extent.

"What do I owe you?" Dad asked. The meter read $10.25.

"Nothing," the cabbie replied. "You don't owe me anything. I am sorry."

The return from Pluto at times can be swift for my dad. Realizing he had been "out-of-body," my father gave the driver a twenty-dollar bill. "I'm not a bad guy," he told the cab driver. "I'm the one who needs to apologize here. I just have some issues. And I'm sorry."

Dad then shook the stunned cabbie's hand, gave him what he calls a "manly" hug, and the cabbie, probably wondering what the hell had just happened, drove off. Now we were standing on Broadway in a crush of rush hour humanity with our luggage and no ride. When I suggested that we call another cab or an Uber, Dad, who apparently had crash landed from Pluto, slipped into rage again, grabbed his oversized bag, handed me cash for a cab, then vanished into the masses.

"I'm done," he said. "I'm done…"

Our family has learned that when Dad hurls into an Alzheimer's rage to let out some rope, like the spool of a fishing rod. I couldn't stop him, a hail of bullets couldn't stop him, so with great reluctance I let him go. Except this time, Dad had cut the line. Seconds later, reality hit me: Oh my God, Dad is lost in New York, dragging a heavy oversized bag with a bewildered demeanor that says he's bait. I was in a full-blown panic. The only saving grace was that he had the hotel address in his pocket.

Later Dad told me that he was in such a fury, hauling his heavy bag along Broadway, that he had hoped, actually prayed, to be accosted by a street gang so he could liberate his anger. He had even decided what to tell his imagined attackers:

"This is NOT going to be a good day for you!"

Dad said he practiced the line for several city blocks.

Greatly concerned, I immediately hailed a cab to the hotel and tried to call my father. He wouldn't answer. The cabbie was an extremely friendly and engaging guy from Ireland. I don't come across a lot of Irish cabbies in New York City. We talked. Instantly, I felt reassured. I thought it was a sign from God that Dad was OK. We spoke about our family trip to Ireland for Dad's 60th birthday, about time spent in Dingle, Galway, and Ring of Kerry. I was at ease. Still my father wouldn't accept a call. In angst again, I began thinking of Michael Scott, a.k.a. Steve Carrell, hopelessly lost in New York in an episode of *The Office*.

So I phoned my mother.

"You need to call Dad immediately," I said. "He's not answering his phone. Call him now, now, now!"

"Where is he?" she asked, building up to a panic herself.

"He's lost on Broadway..."

"He's WHAT?"

You can imagine the exchange from here.

So Mom started speed-dialing Dad, but still he wouldn't answer. He was chumming for would-be attackers. Upon my arrival at the hotel lobby, I called him. He finally answered, then I saw him off in the distance towing his suitcase, like a bulky garbage bag, toward the hotel. He had stopped 15 strangers along the way to get directions, or maybe to pick a fight. I was awestruck.

At first, he refused to talk, but at least he was safe. Another close call. Dad is a survivor.

Not all episodes on the Pluto loop are so intensely charged. One time in Portland, Maine, after speaking before 500 people at an annual Alzheimer's Association conference, my father removed himself from the auditorium to sit alone out in the lobby. He was spent, mentally exhausted, and wondering if anyone was listening. Dad doesn't want pity; he just wants to offer encouragement and perseverance to others.

When he looked up, there were more than a hundred people lined up to talk to him. Those in line didn't want to talk about how Dad was feeling (they knew he wouldn't go there); they wanted, instead, to talk about their families, their journeys. Dad lit up like a candle.

The effort he puts in each day of raising awareness of this disease is remarkable; his passion for those in the same boat is limitless. His words are powerful. Those who come to hear him seem to connect on a certain level with him regardless of whether they have or have not personally met him.

When Dad asks me to speak on the road, often I'm not sure what to say, so I speak from the heart, as he has taught me. I talk about the little things I notice now, such as the rage, confusion, and dislocation that he goes through daily, his day-to-day short-term memory problems, whether he'll be asking where his keys are when they're in his hand, reaching for his Big Bertha driver on the golf green, thinking it's his putter, or calling out for our dog Sox before she died when Sox was sitting at his feet. I'm not sure mentally where Dad is at those times, but those blank stares are so peaceful. He's calm, not stressed, and honestly seems not to have a care in the world. That's the silver lining of this disease: learning to deal with it.

I can't say enough about my father; he has qualities that people would die for. I would take a bullet for him; so would Brendan, Colleen, and my mother. Dad is not only fighting Alzheimer's, but a long list of other serious medical issues. You'd never know it; he's on a mission about this disease, and just busting his ass against all odds to make a living.

One of the hundreds of things I love about my dad is his sense of humor. He still has it, and I pray every day that he doesn't lose it. He can take a joke like no one else. If you look in the dictionary for the meaning of self-deprecating humor, it will likely say: see also Greg O'Brien. Dad relishes the mockery. His humor, passion, and love for his family and friends is all he needs now. That's not going anywhere for the moment, though the constant Alzheimer's progressions we, as a family, will never fully understand. Dad won't let us in. He is still the man of the family, whether he can act like it or not. Dad can go from complete rage, to laughing it up with family and friends in seconds. Seeing my dad smile warms my heart in so many ways. His sense of humor and a few laughs a day really help in fighting this disease. He takes pride every day in waking up and giving Alzheimer's the finger.

You gotta laugh at life, the Irish way, Dad says, stare down the demons. We all need to do more of that: laugh, cry, think, love, and stare. My time with my father, and who he was, is now fleeting. I know that. Yet I know that the journey I've been on with him will sustain me forever. Through good times and bad, Dad is the same loving father, and he possesses a heartwarming soul that will never leave him.

26

Unforgettable

Brendan McGeorge O'Brien

Alzheimer's is terrifying, but not because I fear the disease itself. Yet I know it could be my future. What I fear most is the menacing wake that Alzheimer's leaves in its path. My father's waning memory will one day erase his perception of who I am, who he is, and of every moment we've shared together. The word *unforgettable* has new meaning for me today. Unforgettable moments in life are truly rare, and in this certain fear, I've learned to cherish every single one of them. Never forget.

The awe of the Cape's vast coastline falling into the wrath of a consuming sea is something my father taught me to never forget. The analogy is not lost on me now, as erosion of my father's memory devours. The attrition of the high bluff above the Great Outer Beach was part of what Dad called our "backyard," and as a first-born son, I was his sidekick in exploring its splendor. The bluff, my dad, continue to slowly slip.

On countless Saturdays, particularly when autumn had thinned the summer crowd, we would pack lunches and fishing rods and haul our canoe down to nearby Lower Mill Pond in Brewster. Barely old enough to bait a hook, I would laughably tell my mom, "We're headed out to do what men do!"

Dad has always been my hero. My mentor. My best friend.

Almost 25,000 years ago, Lower Mill Pond was a lifeless crater, discarded from the clawing drag of the vast Laurentide Ice Sheet. The pond, long-sufferingly, had spent thousands of years transforming itself into a brilliant habitat, one of Cape Cod's historic kettle ponds. In childhood it was a sanctuary to me, a place where I learned of nature's unrelenting force and the marvel at its creation. My dad would always tell me, "It takes time, but nature always finds a way, day by day."

Soon after my father's diagnosis, I found myself just a few miles from that same pond, with power of attorney documents spread across our family oak living room table, wondering where I should sign. Dad had given me everything I ever needed in life, and now had to sign over whatever it was he had left. Wasn't fair, and I wanted no part of it. For two Irish guys who didn't like to talk about their emotions, we kept it business as usual, signing the documents, cracking a few jokes, and deciding it was time for a walk.

It had been close to twenty years since visiting the Mill Pond together, but without debate, we found ourselves at the head of the nature path we knew so well. Everything was just as I had remembered: the crowds were gone; the air was light; and winter was just a few storms away. Except this time, there was no canoe, no fishing rods, no packed lunches—just a deafening silence that stalked us.

Skirting the tip of a large granite boulder at the water's edge, a remnant of the ice sheet, we sat side by side, blankly staring into the distance. Becoming his power of attorney had implications that neither of us wanted to acknowledge. The icy silence of the pond's crater had returned; like a nuclear winter, it pulled us in, and defined the moment.

Tears began to stream down Dad's face. "I'm so fucking scared," he mustered, "I don't know what's happening to me."

I'd never seen him cry. In that moment, I wanted to tell him everything would be okay. But I couldn't. I knew it wouldn't be okay. We buried our heads into the arms of one another, and tried to let it wash away. It was a far cry from early days on the pond "doing what men do," as we let our fears cascade into the pond.

The torment of Alzheimer's doesn't start in a nursing home; far from it. Instead, it's a tireless journey with no predictable direction, and it commences long before one is prepared to embark.

I spent most of my late-twenties growing impatient with my father. His once lovable "artistic quirkiness" had soured into a predictably stubborn, inflammatory character flaw, as I saw it then. As a family, we found it therapeutic to ignore the blatant warning signs of Alzheimer's, not wanting to embrace our inevitable future.

I never expected to escape my thirties without some degree of loss, but Alzheimer's has a perverse way of making one re-live that painful loss every single day, at a glacial speed, but knowing it will never retreat.

No one signs up for this. But the logical step is to forge on, start redefining the loss, and assess how the disease will impact the lives on the edge. Then comes the undeniable ethical dilemma: how much will we let this disease dictate our lives? What kinds of sacrifices will we make, and at what cost?

Whether we bear the disease like a cross, or wear it like a badge, there is peace in walking a chosen path with inherent decisions and inner conviction. Selfishly in the moment, I thought the diagnosis could not have come at a worse time in my life. I was just getting started with my writing and producing career, lots of dreams filled with promise, then the pink slip. Dad has Alzheimer's! I, too, was feeling like George Bailey in *It's a Wonderful Life*. I wanted out of the Bedford Falls of my past, but was getting sucked back in.

I found that reality has no regard for timelines. In my heart, I accepted that Alzheimer's may one day define my own life, but that I would never let the disease dictate it. Though I don't have the GPS coordinates for this disease, I've tried to guide my parents into uncharted financial waters. Financial planning, the gathering of family assets, and advising on long- and short-term options are just the beginning; nothing in life prepares us for the path ahead.

Dad says fighting Alzheimer's is like a board surfer breaking the waves to paddle to the swell. The forces of nature keep crashing down. Dad's first assault against this tide was making it to my sister Colleen's wedding. Like so many families, it was a day we had all dreamt about. We were letting her go, like a firefly, to steady blinks of bright happiness with the kind of guy who would chase down her every dream.

But Alzheimer's brutally exposes the significance of life's precious milestones. Watching my dad's father/daughter dance with Colleen was heart-wrenching. I found myself sobbing.

I'm engaged now to a beautiful woman, Laken Ferreria, the love of my life. I recently proposed to Laken on Martha's Vineyard, at sunset on Menemsha Harbor. I pray my dad can toast us at our wedding. I find peace in knowing his legacy will never leave us. The inconsolable pain comes from knowing that the story of our lives together is drifting away. These unforgettable moments will one day be lost on him, and we'll have to start over. Again, and again. It's the painful reminder of that loss that hurts the most.

It took me a long time to take the leap outside of my own hurt. I had to abandon willfully my perception of reality. Alzheimer's steals memory, family, and realities.

A close family friend and author of *Still Alice,* Lisa Genova put everything into perspective with one swift sentence. She told me, "If your dad thinks the sky is purple one day, just let it be purple." It's agonizing to think that he won't know who I am someday, but there's no solace or gain in frustration from that. He knows when he can't remember something, and when that happens he just needs an embrace, not a harsh reminder of his disease.

This is a war we must all wage together, and the only way to win is to talk about it; take it public, and bring it out of the closet, as we did with cancer and AIDS. With close to 50 million affected across the world, proportionately more women and men, and more to come, we have power in numbers. Wear Alzheimer's like a badge of honor, and make the disease regret the day it ever crossed your path. I've heard my dad's close friend and best-selling writer David Shenk say of my father, "Alzheimer's picked the wrong guy…"

Until local, state, and federal governments truly understand the disease, we'll never get the funding to find a cure. Capitol Hill, on all sides of the political aisle, needs to continue to listen and to act. Alzheimer's is a bipartisan killer. We will never fully, all of us, understand the disease until we collectively listen to the stories of the millions affected. It's the truth, in our vulnerability, that will create real progress.

Our family journey has been filled with challenge, sadness, and fight, but it's also been filled with opportunity—opportunity to share our story, your story, to strengthen relationships, and to cherish the time we spend together.

Breaking the icy silence that day at Mill Pond is what jump-started our family dialogue, and on our collective terms. The gaping crater the ice sheet left behind 25 millennia ago has slowly filled with beauty and life. We find peace in that.

My father may never be able to share the unforgettable moments of my future, but those whom I love will know of the hope he gave to others. That's the legacy my children will someday know. Mom and Dad, I'll always be right there with you guys, fighting dementia with all I have. Everything you've taught me will live far beyond our years, and I wouldn't trade that for anything in the world. Our love is unforgettable. Here and on Pluto…

27

Walking in Faith

Colleen (O'Brien) Everett

*"Now faith is confidence in what we hope for
and assurance about what we do not see."*
—HEBREWS 11:1

Faith is a stretch at times. It is believing in something one cannot see, desperately reaching out at times into a void. Faith is the only thing stronger than fear.

My father has always been a man of faith. Some of my earliest memories of him are watching him kneel by his bedside with eyes closed, clutching a tattered Bible that was peppered with personal notes in his scratchy handwriting. A perfectly imperfect man, by his own admission, he would be so deep in thought and prayer that he would never even hear you enter the room. At the time, I was too young to understand the worries weighing on his heart, but I grew up learning that when life is difficult, or even when it is wonderful, or when one sins, as my father can with the best of them, one needs to close their eyes and talk to God.

Everything was less scary to me as a kid, and eventually as an adult, because I saw the power of faith through my father's eyes: that no matter what life puts in front of you, God is already one step ahead of you. The Lord has a plan.

Well, I'm pissed off today about God's plan for my dad. Yet, I try in faith to listen.

Looking back, I don't ever remember my father yelling in torrents. He hardly ever lost his cool. When he coached my youth softball team, he would gently guide me to focus on fly balls, instead of picking dandelions in centerfield with my childhood friend Liz Seymour. Or when our team cheered wildly after a member of the opposing team hit a home run—anathema to my sports-minded father—he would just smile. Or when as young kids, Brendan, Conor, and I found ourselves on Saturday mornings, beyond stated boundaries, playing hide and seek by the printing press at the *Cape Codder* newspaper where Dad was editor and publisher, my father jokingly would get on the public address system and loudly announce: "Brendan, Colleen, and Conor, to the Principal's Office! Brendan, Colleen, and Conor, to the Principal's Office!!"

Later, when I began dating, Dad welcomed boyfriends into the house with a hug instead of an intimidating glare. My older brother, Brendan, often had to take on the responsibility of scaring off rogue teen suitors. Dad rarely swore in front of us then, and treated everyone with respect; he saw the good in everyone—no matter their story, their look, or their past. Still does. He has always been one to reach out in gut instinct to help and mentor those in need, usually outside of the view of others.

Today is a different narrative in our journey with Alzheimer's. Now Dad has violent outbursts and eruptions of profanity. When he gets confused, which is often these days, he lashes out—usually at the people who love him the most. Outings with him can become uncomfortable, painful actually. At times, for example, I want to grab the waitress or cab driver, or whoever he's yelling at, and let them know it's not them, it's not him. It's Alzheimer's.

A few years ago, my father was invited to speak in San Francisco. The trip happened to coincide with my spring break as a teacher in Baltimore City, so I agreed to go as his caretaker. He doesn't travel alone. I remember my mother asking if I was sure I could handle it. Living now several hundred miles away from the Cape, I don't get to witness the full picture of my father. When he only sees me for a short period of time, he is able to use up all of his energy to be in the present with me. I don't always see the darker side of the disease that my mother and brothers do. Until I spent a week as his caregiver, I had no idea how much of my father this disease has consumed.

Going through airport security without a second thought, I took my shoes off, put my bags on the conveyor, and walked through the AIT machine. I then heard someone spewing profanity behind me, and my stomach dropped. My father couldn't figure out how to take his belt off, and the TSA officer wouldn't let him through until he did. In that moment, nothing made sense to my father. He knew that he should be able to take his own belt off, yet couldn't. From 30 feet away, I had to watch the man who raised me to be a kind soul and taught me to field ground balls break down over his belt, as crowds of people stared in judgmental confusion over his confusion. In that moment, we switched roles. I became the parent. I closed my eyes, and asked the Lord for the strength to calm my dad. I made eye contact with him from the other side of the security screening, and coached him through the rest of the security line, like I would with one of my young students. I felt embarrassed and then immediately guilty for feeling that way. I knew that it was Alzheimer's, not my father. But that's the thing with Alzheimer's; it strips the person you love of all elements that make them who they are. There are many things that define my father—he is a devoted husband, a loyal friend, a loving father, an avid sports fan, and stubborn Irish. Alzheimer's does not define my father, but it does slowly strip away all of the things that do define him. All of the things that make him who he is.

My father today has become more childlike; the disease takes you there. And maybe that's a good thing toward the end of one's life. We all are so busy being adults that we forget the beauty and innocence of being a child, reinforced in me now as a young mother. Dad, in his disease, has found the balance sought in the Gospel of Matthew 18:2-4, "I tell you the truth. You must change and become like little children (in your hearts)…The greatest person in the Kingdom of Heaven is the person that makes himself humble as a child."

Dad is now a child in so many ways.

Each Father's Day, I can't help but wonder how many more I'm going to have left with my dad. And not just physically, but mentally— where my dad remembers me, and remembers my daughter, Adeline. It's a terrible thought, but one I can't seem to get off my mind. Watching him slip away has been one of the most painful things I've ever had to experience.

While I can't help these thoughts from flooding my mind, I also think of the wonderful memories that I do have: baseball games in the front yard; father/daughter trips to Fenway Park; ice cream at the Smuggler; and summer walks on the Brewster flats on the Cape. My father coached my little league softball team; as school committee chairman, gave the commencement speech at my high school graduation and handed me my diploma; surprised me with a yellow lab puppy for my 16th birthday; and walked me down the aisle on the most important day of my life. Alzheimer's may take a lot from my family, but it will never take those memories away from me.

It's really incredible to watch my father with my infant daughter. It's a moment I wasn't sure if I would ever get to have. I've read that children can reach those in the throes of Alzheimer's at a deep emotional level—a level that most adults can't. That's the grace of being a child, for Adeline and for my dad. I've seen it in the way that Adeline looks at my dad. She looks past his temper and his confusion, and only looks at him with adoration and love. When she smiles, she smiles with her whole face. She can't help but be all smiles when she's with my father.

She is in awe of him, as I am, too.

My father today has a short commute to work. The path from our home's back deck to his writing studio on the Outer Cape is lined with broken clam shells that mark the path like airport runway lights as he comes in for a safe landing. He can't get lost there.

Halfway up the narrow path, at the base of an old oak tree, is a yellow Tonka toy truck, weathered with age. Conor and I used to play with it. The wheels, ironically, are now off; the plastic toy truck has been parked by the tree in solitude for close to 20 years. Dad put it there as a memory of our childhood, not far from what he calls "Christmas Tree Heaven," a patch of woodland on our property piled with the bones of family Christmas trees from all these years of our childhood. My father is a sap, excuse the pun.

The yellow truck, angels, and the color yellow are driving forces in his life; they give my father great comfort. It brings him back in faith to an innocent time, to childhood, and to his own young fatherhood. On his way to the office, he religiously touches the top of the toy truck and says a prayer, as if to reassure himself that he has a past. We often quietly witness the exchange from behind the sliding door of the family room.

In Baltimore, which I now call home, my husband, Matt, and I discovered a little more than a year ago that "we" were pregnant. I was carrying the baby; and Matt was carrying me. I had always wanted to be a mom; it's been something I've looked forward to my entire life. But as I sat on the floor with our new yellow baby lab, Crosby, awaiting the test results, a crushing feeling of anxiety swept over me: I was anxious about having to leave my six-year-old students a third of the way through the school year; I was anxious about being a good-enough mother; I was anxious about giving my students, my husband, my child, and our new puppy all of me. How does one even do that? I was far more fearful about passing the Alzheimer's gene on to our child. I was scared that if I had the gene, like my dad, I'd leave my baby too soon.

I woke up early one Saturday morning a few weeks later, then almost 12 weeks pregnant, and decided to go for a run—a route I've been running since we moved to our neighborhood in Baltimore.

There is a house on my route where three young kids live. They're always outside playing with chalk or games in the yard, and when I'm running by or walking Crosby, they love to say hi. When I ran by the house early that morning, no one was awake yet, but something caught my eye. By the big tree on the front lawn was a yellow Tonka truck—just like the one we grew up with. I stopped, held my hand over it, and felt a rush of calm. Faith told me everything was going to be right in God's plan.

This past Christmas Eve, I introduced my healthy baby girl, Adeline, to my father, a moment I never knew I would have. He held my angel tightly, and they danced slowly, grandfather to granddaughter. All was good in that moment. While we do not know what the future holds for all of us, I've come to understand that we can have faith in God's plan. No matter what you choose to believe in, a personal choice for all, I've learned in this trial that one needs to have faith in something.

I have renewed faith today in angels, and in yellow Tonka trucks.

EPILOGUE

Ready, Set, Action

David Shenk

You can't go back now. You can't un-know Greg O'Brien's fearlessness, or his family's heartache. Alzheimer's has too young a face now, and a warm, lovely cottage on Cape Cod. It has a gentle wife and three loving kids who aren't nearly ready to say goodbye to their dad. It has a story that won't ever leave you, or me ... unless we stop Alzheimer's.

This is just a simple truth.

So what now? What are you going to do with this knowledge? For this Epilogue, my friend Greg asked me to address what specific action the reader can or should take. You've already opened up your heart and let Greg in—that's the most important thing. But what else can you do?

We have to stop Alzheimer's. We have to. That's why Greg wrote this book, and allowed filmmakers into his home, and why he travels around the world giving speeches, and occasionally embarrasses himself on the radio, and gets lost, and sometimes feels like an idiot. He does it because he wants to knock us into action and stop this goddamned disease. Now!

We can do it. A good argument could be made that Alzheimer's still exists today only because we haven't yet stepped up to fight it hard enough. Smart researchers have been at it for decades, but we've only given them a fraction of the money they need to do the job.

This is a disease that has been afflicting the elderly throughout history. Ralph Waldo Emerson had it. Jonathan Swift had it. The Greek legislator Solon wrote about it in 500 BC. But only in recent decades, due to dramatic gains in human longevity, has Alzheimer's emerged as a true social health catastrophe. People are living longer than ever before, thanks to modern nutrition and medicine, and are thus paradoxically exposed to increasing risks of Alzheimer's.

Currently afflicting 5.5 million Americans at an annual cost of more than $200 billion, these numbers will triple by 2050. The global picture is quite similar: already, 34 million people worldwide have Alzheimer's or a related dementia. If left unchecked, Alzheimer's could bankrupt health systems everywhere. You've heard it before. This is no exaggeration. Perhaps in this disease we learn by rote.

More to the point, unless you plan on dying young, there is a strong chance *you* will get Alzheimer's. Or your spouse. Or your best friend. There's no shame in selfishness. We should all feel compelled to stop this disease for the most selfish of reasons.

Researchers have made great recent strides, but we are not moving fast enough. Federal research funding stands at a paltry amount considering the scope of the problem and what the U.S. government spends on other challenges of this magnitude. This is augmented by smaller, but significant private efforts. After years of getting to know the Alzheimer's research community, I have recently come to support the Cure Alzheimer's Fund (CAF), an exemplary consortium of top Alzheimer's scientists led by renowned geneticist Rudolph Tanzi, PhD of Massachusetts General Hospital and Harvard University, and connected to researchers at the Icahn School of Medicine at Mount Sinai in New York City, Washington University, University of Chicago, University of Pennsylvania, University of Southern California, Stony Brook, Stanford University, Rockefeller University, Johns Hopkins University School of Medicine, and many other great institutions.

CAF's current annual research budget, all from private citizens like you and me, is approximately $10 million. They've already scored several important breakthroughs in genetics, diagnosis, and drug discovery. Greg and I know them well (and I assist them in educating the public). We trust them. See for yourself (curealz.org).

Here's what we should do soon, you and I: I'd like to introduce you to Greg in person. He's even more real and inspiring, and funnier. I'd also love for you to meet Dr. Tanzi, another extraordinary person. The four of us could have a nice glass of wine and revel in life's richness and sadness.

But in the meantime, please consider playing a direct role in the fight to halt this urgent epidemic. Call your congressional representatives, and let them know Alzheimer's is a priority for you and your family; that they are letting Americans down if they aren't fighting hard for more research. Also, donate a little something, or half your net worth, to the Cure Alzheimer's Fund—or to any Alzheimer's research foundation you admire.

If you like to help the caregiving world, consider a donation to, or volunteering some time at, the Alzheimer's Association (alz.org). They do incredible work in every state in the U.S.

Don't do this for Greg. Do it for yourself!

David Shenk is author of The Forgetting, *creator of the* Living With Alzheimer's *film project (LivingWithAlz.com), and a senior advisor to Cure Alzheimer's Fund (CureAlz.org).*

ALZHEIMER'S
RESOURCES

Alzheimer's is an insidious disease that slowly unravels the mind, the body, and the self. It shakes families to the core, and forces them to adapt in smart and meaningful ways.

While scientists work feverishly to stop Alzheimer's, there is much to be done for families right now. With funding from MetLife Foundation and in partnership with Cure Alzheimer's Fund, executive producer David Shenk recruited four world-class filmmakers to produce short films, true-life stories, about how individuals and families cope. Greg O'Brien and his family were the subject of a short film produced by renowned documentary producer Steve James. The film is titled *A Place Called Pluto*, and can be viewed online at: livingwithalz.org.

Other Living With Alzheimer's filmmakers include: Oscar-winning producer Roger Ross Williams; Oscar-winning director Megan Mylan; and Emmy-winning producer Naomi Boak.

This resource guide is courtesy of David Shenk and the Living With Alzheimer's project.

Learning about Alzheimer's

DISEASE OVERVIEW
A Quick Look At Alzheimer's Disease: Five 'Pocket' Films to Increase Understanding of a 21st Century Epidemic: http://aboutalz .org

NIH—What is Alzheimer's Disease?: http://nihseniorhealth.gov/ alzheimersdisease/toc.html

The Forgetting, by David Shenk: http://www.amazon.com/The-Forgetting-Alzheimers- Portrait-Epidemic/dp/0385498381

Alzheimer's Association—What Is Alzheimer's?: http://www.alz .org/AboutAD/WhatIsAD.asp

Understanding Alzheimer's: A guide for families, friends, and health care providers

STATISTICS AND DATA

Alzheimer's Disease, National Center for Health Statistics: http:// www.cdc.gov/nchs/fastats/alzheimr.htm

Statistics about Alzheimer's Disease, Alzheimer's Association: http://www.alz.org/AboutAD/statistics.asp

The Silver Book, Alliance for Aging Research: http://www .silverbook.org

CLINICAL TRIALS

ADEAR Clinical Trials Database, National Institute on Aging http://www.nia.nih.gov/Alzheimers/ResearchInformation/ ClinicalTrials/

Clinical Trials, The Alzheimer's Information Site: http://www .alzinfo.org/treatment/clinicaltrial/default.aspx

Alzheimer's Association alz.org

UsAgainstAlzheimer's usagainstalzheimers.org

LATEST NEWS AND RESEARCH

Alzheimer's Association Research Center: http://www.alz.org/ Research/overview.asp

Alzheimer's Research Forum: http://www.alzforum.org/

Updates from Cure Alzheimer's Fund: http://www.curealz.org/ news

Key Research Findings in 2012, by Rudolph E. Tanzi, PhD: http:// www.curealz.org/message-research-consortium-chairman

FILMS

Glen Campbell...I'll Be Me, award-winning documentary directed by actor-filmmaker James Keach, produced by Trevor Albert

Understanding Alzheimer's: Five 'Pocket' Films, directed by David Shenk: aboutalz.org

PBS's *The Forgetting,* directed by Elizabeth Arledge: http://www.pbs.org/theforgetting

Away from Her, directed by Sarah Polley

DOCUMENTARIES
Prevention

Can Alzheimer's Be Stopped, NOVA/PBS, producer, Sarah Holt

Alzheimer's: Every Minute Counts, PBS/WGBH, producer, Elizabeth Aldredge

TREATMENT AND PREVENTION
Prevention

Maintain Your Brain, Alzheimer's Association: www.alz.org/maintainyourbrain/overview.asp

Treatment Options

Alzheimer's Disease Medications Fact Sheet, National Institute on Aging: www.nia.nih.gov/Alzheimers/Publications/medicationsfs.htm

Alzheimer's Disease: Treatment Overview, WebMD: www.webmd.com/content/article/71/81399.htm

Medications for Memory Loss, Alzheimer's Association: www.alz.org/AboutAD/Treatment/Standard.asp

Alternative Treatments for Alzheimer's: www.alz.org/AboutAD/Treatment/Alternative.asp

CAREGIVING
Caregiving Resources
Caregiving strategies: www.alzfdn.org/EducationandCare/strategiesforsuccess.html

Find an in-person support group in your area: www.alz.org/apps/we_can_help/support_groups.asp

Online support groups: www.alzconnected.org/discussion.aspx

Live contact: phone, chat, or skype with a licensed social worker: carecrossroads.org/cms/index.php?option=com_content&view= article& id=58&Itemid=19

FIGHTING ALZHEIMER'S
Calls to Action
Short Film: *Let's Stop Alzheimer's Now*: vimeo.com/31089084

"Memory Hole," *The New York Times* Op-Ed by David Shenk: www.nytimes.com/2006/11/03/opinion/03shenk.html

Advocacy Organizations
Alzheimer's Association: www.alz.org

Cure Alzheimer's Fund: www.curealz.org

Accelerate Cure/Treatments for Alzheimer's Diseases: www.act-ad.org

Alzheimer's Foundation of America (AFA): www.alzfdn.org

Additional Resources:

USAGAINSTALZHEIMER'S

Alzheimer's is among the only top 10 cause of death in the United States with no treatment or means of prevention, yet federal research funding is a fraction of that for other major diseases. New research says Alzheimer's is America's third leading cause of death—claiming 500,000 lives in 2010—with more than 5 million people slowly dying of it. Worldwide, today, 44.4 million battle some form of dementia. They are cared for by 15 million caregivers in the U.S. and an estimated 100 million worldwide. The direct care costs for Alzheimer's exceed those for cancer and heart disease.

UsAgainstAlzheimer's (usagainstalzheimers.org) is an innovative advocacy organization demanding—and delivering—a solution to Alzheimer's. Driven by the suffering of millions of families, we press for and are achieving greater urgency from government, industry and the scientific community in the quest for an Alzheimer's cure—accomplishing this through effective leadership, collaborative advocacy and strategic investments.

We mobilize the most deeply affected communities, united under the relentless force of UsAgainstAlzheimer's, to stop Alzheimer's and those touched by it.

AFRICAN AMERICANS

AfricanAmericansAgainstAlzheimer's is the preeminent voice in and for the African- American community on Alzheimer's and its disproportionate impact. We reach communities nationwide to build participation in clinical trials by African Americans. Contact: Stephanie Monroe, smonroe@usagainstalzheimers.org

BUSINESS & ORGANIZATIONS

The Global CEO Initiative on Alzheimer's (CEOi) is a coalition of 13 corporate members and partnerships globally with public authorities. Contact: Drew Holzapfel, dholzapfel@ highlanterngroup.com

Leaders Engaged on Alzheimer's Disease is a growing national coalition of 80 diverse organizations that work collaboratively to focus the nation's strategic attention on Alzheimer's disease and related disorders and to accelerate transformational progress in care and support, detection and diagnosis, and research leading to prevention, effective treatment and eventual cure. Contact: Ian Kremer, ikremer@leadcoalition.org

AD-PACE (Alzheimer's Disease and Caregiver Engagement): A patient and caregiver-led initiative, AD-PACE will develop a range of patient-focused drug development tools and resources to support Alzheimer's drug development and regulatory and payment review. Contact: Terry Frangiosa, tfrangiosa@usagainstalzheimers.org

CAREGIVERS & ACTIVISTS

ActivistsAgainstAlzheimer's engages caregivers and others on the frontlines of national and community efforts to fight this disease—including an online caregiver support group. Contact: Virginia Biggar, vbiggar@usagainstalzheimers.org

CLERGY & FAITH LEADERS

ClergyAgainstAlzheimer's is a diverse, multi-faith network of ordained clergy working to focus our nation's attention on Alzheimer's and related dementias. Contact: Virginia Biggar, vbiggar@usagainstalzheimers.org

Faith United Against Alzheimer's is a diverse coalition of faith leaders and organizations, in partnership with the United Methodist Church, mobilizing the faith community against Alzheimer's and related dementias. Contact: Virginia Biggar, vbiggar@usagainstalzheimers.org

CLINICAL TRIALS

GAP (Global Alzheimer's Platform) Foundation is building a standing global trial-ready platform to drive quality, efficiency and innovation in Alzheimer's clinical trials. Contact: Joni Henderson, info@globalalzplatform.org

LATINOS

LatinosAgainstAlzheimer's works to raise the profile of Alzheimer's disease as an urgent Latino health care issue. Contact: Jason Resendez, jresendez@usagainstalzheimers.org

LatinosAgainstAlzheimer's Coalition is the first national coalition of Hispanic-serving organizations dedicated to raising awareness of Alzheimer's within the Latino community. Contact: Jason Resendez, jresendez@usagainstalzheimers.org

RESEARCHERS

ResearchersAgainstAlzheimer's is a network of top Alzheimer's researchers that informs policymakers on the importance of increasing federal research funding and instituting reforms, such as accelerating the drug pipeline. Contact: Yael Miller, miller@highlanterngroup.com

VETERANS/MILITARY

VeteransAgainstAlzheimer's is a coalition of military leaders, veterans service organizations, researchers, clinicians, and veterans with/at risk of cognitive impairment and their families, raising the profile of Alzheimer's as an urgent veterans/service member health issue. Contact: Virginia Biggar, vbiggar@usagainstalzheimers.org

WOMEN

WomenAgainstAlzheimer's brings Alzheimer's out of the shadows as a women's health and financial crisis, given its heavy impact on women as patients and caregivers. Contact: Brooks Kenny, bkenny@usagainstalzheimers.org

On the UsAgainstAlzherimer's front:

Driven by the vision and leadership of UsAgainstAlzheimer's board member Meryl Comer, an Alzheimer's caregiver for more than 20 years, GALAXY is a virtual gateway to a constellation of innovative initiatives that makes it easy for people to participate in Alzheimer's research. GALAXY showcases partnerships and projects that focus on modeling new online platforms to support those living with dementia and their families, aligning with the goals of the National Alzheimer's & Dementia Patient & Caregiver-Powered Research Network (AD-PCPRN), which aims to amplify the patient and caregiver voice to accelerate development of effective treatments for Alzheimer's disease.

GALAXY is the launch pad for the *A-List*, an online community of those living with Alzheimer's, other dementias and mild cognitive impairment, care partners and anyone with memory concerns, who are using their collective voice to speed the search for a treatment, prevention or cure for this devastating disease. The *A-List* will communicate with researchers and clinicians, test new technologies, and increase participation in prevention studies to speed cures.

UsAgainstAlzheimer's, a partner of the AD-PCPRN and GALAXY, is committed to speeding cures by strengthening research and supporting the physical and emotional needs of caregivers. GALAXY, shaped by Comer's guidance and caregiver perspective, is a significant step to overcome scientific skepticism about patient-reported data, and inform and advance research.

Alzheimer's Association

The Alzheimer's Association, Alz.org, was founded in 1980 by a group of family caregivers and individuals interested in research. Jerome H. Stone was our founding president.

Resources below courtesy of Alzheimer's Association (alz.org).

Today, the Association reaches millions of people affected by Alzheimer's across the globe through our headquarters in Chicago, a public policy office in Washington, D.C., and a presence in communities across the country. We are the leading voluntary health organization in Alzheimer's care, support and research.

Together, we can change the future of Alzheimer's.

- The Alzheimer's Association, as noted on alz.org, works on a global, national and local level to provide care and support for all those affected by Alzheimer's and other dementias. We are here to help.

- We have local chapters across the nation, providing services within each community. Find a chapter near you.

- Our professionally staffed 24/7 Helpline (1.800.272.3900) offers information and advice to more than 300,000 callers each year and provides translation services in more than 200 languages.

- We host face-to-face support groups and educational sessions in communities nationwide.

- We connect people across the globe through our online message boards, ALZConnected. Our online community is ready to answer your questions and give you support.

- We provide caregivers and families with comprehensive online resources and information through our Alzheimer's and Dementia Caregiver Center, which features sections on early-stage, middle-stage and late-stage caregiving.

- Our free online tool, Alzheimer's Navigator, helps those facing the disease to determine their needs and develop an action plan, and our online Community Resource Finder is a comprehensive database of programs and service, housing and care services, and legal experts.

- We house the Alzheimer's Association Green-Field Library, the nation's largest library and resource center devoted to increasing knowledge about Alzheimer's disease and related dementias.

- *Our safety service, MedicAlert + Alzheimer's Association Safe Return*, is a 24-hour nationwide emergency response service for individuals with Alzheimer's or a related dementia who wander or have a medical emergency.

WE ACCELERATE RESEARCH AND CREATE A PATH FOR GLOBAL PROCESS

- As the largest nonprofit funder of Alzheimer's research, the Association is committed to accelerating the global progress of new treatments, preventions and ultimately, a cure. Visit our online Research Center.

- We advance the understanding of Alzheimer's through our peer-reviewed research grant program, has invested over $385 million in more than 2,500 scientific investigations since 1982.

- Our annual Alzheimer's Association International Conference (AAIC) is the world's largest conference of its kind, bringing researchers together to report on groundbreaking studies.

- We bring researchers together worldwide to advance scientific data sharing through GAAIN, the Global Alzheimer's Association International Network, a first-of-its-kind database with advanced analytical tools to accelerate discoveries.

- Our scientific journal, *Alzheimer's & Dementia*, provides a single publication for the global scientific community to share its diverse knowledge.

- Our professional society, Alzheimer's Association International Society to Advance Alzheimer's Research and Treatment (ISTAART), is the only professional society designed exclusively for individuals dedicated to Alzheimer's and dementia science.

- We accelerate clinical studies by connecting healthy volunteers, people with the disease and caregivers to current studies through Alzheimer's Association TrialMatch, a free, easy-to-use clinical studies matching service.
- We play a pioneering role in increasing knowledge about prevention. The Association has invested in projects revealing that what's good for the heart is good for the brain, and that eating a healthy diet, staying physically active and not smoking will help reduce risk of cognitive decline.
- Sign up for our weekly e-newsletter.
- Stay up-to-date on the Alzheimer's Association latest advances in Alzheimer's treatments, care and research.

WE ADVOCATE

The Association is the leading voice for Alzheimer's disease advocacy, fighting for critical Alzheimer's research, prevention and care initiatives at the state and federal level. We diligently work to make Alzheimer's a national priority. Join our cause.

- We develop policy resources, including Alzheimer's Disease Facts and Figures and Changing the Trajectory of Alzheimer's Disease, to educate decision makers on the economic and emotional toll that Alzheimer's takes on families and the nation.
- Our advocates engage elected officials at all levels of government and participate in our annual Alzheimer's Association Advocacy Forum, a march on Capitol Hill to meet with elected representatives.
- With our chapters, we work to pass legislation at the federal, state and global level. Our advocacy victories include passage of the National Alzheimer's Project Act (NAPA), which mandated the creation of a national plan to fight Alzheimer's.

JOIN THE CAUSE

- Volunteer with the Alzheimer's Association. Plan an event, facilitate a support group or sign up for another opportunity to advance the cause.
- Advocate for those affected by Alzheimer's and urge legislators make the disease a national priority.
- Participate in Walk to End Alzheimer's, the world's largest event to raise awareness and funds for Alzheimer's disease care, support and research.
- Start a team for The Longest Day. Honor the strength, heart and endurance of those facing Alzheimer's with a day of activity June 21—the summer solstice.
- Donate to advance vital research and provide care and support programs.
- Register for Alzheimer's Association TrialMatch, a free, easy-to-use clinical studies matching service that connects individuals with Alzheimer's, caregivers, healthy volunteers, and physicians with current studies.

ABOUT THE AUTHOR

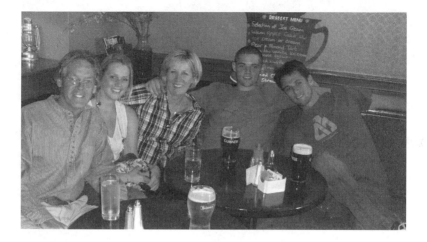

At a tavern on the Dingle Peninsula, west coast of Ireland, August 2010: (from left to right), author Greg O'Brien; daughter, Colleen; wife, Mary Catherine; son Conor; son Brendan.

Greg O'Brien has more than 35 years of newspaper and magazine experience as a writer, editor, investigative reporter, and publisher. Over the years, he has contributed to the *Huffington Post, Psychology Today, Washington Post, Chicago Tribune, Runner's World, Time, Denver Post, Associated Press, UPI, USA Today, The Arizona Republic, Boston Herald American, Boston Metro, New York Metro, Philadelphia Metro,* the *Providence Journal, Cape Cod Times, Boston Irish Reporter,* and *Boston Magazine,* where he was a senior writer. The author/editor of several books, O'Brien has published 17 books by other writers, and was a founding managing director of Community Newspaper Company, initially headquartered in Boston. He is president of Stony Brook Group, a political and communications strategy company, and lives in West Brewster on Cape Cod with his wife, Mary Catherine. The couple has three children: Brendan, Colleen, and Conor, and one grandchild, Adeline Mae Everett.